Aphasia: A Cognitive Neuropsychological Approach

Aphasia: A Cognitive Neuropsychological Approach

Editor: Adlan Brooks

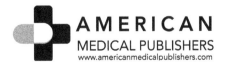

AMERICAN
MEDICAL PUBLISHERS
www.americanmedicalpublishers.com

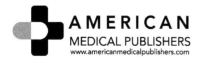

Cataloging-in-Publication Data

Aphasia : a cognitive neuropsychological approach / edited by Adlan Brooks.
    p. cm.
Includes bibliographical references and index.
ISBN 978-1-63927-573-1
1. Aphasia. 2. Neuropsychology. 3. Cognitive neuroscience. 4. Aphasia--Treatment.
5. Brain--Diseases. 6. Language disorders. 7. Speech disorders. I. Brooks, Adlan.
RC425 .A64 2023
616.855 2--dc23

American Medical Publishers,
41 Flatbush Avenue,
1st Floor, New York,
NY 11217, USA

ISBN 978-1-63927-573-1 (Hardback)

Contents

Preface

The purpose of the book is to provide a glimpse into the dynamics and to present opinions and studies of some of the scientists engaged in the development of new ideas in the field from very different standpoints. This book will prove useful to students and researchers owing to its high content quality.

Damage to the language dominant side of the brain usually results in a condition called aphasia. In aphasia, the speech of a person is impaired. Although, any type of damage can cause aphasia, it is primarily caused by stroke. Cognitive neuropsychological techniques aim to identify the essential language skills or modules that are not functioning properly in each individual rather than putting them into a specific subtype. A person may struggle with a single module or a number of modules. These methods necessitate a framework or theory for determining which skills/modules are required to execute various types of language activities. Different types of speech and language therapies, such as visual communication therapy (VIC), functional communication therapy (FCT) and melodic intonation therapy (MIT) are helpful in managing aphasia. This book is compiled in such a manner, that it will provide in-depth knowledge about the cognitive neuropsychological approach to aphasia. The topics covered herein offer the readers new insights in this condition. This book includes contributions of experts and scientists which will provide innovative insights into aphasia.

At the end, I would like to appreciate all the efforts made by the authors in completing their chapters professionally. I express my deepest gratitude to all of them for contributing to this book by sharing their valuable works. A special thanks to my family and friends for their constant support in this journey.

Editor

Changes in Resting-State Connectivity following Melody-Based Therapy in a Patient with Aphasia

Tali Bitan (ID),[1,2] Tijana Simic,[2,3,4] Cristina Saverino,[3] Cheryl Jones,[2] Joanna Glazer,[3] Brenda Collela,[3] Catherine Wiseman-Hakes,[2,3] Robin Green,[2,3] and Elizabeth Rochon[2,3,4]

[1]University of Haifa, Haifa, Israel
[2]University of Toronto, Toronto, ON, Canada
[3]Toronto Rehabilitation Institute, Toronto, ON, Canada
[4]Canadian Partnership for Stroke Recovery, Heart and Stroke Foundation, Ottawa, ON, Canada

Correspondence should be addressed to Tali Bitan; tbitan@research.haifa.ac.il

Academic Editor: Wenhua Zheng

Melody-based treatments for patients with aphasia rely on the notion of preserved musical abilities in the RH, following left hemisphere damage. However, despite evidence for their effectiveness, the role of the RH is still an open question. We measured changes in resting-state functional connectivity following melody-based intervention, to identify lateralization of treatment-related changes. A patient with aphasia due to left frontal and temporal hemorrhages following traumatic brain injuries (TBI) more than three years earlier received 48 sessions of melody-based intervention. Behavioral measures improved and were maintained at the 8-week posttreatment follow-up. Resting-state fMRI data collected before and after treatment showed an increase in connectivity between motor speech control areas (bilateral supplementary motor areas and insulae) and RH language areas (inferior frontal gyrus pars triangularis and pars opercularis). This change, which was specific for the RH, was greater than changes in a baseline interval measured before treatment. No changes in RH connectivity were found in a matched control TBI patient scanned at the same intervals. These results are compatible with a compensatory role for RH language areas following melody-based intervention. They further suggest that this therapy intervenes at the level of the interface between language areas and speech motor control areas necessary for language production.

1. Introduction

The goal of the current study was to examine changes in functional connectivity within the right and left hemispheres following melody-based treatment in a patient with aphasia. The long-held notion that recovery from aphasia following LH damage involves compensatory recruitment of the RH [1–4] has been challenged in the last two decades [5]. Many neuroimaging studies showed the effect of treatment-related changes in aphasia predominantly in LH language areas [6–9], and some even suggest that long-lasting RH recruitment is maladaptive for language performance [10–14]. However, melody-based treatments, which have been used for several decades, were developed specifically to harness preserved abilities of the RH in patients with left hemisphere (LH) damage and to facilitate the recovery of speech through RH compensation. Nevertheless, despite evidence for the effectiveness of melody-based therapies in improving speech production in patients with aphasia, the involvement of the RH in this improvement remains an open question [15–19]. While previous neuroimaging studies have examined structural changes and changes in local brain activation following melody-based interventions [20, 21], the current case study focused on changes in functional connectivity within the language network bilaterally. We examined the question whether compensatory processes following melody-based treatment involve changes in connectivity among the right or left hemisphere regions.

1.1. Melody-Based Therapy for Aphasia. The use of melody in aphasia treatment is based on the observation that singing and the production of melodic speech are often intact, even when standard speech is impaired in patients with nonfluent aphasia [22–24]. In Melodic Intonation Therapy (MIT), the most commonly used melody-based therapy, participants repeat phrases with a simplified and exaggerated prosody, characterized by a melodic component of two notes and a rhythmic component of two durations [16, 25]. The protocol of MIT also includes tapping the rhythm with the left hand while repeating the melodic phrases [18]. Other melody-based therapies modify the melodic structure of the phrases or expand some of the musical elements [16, 26]. MIT has been recommended for use with nonfluent aphasia patients with poorly articulated speech, severe disorders in repetition, and relatively good auditory comprehension [19]. MIT has been employed primarily with patients with aphasia due to stroke; however, MIT or similar therapies have also been administered to patients with other neurologically based speech and language disorders, such as traumatic brain injury (TBI, e.g., [26]). Two review papers of MIT and other melody-based therapies [16, 19], which together include over 600 patients, concluded that there is positive evidence for the benefit of these therapy methods (although many studies did not measure generalization to spontaneous communication). The efficacy of these treatment methods was evident in both subacute [27] and chronic [16] patients. Nevertheless, a recent randomized control trial, with 17 chronic patients that received MIT, did not find stable maintenance of the effects at 6-week follow-up and no generalization to untreated items [28].

1.2. Mechanism and Lateralization. Despite the common use of melody-based therapies, and the positive evidence for their effectiveness, the underlying mechanisms and the role of the melodic component in language recovery are still unresolved [16, 19]. Other critical ingredients may be the rhythmic cueing provided during treatment [29] or the slow articulation of connected syllables which enhances auditory-motor feedback and increase inner rehearsal [23, 25]. Processing of music and prosody, and spectral processing more generally, have traditionally been associated with the RH [30–33]. RH regions have also been associated with the production of sung versus spoken output [34–37]. The preserved ability of patients with aphasia to sing, despite difficulty in producing spoken output, underlies the assumption that melody-based treatments should recruit RH regions [22].

The current evidence, from functional imaging studies, for the involvement of the RH in melody-based treatment is mixed. An early PET study ([38], $N = 7$) and several smaller fMRI studies ([39–41]; total N (across studies) = 5) showed an increase in LH activation and decrease in RH activation in patients who benefitted from melody-based treatments. However, some interpreted such a decrease in RH activation as reflecting greater efficiency of the RH language processing [42], and others ([17, 18]; total $N = 4$) showed bilateral increases in activation with a more prominent increase in right frontal activation. Recently, a case series with patients with aphasia showed increases in right lateralization in four out of five subacute patients (i.e., within three months poststroke) following MIT but no right lateralization in chronic patients (i.e., greater than 1 year postonset; [43]).

Structural-imaging studies show more consistent evidence for the involvement of the RH in melody-based therapy. 11 patients undergoing MIT showed an increase in RH white matter volume and a correlation of behavioral improvement with changes in the right IFG pars opercularis [44]. Diffusion tensor imaging (DTI) measures show an increase in the number of fibers in the right arcuate fasciculus in 7 patients undergoing MIT [20, 21] and showed a marginally significant correlation with improvement [20]. In addition to the effects of melody, this can be the result of the left hand tapping that accompanies treatment [20], as was also shown in naming treatment studies that do not involve melody [45, 46].

Finally, two transcranial brain stimulation studies showed that excitatory stimulation of the right posterior IFG has improved the effects of MIT in some of the participants [15, 47]. It should be noted that although these studies show a role for right frontal areas in treatment improvement, they do not compare it to the role played by the LH.

1.3. The Current Study. The current study aims to examine the underlying brain mechanisms associated with melody-based treatment by looking at changes in the functional connectivity in the language network. In contrast to the ambiguous interpretation of local activation changes (in which a decrease in activation in the RH may reflect less reliance on the RH or more efficient processing in the RH), functional connectivity with RH regions is more clearly associated with increased involvement of the RH. We examined the changes in resting-state connectivity in the language network of a patient with chronic nonfluent aphasia associated with melody-based treatment. Resting-state measures do not depend on the patient's level of language performance, while still depicting connectivity in the language network [48–52]. Treatment-related changes in resting-state connectivity have been shown following motor recovery in motor areas [53] and following aphasia treatment in both the default mode [54] and language [55] networks. Patient connectivity analyses were compared to a control patient who did not receive therapy during the same time interval. We predicted that melody-based treatment would enhance the connectivity among right frontal language areas (i.e., language production homologues), as well as between these areas and motor regions associated with planning and execution of speech. We did not expect to find such enhancement of connectivity among LH language areas in our patient or in the untreated control patient.

2. Methods

2.1. Participants. JV was a 48-year-old right-handed female at the time of injury, with 16 years of education. She is a native speaker of Tagalog, and was a fluent speaker of English as a second language. She sustained a moderate-severe traumatic brain injury (TBI) secondary to a fall from a ladder onto a concrete floor. A CT scan performed on the day of the injury indicated left frontal and temporal subdural hematomas

(Glasgow Coma Scale (GCS) score not available), which were evacuated in an urgent craniotomy. JV was in a coma for five to six weeks. Unfortunately, she sustained a second TBI three months later, as a result of another fall while in hospital, at which time her language symptoms worsened. MRI at the time of the second TBI showed evidence of a new subarachnoid hemorrhage in the left medial temporal sulcus, in addition to underlying encephalomalacia in the left frontal and left temporal lobes associated with the initial hematomas (see Figure 1). The results of neuropsychological assessment conducted 25 months after the second injury and language assessment conducted 36 months after the second injury (immediately before therapy) show moderate-severe nonfluent aphasia, characterized by limited spontaneous speech output, stereotypical utterances, moderate comprehension deficits, and good use of gestures and facial expressions to support communication. The patient also presented with moderate apraxia of speech (based on tasks for assessing apraxia of speech [56]), characterized by audible groping, sound distortions and substitutions, articulatory self-corrections, difficulty with words of increasing length, delayed response initiation, and slow rate of speech. She had normal visuoperceptual and hearing abilities. She appeared to respond well to musical stimulation, including melodic and rhythmic cueing, during informal diagnostic testing. Detailed language and neuropsychological assessment findings are presented in Tables 1 and 2.

The control TBI patient, GB, was a right-handed female, native speaker of English, with 13 years of education who was 54 years of age at the time of injury. She had sustained a moderate to severe TBI secondary to a motor vehicle accident. Her GCS at the scene was 5 and declined to 3 at the time of admission to the emergency department. A CT scan performed on the day of injury indicated a left temporal subarachnoid hemorrhage as well as an intraventricular hemorrhage. GB was in a coma for approximately 1 week following the accident. Neuropsychological assessment at 28 months postinjury did not indicate any persistent language deficits. Although the control patient is a native English speaker, while the treated patient speaks English as a second language, we do not expect this to affect the results because we are not comparing between them on language performance or on a language task-related functional imaging. Ethics approval was granted for the study, and both participants had signed an informed consent.

2.2. Treatment Description. Thirty-six months after her second injury, as part of the current study, JV started receiving a melody-based treatment, which was a modified version of MIT [25, 28]. Therapy was developed jointly by a speech language pathologist and music therapist and administered in English, remotely via Skype® by the accredited music therapist (coauthor Cheryl Jones), specialized in Neurologic Music Therapy [60]. All treatment stimuli were trained using the musical elements of melody and rhythm. A unique melody, distinct in shape and rhythmic pattern, was assigned to each target phrase and served as a timing template to support word retrieval and the fluency of word production. This is in contrast to the standard MIT protocol, which

uses only two to three tones for all phrases. Rhythmic cues served to support oral motor timing impairments and word fluency [60].

Each target phrase, and its associated unique melody, was presented following the standard MIT hierarchy (e.g., [25]): the clinician, accompanied by an electric keyboard, first played and hummed the melody and then sang the target words. The participant then sung the phrase in unison with the therapist for a number of repetitions, with the therapist gradually omitting words until the participant was singing independently. These steps were repeated until the patient could sing the target phrase without support. The participant's son or daughter, present at every session, tapped her left hand, as per the MIT protocol.

Melody served as the primary cue to support word production within the target phrase, and the unique melody was played up to five times, as required, allowing the participant to gradually fill in the melody with the target words. Initially, the participant required maximal melodic cueing (i.e., 5 cues), but this need decreased (i.e., to 1-2 cues) over the course of treatment. Rhythm served as the secondary cue, whereby the rhythm of the target phrase was tapped on her left arm in order to help the participant overcome hesitations or sustained pauses during a phrase. Additional cues included modelling of oral-motor placement and providing the first word in the target phrase. The need for these cues, however, significantly reduced as treatment progressed. In addition to the hierarchical progression of cues, the treatment was designed to enhance generalization, by gradually decreasing the structure of the target phrases, thereby increasing the linguistic difficulty. Namely, the treatment involved progressing through 5 steps: steps 1 to 3 primarily involved repetition; step 4, sentence completion; and step 5, phrase production (in response to target questions). Novel responses were encouraged in steps 4 and 5.

The primary goal of steps 1 to 3 was to use melodic and rhythmic cues to encourage word retrieval and fluency in sentences of increasing length and complexity. The participant was required to produce target phrases with and without melodic intonation. The primary goal of step 4 (sentence completion task) was to encourage generalization beyond trained phrases, by asking the participant to generate novel words at the end of each rehearsed target phrase. In step 5, the primary goal of treatment was for JV to produce fully self-generated phrases, using two tones to produce nonrehearsed responses to target questions. Untreated items were also created and matched to all treatment stimuli in terms of number of syllables, syntactic complexity, and relevance to the participant's life and interests. These items were not treated and served for testing before, immediately after, and eight weeks following treatment (see outcome measures).

2.3. Treatment Stimuli. Treatment stimuli were created based on an "interest" inventory completed by JV and her family, whereby the participant listed her primary hobbies and interests, important members of her family and friend groups, details from her past, and her speech-related goals. Treatment stimuli were phrases on a continuum of difficulty in terms of syllable length and syntactic complexity. Shorter,

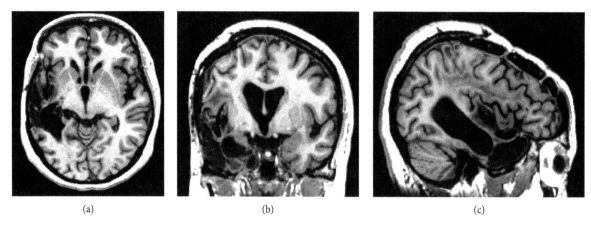

FIGURE 1: MR T1-weighted image of the patient's brain in (a) axial, (b) coronal, and (c) sagittal views. The patient presents with an extensive area of encephalomalacia within the left cerebral hemisphere involving the temporal and frontoparietal lobes with volume loss.

TABLE 1: JV's language assessment 36 months postinjury.

Language assessment	Pretreatment		Posttreatment	
	Raw score	Percentile	Raw score	Percentile
Boston Naming Test (BNT)—short form				
BNT—number of spontaneously given correct responses	2/15	30	0/15	30
BNT—number of correct responses following phonemic cue	4/11	NA	4/13	NA
BNT—number of correct choices	3/9	NA	6/11	NA
BDAE—short form				
I.A. simple social responses	6/7	50	6/7	50
Aphasia Severity Rating Scale	1/5	40	2/5	50
II.A. word comprehension	8/16	<10	10/16	10
II.B. commands	8/10	40	8/10	40
II.C. complex ideational material	3/6	30	4/6	50
III.B. automatized sequences	1/4	10	1/4	10
III.B. repetition single words	4/5	60	4/5	60
III.B. repetition sentences	1/2	60	1/2	60
III.C. responsive naming	0/10	10	4/10	30
III.C. naming—screening of special categories	7/12	20	7/12	20
IV.C. oral word reading	3/15	<20	3/15	<20
IV.C. oral sentence reading	0/5	30	0/5	30
IV.C. sentence comprehension	0/3	10	0/3	10
IV.D. reading comprehension—sentences and paragraphs	2/4	40	1/4	10
PPTT (3 pictures)	40/52	NA	DNT	
PALPA 7 syllable length repetition	22/24	NA	22/24	NA

BDAE = Boston Diagnostic Aphasia Examination [57]; PPTT = Pyramids and Palm Trees Test [58]; PALPA = psycholinguistic assessments of language processing in aphasia [59]; NA = percentiles not available.

simpler (e.g., imperative and wh-question) phrases were used initially, followed by longer, declarative present- and past-tense phrases (based on HELPSS hierarchy, [61]). The target phrases were categorized into five distinct treatment steps: (1) 2–4 syllables (e.g., "How are you?"); (2) 5–7 syllables (e.g., "Please do the dishes"); (3) 8–10 syllables (e.g., "I drink coffee every morning"); (4) sentence completion cues (e.g., "For dinner I will make…"); and (5) question probes (e.g., "What did you do yesterday?"). There were seven target

phrases in steps 1 to 3, nine target phrases in step 4, and 10 target questions in step 5.

2.4. Treatment Schedule/Protocol. JV started receiving treatment 36 months after her second injury and received treatment three days a week for 16 weeks, for a total of 48 sessions. Each session lasted approximately 30 minutes. At the beginning of each session, three previously learned phrases were rehearsed, to encourage maintenance and

TABLE 2: JV neuropsychological assessment 25 months postinjury.

Domain/test	Raw score	Standard score	Classification
Manual motor/psychomotor functioning			
Grip strength (dom)	25 kg	$T = 41$	Low average
Grip strength (non-dom)	22.5 kg	$T = 45$	Average
Grooved pegboard (dom)	119 sec (0 drops)	$T = 19$	Severely impaired
Grooved pegboard (non-dom)	80 sec (0 drops)	$T = 42$	Low average
Attention/speed of processing			
Visual span forwards	8	$SS = 9$	Average
Symbol Digit Modalities Test—W	42 items (0 errors)	$z = -1.2$	Mildly impaired
Trail Making Test A	40 sec	$T = 38$	Mildly impaired
Trail Making Test B	179 sec (2 errors)	$T = 23$	Moderately impaired
Language functions			
MAE Token Test	9/44		Very defective
Peabody Picture Vocabulary Test-III	126	1st %ile	Impaired (age equivalent = 9 years, 9 months)
Visuospatial functioning			
Visual Form Discrimination	32/32		Intact
WAIS—Block Design	24/68	$SS = 7$	Borderline impaired
RVDLT—copy	32/36	6–10%ile	Mildly impaired
RVDLT—time to complete (copy)	361 sec	2-5th %ile	Mildly impaired
RVDLT—copy organizational quality	1/5		Extremely piecemeal; drawn rotated 90 degrees
Memory			
RVDLT—total trials 1–5	46 Figures (26 intrusions)	$z = 0.13$	Average
RVDLT—immediate recall	14.5/36	$T = 37$	Mildly impaired
RVDLT—highest number of figures recalled	12/15		
RVDLT—delayed recall	11/15 (4 intrusions)		
RVDLT—delayed recognition	10/15 (2 false alarms)	$z = -4.7$	Severely impaired
BVMT Total Immediate Recall	17/36	$T = 36$	Mildly impaired
BVMT Total—Delayed Recall	8/12	$T = 44$	Average
BVMT Recognition	6/6 (0 false alarms)	>16th %ile	Intact
Executive functioning			
Visual span backwards	7	$SS = 10$	Average
WAIS—matrix reasoning	11/26	$SS = 9$	Average
WCST—total administered	128 (full WCST)		
WCST—errors	40	$T = 33$	Mildly impaired
WCST—perseverative responses	27	$T = 31$	Mildly impaired
WCST—perseverative errors	23	$T = 31$	Mildly impaired
WCST—nonperseverative errors	17	$T = 37$	Mildly impaired
WCST—conceptual level responses	45	$T = 31$	Mildly impaired
WCST—categories	4	11-16th %ile	Mildly impaired
Trials to complete 1st category	12	>16th%ile	Intact

MAE Token Test = Multilingual Aphasia Examination Token Test; WAIS = Wechsler Adult Intelligence Scale; RVDLT = Rey Visual Design Learning Test; BVMT = Brief Visuospatial Memory Test; WCST = Wisconsin Card Sorting Test; W = written.

continued practice of all treated items. Progression through steps 1 to 5 occurred if either (a) the participant produced 80% of the target phrases with 80% accuracy on two consecutive sessions or (b) the participant completed 9 sessions of therapy within a single step. Target accuracy was measured as the proportion of syllables correctly produced within the target phrase (for steps 1 to 3) and the appropriateness of the responses given to sentence completion and question probes (for steps 4 and 5). Each melody and phrase was notated and emailed to the participant, who was instructed to practice the target phrases between sessions for 30 minutes, three times per week. The participant was also required to sing personally significant songs for ten minutes a day, five days a week, in an attempt to reinforce word retrieval through familiar melody and word associations. These activities were monitored by the patient using a "homework log." These logs indicated very good compliance of the patient with the homework.

2.5. Primary Outcome Measures. Both treated and untreated items were administered pretherapy, immediately posttherapy, and at eight weeks posttherapy by a registered speech-language pathologist who was not involved in the treatment (coauthor Tijana Simic). The primary outcome measure for steps 1 to 3 was the ability to repeat target phrases accurately (measured as the *proportion* of correctly produced syllables in each phrase). In steps 4 and 5, the primary outcome measures were the *raw number* of syllables produced in appropriate responses to sentence completion cues (step 4) and questions (step 5). Syllables produced in inappropriate responses (e.g., that did not fit the context of the cue or question probe) were discarded and not included in the raw counts. All outcome measures were taken using spoken, not melodic, cues.

2.6. MR Image Acquisition Protocol. Whole head MR scans were acquired on a General Electric (GE) Signa-Echospeed 1.5 Tesla high-definition scanner, located at Toronto General Hospital—University Health Network, using an eight-channel head coil. The high-resolution 1 mm isotropic T1-weighted, three-dimensional radio-frequency spoiled-gradient recalled-echo (SPGR) images were acquired in the axial plane utilizing a 25 cm field of view (FOV) (TR/TE/TI = 12/5/300 ms), flip angle = 20°, slice thickness = 1 mm no gap, 160 slices, and matrix 256×256. Resting-state BOLD fMRI data were acquired with the following imaging parameters: TR/TE = 2000/40 ms, flip angle = 85°, FOV = 22, slice thickness 5 mm with no gap, 32 slices with 4800 images, and matrix 64×64. Resting-state data were collected at three time points. For JV, this was at 25 months, 35 months, and 39 months after the second injury, with treatment occurring between 36 and 39 months postinjury. Resting-state data for the control patient GB was collected at 28 months, 32 months, and 36 months postinjury, with no speech and language treatment. Additional sequences include DTI and axial fast spin-echo PD/T2-weighted images, which are not presented here. All sequences were obtained with a 22 cm FOV. The entire scanning session lasted approximately 55 min.

2.7. Resting-State Connectivity Analysis

2.7.1. Preprocessing. The preprocessing of resting-state data was performed using SPM12 (Wellcome Department of Imaging Neuroscience, London, UK; http://www.fil.ion.ucl.ac.uk/spm). The preprocessing steps included removal of the first five scans, slice-timing correction, rigid-body motion correction and unwarping, spatial normalization to the Montreal Neurological Institute (MNI) space, and smoothing with an 8 mm FWHM Gaussian kernel.

2.7.2. Functional Connectivity. Functional connectivity analysis was performed using a region of interest (ROI) to ROI approach within CONN's functional connectivity toolbox (Whitfield-Gabrieli and Nieto-Castanon 2012; http://www.nitrc.org/projects/conn). We selected anatomical ROIs in bilateral frontal areas: inferior frontal gyrus (IFG) pars opercularis (Operc), pars triangularis (Tri), and pars orbitalis (Orb); precentral gyrus (PreC), insula, and supplementary motor area (SMA). Subregions within left IFG (opercularis, triangularis, and orbitalis), known to be involved in language production [62], were previously used as seed regions for the language network in resting-state studies [48, 51, 52]. Their homologous regions in the right IFG were shown to be involved in melody-based treatments, in structural-imaging and brain stimulation studies [15, 44, 47]. The left precentral gyrus, insula, and SMA are typically involved in motor sequence planning for articulation and initiation of speech [63–65], and the right SMA was also shown to be involved in melody-based treatments [21]. A mask was created to encompass these ROIs using the automated anatomical labeling (AAL) atlas [66].

Sources of physiological noise (based on white matter and cerebrospinal fluid segmentation) and movement covariates (motion correction and scrubbing using Artifact Detection Tools; ART http://www.nitrc.org/projects/artifact_detect) were regressed out of the data. Data was also bandpass filtered to retain low-level frequencies $(0.009 < f < 0.08 \text{ Hz})$. Semipartial correlations were then computed using the residual data across all ROIs, for each time point (T1-baseline, T2-pretreatment, and T3-posttreatment) and participant (treated versus control patient). In semipartial correlations, the effects of all other regions on the *target* region alone are held constant while computing the correlation between the source and the target region. Therefore, semipartial correlation between two regions is not symmetric and depends on which region is the target. The correlations were then transformed into *z*-scores using Fisher's *r* to *z* transformation.

Similar to the approach taken by Sandberg et al. [67], difference matrices were computed to determine the level of increase and/or decrease in functional connectivity across time points. A difference matrix was calculated by subtracting post- minus pretreatment functional connectivity to identify changes during the "treatment period" (or its equivalent in the control patient; T3 – T2) and by subtracting pretreatment minus baseline functional connectivity to identify changes during the "baseline period" (T2 – T1). Significant differences in correlational changes across time points (treatment versus baseline period; separately for each participant; $p < 0.05$ (FDR corrected for 66 comparisons)) were determined using Fisher's test.

3. Results

3.1. Treatment Outcomes/Behavioral Results. The proportions of correctly produced syllables before and immediately posttreatment, for both treated and untreated phrases, are presented in Table 3(a) for the repetition task (steps 1 to 3, collapsed). The *number* of syllables produced in appropriate

TABLE 3: Treatment outcome measures for JV.

(a)

| | Sentence repetition (steps 1 to 3) | |
| | Mean % correctly produced syllables (SD) | |
	Treated phrases ($N = 21$)	Untreated phrases ($N = 21$)
Pre-	71.34 (28.79)	64.60 (32.59)
Post-	96.78 (8.05)	61.55 (33.15)
8-week	93.33 (13.30)	74.11 (30.88)

| | p values (Wilcoxon signed-rank test for related samples) | | |
	Treated post	Treated 8 weeks	Untreated post
Treated pre	$p = 0.002^*$	$p = 0.011^*$	
Treated post			$p = 0.001^*$

*Alpha = 0.0167 (Bonferroni correction).

(b)

| | Sentence completion (step 4) | |
| | Mean number of syllables produced (SD) | |
	Treated phrases ($N = 9$)	Untreated phrases ($N = 9$)
Pre-	1.44 (1.88)	1.78 (1.20)
Post-	4.22 (2.44)	4.78 (2.28)
8-week	2.78 (2.04)	3.78 (1.72)

| | p values (Wilcoxon signed-rank test for related samples) | | | |
	Treated post	Treated 8 weeks	Untreated post	Untreated 8 weeks
Treated pre	$p = 0.02^\wedge$	$p = 0.114$		
Treated post			$p = 0.481$	
Untreated pre			$p = 0.048$	$p = 0.026^\wedge$

$^\wedge$Approaching significance of Alpha = 0.01 (Bonferroni correction).

(c)

| | Answering questions (step 5) | |
| | Mean number of syllables produced (SD) | |
	Treated phrases ($N = 10$)	Untreated phrases ($N = 10$)
Pre-	0.50 (1.08)	0.40 (0.97)
Post-	6.20 (2.90)	2.10 (3.03)
8-week	4.60 (3.06)	2.40 (3.13)

| | p values (Wilcoxon signed-rank test for related samples) | | | |
	Treated post	Treated 8 weeks	Untreated post	Untreated 8 weeks
Treated pre	$p = 0.005^*$	$p = 0.007^*$		
Treated post			$p = 0.010^*$	
Untreated pre			$p = 0.068$	$p = 0.066$

*Alpha = 0.01 (Bonferroni correction).
Performance on treated and untreated phrases at pre-, post- and 8-week follow-up tests. Sentence repetition (steps 1–3; (a)), sentence completion (step 4, (b)), and probe questions (step 5, (c)) are presented. Statistical comparisons with Wilcoxon signed-rank test are indicated at the bottom of each panel.

responses to sentence completion and question probes (steps 4 and 5, resp.) are presented in Tables 3(b) and 3(c), respectively. The Wilcoxon signed-rank test for the comparison of two related samples showed no significant difference in pretreatment performance between the treated and untreated phrases for the repetition ($Z = -0.967$, $p = 0.333$), sentence completion ($Z = 0.853$, $p = 0.394$), and probe question ($Z = -0.272$, $p = 0.785$) tasks. Given the varying task demands, analyses for these three tasks were completed separately.

The Wilcoxon signed-rank test for related samples was used to assess the treatment effect on syllable production when repeating sentences of increasing length and complexity (steps 1 to 3) and compared to performance on untreated stimuli sets. Three comparisons were made with these data; using the Bonferroni correction, alpha was set at 0.017. JV's ability to repeat syllables within treated phrases significantly improved pre- to posttreatment ($Z = 3.061$, $p = 0.002$) and was significantly better than her ability to repeat syllables in matched untreated phrases posttreatment ($Z = -3.313$, $p = 0.001$); this treatment effect was maintained at eight-week follow-up ($Z = 2.552$, $p = 0.011$).

In the sentence completion task (step 4), five comparisons were made using the Wilcoxon signed-rank test for related samples; thus, alpha was set at 0.01 (Bonferroni correction). The difference between pre- and posttreatment tests in the number of syllables produced by JV when given a sentence completion cue approached, but did not reach, significance ($Z = 2.319$, $p = 0.020$); no significant increase was seen from pretreatment to the eight-week follow-up either ($Z = 1.582$, $p = 0.114$). Visual inspection of the data for untreated phrases suggested a generalization effect to untreated items in this task. Indeed, when comparing treated and untreated items posttreatment, no significant difference was found ($Z = 0.704$, $p = 0.481$), indicating overall improvement of both treated and untreated items over time. We therefore also compared improvement in untreated items pre- to posttreatment ($Z = 1.975$, $p = 0.048$) and pre- to eight-week follow-up ($Z = 2.232$, $p = 0.026$). These comparisons approached, but did not reach, significance.

Finally, JV's ability to answer questions (step 5) was also assessed using the related-sample Wilcoxon signed-rank test; five comparisons were again made here; thus, alpha was set at 0.01. JV's ability to answer treated questions significantly improved pre- to posttreatment ($Z = 2.814$, $p = 0.005$), and this was maintained at eight-week follow-up ($Z = 2.692$, $p = 0.007$). In addition, her ability to answer trained questions compared to untreated questions posttreatment was significantly better ($Z = -2.561$, $p = 0.010$). As in the sentence completion task (step 4), we assessed whether generalization to untreated items occurred but did not find significant improvements in performance on untreated stimuli pre- to posttreatment ($Z = -1.826$, $p = 0.068$) and pretreatment to eight-week follow-up ($Z = 1.841$, $p = 0.066$).

JV was reassessed on various language measures following treatment (Table 1) but, apart from better performance on the BDAE responsive naming task, did not show notable improvements on these tasks.

3.2. Resting-State Connectivity. Changes in resting-state connectivity during the treatment interval in the treated patient and the equivalent interval in the control patient are presented in Figure 2 and in the upper half of Tables 4 (for the treated patient) and 5 (for the control patient) in the Supplementary Materials. The values in Figure 2 represent differences in semipartial correlations in T3 – T2. These changes were compared to the changes during the baseline interval (T2 – T1), which are presented in the lower halves of Tables 4 and 5 (in the Supplementary Materials). Only changes that are significantly different between the treatment and baseline intervals are presented in Figure 2. Significance is determined with FDR correction for 66 comparisons ($p < 0.05$ and $*p < 0.01$). The results for the treated patient show an increase in the connectivity during the treatment period between regions involved in speech motor control (bilateral SMA and insula) and right frontal language areas. These connections include R.Operc–L.SMA, R.Tri–R.SMA, and R.Tri–L.Insula. There was also an increase in connectivity within the right frontal language areas (R.Orb–R.Operc). These increases were significantly larger than the changes that occurred during the baseline period. Importantly, no increase in connectivity was found for the left language area. In addition to these increases in connectivity, there were also connections showing a decrease in connectivity during the treatment period, and these were for both the left and right language areas (see Figure 2(a)). The pattern of results is altogether different in the control patient, who did not undergo treatment. In this patient, there was no increase in connectivity in the right frontal language areas. Instead, increase in connectivity for the control patient was found between the left frontal language areas and regions involved in speech motor control (L.SMA–L.Operc) and within the left frontal language areas (L.Orb–L.Operc). Finally, both patients showed increases in connectivity between bilateral regions involved in speech motor control, that is, R.Insula–L.Insula in the treated patient and L.PreC–R.PreC and L.PreC–R.Insula in the control patient (see Figures 2(a) and 2(b)).

4. Discussion

This study examined the effect of melody-based treatment on a chronic patient with moderate to severe aphasia due to extensive left frontotemporal lesions following two temporally proximal brain injuries three years earlier. The patient's performance on treated and untreated phrases was examined before, immediately after, and eight weeks following treatment. Resting-state connectivity was examined at three time points: T1—baseline (25 months postinjury), T2—pretreatment (36 months postinjury), and T3—posttreatment (39 months postinjury). This was compared to a control patient, who did not receive treatment during the same time period. We expected that improvement in language performance following treatment would be associated with an increase in functional connectivity between right frontal homologues of language areas and regions involved in motor speech control.

Behavioral measures of performance on treated phrases showed improvement in the repetition of sentences of varying lengths and complexity. Likewise, JV's ability to

answer question probes improved following treatment, with more appropriate and longer answers; these improvements were maintained at the eight-week follow-up, and similar improvements were not seen in the untreated phrases and/ or question probes. Performance on the sentence completion task improved numerically during treatment, but improvement was only marginally significant. Moreover, visual inspection of the data indicated similar levels of improvement in both treated and untreated phrases in the sentence completion task, with no difference between treated and untreated phrases posttreatment. These results, together with improved performance on the responsive naming subtest of the BDAE (a task similar to sentence completion), suggest that treatment effects generalized to untreated stimuli in the sentence completion task (step 4). However, the small number of phrases in step 4 may have underpowered the analysis and masked this effect. Alternatively, the marginal treatment effect for treated phrases in the sentence completion task may suggest that relative to the more open-ended nature of the probe questions, the constrained sentence completion task may have proven especially difficult.

Resting-state connectivity measures for the treated patient showed increases in connectivity between right frontal language areas (R.Tri and R.Operc) and regions involved in speech motor control (bilateral SMA and L.Insula) during the treatment period. There were also significant increases in connectivity within the right frontal language areas (R.Orb–R.Operc), compared to the baseline period. Moreover, these changes were specific to the RH and to the treated patient. In contrast, the control patient, who did not receive treatment, showed increases in connectivity between the left frontal language (L.Operc) and speech motor control area (L.SMA) and within the left frontal language areas (L.Orb–L.Operc) during the same time period.

4.1. Behavioral Effect of the Melody-Based Treatment. The behavioral improvements observed in the repetition of treated phrases in the current study are consistent with previous research showing the effectiveness of melody-based treatments for patients with nonfluent aphasia [16, 19]. Although patient JV had focal lesions, she had also suffered from TBI. Except for the two patients reported by Baker [26], other patients reported in the literature who have been treated with MIT or modified versions of MIT have had an etiology of stroke. Our findings extend those of Baker [26] in showing that melody-based therapy can be successful in patients with an etiology other than stroke, which may involve different physiological recovery mechanisms [68]. In addition, the patient's comprehension deficit do not fit the optimal profile for melody-based therapy [18]. Nevertheless, the patient's substantial improvement from the treatment is in keeping with other studies [25, 69] which suggest that relatively intact comprehension ability is not a critical inclusion criterion.

In addition to improvement on treated phrases, our findings also show some evidence for generalization of treatment effects to untreated phrases with the sentence completion task (step 4) and a nonsignificant trend for improvement on the untreated question (step 5). These tasks, which are

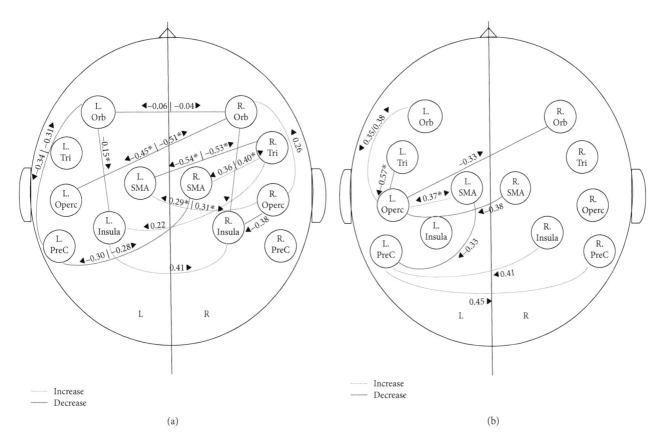

FIGURE 2: Changes in resting-state connectivity during the treatment interval in the treated patient JV (a) and control patient GB (b). Increase: green; decrease: red. Values represent differences (T3 – T2) in the semipartial correlation. Arrows point to the target region in the calculation of semipartial correlations. Only changes in T3 – T2 which were significantly greater than changes during the baseline period (T2 – T1) are shown. Significance is determined with FDR correction for 66 correlations with $p < 0.05$ or $p < 0.01$ (marked by*). L: left; R: right; Orb: orbitalis; Tri: triangularis; Operc: opercularis; PreC: precentral; SMA: supplementary motor area.

not typically included in melody-based treatment protocols, such as the standard MIT [19], were introduced in the present study, in order to encourage generalization in the later stages of treatment by practicing the generation of novel words during treatment. That these tasks, and especially the response to questions in stage 5, are similar to natural spontaneous speech is worth noticing. The relatively scarce evidence for generalization to untreated phrases [70] or to spontaneous speech [18, 20, 71] in other MIT studies points to the potential benefit of the sentence completion task in enhancing generalization of treatment effects.

4.2. The Effect of the Melody-Based Treatment on the Language Network. Analyses of resting-state connectivity, which show an increase in connectivity within the right frontal language areas, and between these areas and regions involved in speech motor control during treatment, are consistent both with our hypothesis and with the underlying assumptions of melody-based treatment approaches, namely, that musical abilities typically associated with RH areas [22] are preserved in patients with LH lesions and may therefore be recruited to successfully compensate for damaged LH language areas. The current results show that indeed the language network in the RH and specifically the right frontal regions are contributing to improvements seen after treatment.

Our findings are consistent with a number of functional imaging studies, showing a greater increase in activation in the right compared to the left frontal cortex following MIT ([17, 18]; total $N = 4$) although lateralization was not consistent across all functional activation studies ([38–41]; total $N = 12$). The results of the current study extend previous functional imaging findings by showing an increase in the right lateralization at the level of the network. While decreases in RH local activation is ambiguous because it may indicate either greater neural efficiency in the RH or less reliance on the RH [42], the results of functional connectivity measures are more clearly interpretable. Even if local activation decreases due to increased neural efficiency, the coupling between these regions and downstream regions is expected to be enhanced.

By using resting-state data, the current results further demonstrate that these treatment effects are not solely task dependent. Treatment-related changes in resting-state connectivity were previously shown with other types of aphasia therapies [54, 55], and the current study extends them to melody-based therapy. Our results are also consistent with brain stimulation studies showing that excitatory stimulation of the right posterior IFG as an adjuvant to MIT improves the effect of aphasia treatment [15, 47]. In relation to these findings, the current study has further shown that treatment effects are specific to the right hemisphere and to a patient that underwent melody-based therapy. Similar RH language network changes were not seen in the control patient, who showed an increase in connectivity only in LH language areas, and the connections between the LH language network and bilateral areas involved in speech motor control. These increases in connectivity in the control patient, who did not undergo any treatment during the relevant period, may be a result of everyday language experiences this patient may have encountered.

In contrast to functional imaging measures, structural-imaging results indicate a more stable change, which is not task dependent. The evidence, for the involvement of the RH in melody-based treatment in the current study, is broadly consistent with findings from DTI studies showing an increase in the number of fibers in the right arcuate fasciculus in patients following MIT [20, 21]. More specific to the location of the effects within the RH, the increase in connections with the right opercularis (R.Operc–L.SMA; R.Operc–R.Orb) in the current study is consistent with volumetric measures showing a correlation between improvement in intonation-based therapy and increases in white matter volume in the right opercularis [44]. The IFG pars opercularis, which roughly occupies BA 44, serves as the intermediate region between language areas involved in retrieval and the precentral gyrus which is part of the speech motor control system involved in articulation [72, 73]. Within the speech motor control system, SMA plays a critical role in controlling the initiation of speech motor commands [74, 75] and the insula is implicated in articulatory coordination and control [76, 77]. The increase in connectivity between language areas and speech motor control regions (R.Operc–L.SMA; R.Tri–R.SMA; R.Tri–L.Insula), and specifically the convergence on the right opercularis (R.Operc–L.SMA; R.Operc–R.Orb), suggests that the treatment changes the interface between language retrieval and speech motor control. These results are also consistent with studies pointing to slow articulation of connected syllables and auditory-motor integration as the critical ingredient in the effect of MIT [23, 25]. An intriguing suggestion based on these findings is that therapy-induced changes that occur at the interface of the language and speech motor control networks may be more readily generalized to untreated stimuli, as compared to higher-level changes (e.g., word-retrieval processes) within the language network, which may be associated with item-specific learning.

A significant limitation of this study is its single-case design, which does not allow for the correlation of changes seen in brain connectivity and language behaviors. Nevertheless, we believe that the comparison to a baseline period, as well as testing of a control patient enabled us to make conclusions about the specificity of the results to the treatment administered. Lastly, although the measurable focal lesions of this patient were in the left hemisphere and secondary to hemorrhages, the probable presence of diffuse axonal injury secondary to traumatic injury does not allow us to rule out the presence of RH damage; indeed, impairments on measures of visuospatial measures are likely attributable to such damage. Arguably, the RH changes and response to treatment may have been more robust in the absence of these putative changes.

5. Conclusions

Our results show the benefit of melody-based treatment for a patient with moderate-severe nonfluent aphasia, more than three years following traumatic brain injury with focal lesions in the left frontotemporal areas due to hemorrhages. The patient's ability to repeat sentences and answer question probes improved on treated items, and this treatment effect was maintained eight weeks following treatment. Improvement in sentence completion was marginally significant and similar for treated and untreated phrases, suggesting generalization. The results of the resting-state imaging suggest that the effect of melody-based treatment is right lateralized. This effect was stable and found at the level of the functional network even during rest and not only in localized task-dependent activation. Our results further show that the effects are treatment specific and are not shown in a patient that did not receive therapy during the relevant period. Beyond the lateralization of treatment, our results further show that melody-based treatment affects the interface between language retrieval and motor speech control and articulation. A treatment affecting this level of processing may be a good basis for generalization to untreated stimuli. Further research is needed in a larger sample of patients with discrete LH focal lesions.

Supplementary Materials

Tables 4 and 5 in the supplementary material show changes in resting-state connectivity in the treated and control patients separately for the treatment and baseline periods. These were used to compute the differences in Figure 2. Table 4: changes in resting-state connectivity in the treated patient (JV) during the treatment and baseline periods. Values represent difference in semipartial correlations during the treatment period (T3 – T2 in the upper half) and baseline period (T2 – T1 in the lower half). Rows represent source regions and columns represent target regions in the calculation of semipartial correlations. Values in boldface indicate significant differences between the treatment and baseline periods after FDR correction for 66 comparisons $p < 0.05$ (or $p < 0.01$ in larger font size). L: left; R: right; PreC: precentral; Orb: orbitalis; Tri: triangularis; Operc: opercularis; SMA: supplementary motor area. Table 5: changes in resting-state connectivity in the control patient (GB) during the equivalent of the treatment period and the baseline period. Values represent the difference in semipartial correlations during the equivalent of the treatment period (T3 – T2 in the upper half) and the baseline period (T2 – T1 in the lower half). Rows represent source regions, and columns represent target regions in the calculation of semipartial correlations. Values in boldface indicate significant differences between the equivalent of the treatment period and the baseline periods after FDR correction for 66 comparisons $p < 0.05$ (or $p < 0.01$ in larger font size). L: left; R: right; PreC: precentral; Orb: orbitalis; Tri: triangularis; Operc: opercularis; SMA: supplementary motor area. *(Supplementary Materials)*

References

[1] M. Abo, A. Senoo, S. Watanabe et al., "Language-related brain function during word repetition in post-stroke aphasics," *NeuroReport*, vol. 15, no. 12, pp. 1891–1894, 2004.

[2] V. Blasi, A. C. Young, A. P. Tansy, S. E. Petersen, A. Z. Snyder, and M. Corbetta, "Word retrieval learning modulates right frontal cortex in patients with left frontal damage," *Neuron*, vol. 36, no. 1, pp. 159–170, 2002.

[3] S. F. Cappa, D. Perani, F. Grassi et al., "A PET follow-up study of recovery after stroke in acute aphasics," *Brain and Language*, vol. 56, no. 1, pp. 55–67, 1997.

[4] L. Winhuisen, A. Thiel, B. Schumacher et al., "Role of the contralateral inferior frontal gyrus in recovery of language function in poststroke aphasia: a combined repetitive transcranial magnetic stimulation and positron emission tomography study," *Stroke*, vol. 36, no. 8, pp. 1759–1763, 2005.

[5] H. J. Rosen, S. E. Petersen, M. R. Linenweber et al., "Neural correlates of recovery from aphasia after damage to left inferior frontal cortex," *Neurology*, vol. 55, no. 12, pp. 1883–1894, 2000.

[6] S. Abel, C. Weiller, W. Huber, K. Willmes, and K. Specht, "Therapy-induced brain reorganization patterns in aphasia," *Brain*, vol. 138, no. 4, pp. 1097–1112, 2015.

[7] J. Fridriksson, "Preservation and modulation of specific left hemisphere regions is vital for treated recovery from anomia in stroke," *Journal of Neuroscience*, vol. 30, no. 35, pp. 11558–11564, 2010.

[8] C. Leonard, L. Laird, H. Burianová et al., "Behavioural and neural changes after a "choice" therapy for naming deficits in aphasia: preliminary findings," *Aphasiology*, vol. 29, no. 4, pp. 1–20, 2015.

[9] E. Rochon, C. Leonard, H. Burianova et al., "Neural changes after phonological treatment for anomia: an fMRI study," *Brain and Language*, vol. 114, no. 3, pp. 164–179, 2010.

[10] W.-D. Heiss, A. Thiel, J. Kessler, and K. Herholz, "Disturbance and recovery of language function: correlates in PET activation studies," *NeuroImage*, vol. 20, Supplement 1, pp. S42–S49, 2003.

[11] M. A. Naeser, P. I. Martin, E. H. Baker et al., "Overt propositional speech in chronic nonfluent aphasia studied with the dynamic susceptibility contrast fMRI method," *NeuroImage*, vol. 22, no. 1, pp. 29–41, 2004.

[12] W. A. Postman-Caucheteux, R. M. Birn, R. H. Pursley et al., "Single-trial fMRI shows contralesional activity linked to overt naming errors in chronic aphasic patients," *Journal of Cognitive Neuroscience*, vol. 22, no. 6, pp. 1299–1318, 2010.

[13] C. J. Price and J. Crinion, "The latest on functional imaging studies of aphasic stroke," *Current Opinion in Neurology*, vol. 18, no. 4, pp. 429–434, 2005.

[14] D. Saur, R. Lange, A. Baumgaertner et al., "Dynamics of language reorganization after stroke," *Brain*, vol. 129, no. 6, pp. 1371–1384, 2006.

[15] S. Al-Janabi, L. A. Nickels, P. F. Sowman, H. Burianová, D. L. Merrett, and W. F. Thompson, "Augmenting melodic intonation therapy with non-invasive brain stimulation to treat impaired left-hemisphere function: two case studies," *Frontiers in Psychology*, vol. 5, p. 37, 2014.

[16] J. Hurkmans, M. de Bruijn, A. M. Boonstra et al., "Music in the treatment of neurological language and speech disorders: a systematic review," *Aphasiology*, vol. 26, no. 1, pp. 1–19, 2012.

[17] C. P. M. Orellana, M. E. van de Sandt-Koenderman, E. Saliasi et al., "Insight into the neurophysiological processes of melodically intoned language with functional MRI," *Brain and Behavior*, vol. 4, no. 5, pp. 615–625, 2014.

[18] G. Schlaug, S. Marchina, and A. Norton, "From singing to speaking: why singing may lead to recovery of expressive language function in patients with Broca's aphasia," *Music Perception: An Interdisciplinary Journal*, vol. 25, no. 4, pp. 315–323, 2008.

[19] I. van der Meulen, M. E. van de Sandt-Koenderman, and G. M. Ribbers, "Melodic intonation therapy: present controversies and future opportunities," *Archives of Physical Medicine and Rehabilitation*, vol. 93, no. 1, pp. S46–S52, 2012.

[20] G. Schlaug, S. Marchina, and A. Norton, "Evidence for plasticity in white-matter tracts of patients with chronic Broca's aphasia undergoing intense intonation-based speech therapy," *Annals of the New York Academy of Sciences*, vol. 1169, no. 1, pp. 385–394, 2009.

[21] L. Zipse, A. Norton, S. Marchina, and G. Schlaug, "When right is all that is left: plasticity of right-hemisphere tracts in a young aphasic patient," *Annals of the New York Academy of Sciences*, vol. 1252, no. 1, pp. 237–245, 2012.

[22] M. L. Albert, R. W. Sparks, and N. A. Helm, "Melodic intonation therapy for aphasia," *Archives of Neurology*, vol. 29, no. 2, pp. 130-131, 1973.

[23] A. Racette, C. Bard, and I. Peretz, "Making non-fluent aphasics speak: sing along!," *Brain*, vol. 129, no. 10, pp. 2571–2584, 2006.

[24] R. Sparks, N. Helm, and M. Albert, "Aphasia rehabilitation resulting from melodic intonation therapy," *Cortex*, vol. 10, no. 4, pp. 303–316, 1974.

[25] A. Norton, L. Zipse, S. Marchina, and G. Schlaug, "Melodic intonation therapy shared insights on how it is done and why it might help," *Annals of the New York Academy of Sciences*, vol. 1169, pp. 431–436, 2009.

[26] F. A. Baker, "Modifying the melodic intonation therapy program for adults with severe non-fluent aphasia," *Music Therapy Perspectives*, vol. 18, no. 2, pp. 110–114, 2000.

[27] I. van der Meulen, W. M. E. van de Sandt-Koenderman, M. H. Heijenbrok-Kal, E. G. Visch-Brink, and G. M. Ribbers, "The efficacy and timing of melodic intonation therapy in subacute aphasia," *Neurorehabilitation and Neural Repair*, vol. 28, no. 6, pp. 536–544, 2014.

[28] I. Van Der Meulen, M. W. M. E. Van De Sandt-Koenderman, M. H. Heijenbrok, E. Visch-Brink, and G. M. Ribbers, "Melodic intonation therapy in chronic aphasia: evidence from a pilot randomized controlled trial," *Frontiers in Human Neuroscience*, vol. 10, p. 533, 2016.

[29] M. Kim and C. M. Tomaino, "Protocol evaluation for effective music therapy for persons with nonfluent aphasia," *Topics in Stroke Rehabilitation*, vol. 15, no. 6, pp. 555–569, 2008.

[30] S. Samson and R. J. Zatorre, "Melodic and harmonic discrimination following unilateral cerebral excision," *Brain and Cognition*, vol. 7, no. 3, pp. 348–360, 1988.

[31] S. Samson and R. J. Zatorre, "Contribution of the right temporal lobe to musical timbre discrimination," *Neuropsychologia*, vol. 32, no. 2, pp. 231–240, 1994.

[32] M. Schuppert, T. F. Münte, B. M. Wieringa, and E. Altenmüller, "Receptive amusia: evidence for cross-hemispheric neural networks underlying music processing strategies," *Brain*, vol. 123, no. 3, pp. 546–559, 2000.

[33] R. J. Zatorre, P. Belin, and V. B. Penhune, "Structure and function of auditory cortex: music and speech," *Trends in Cognitive Sciences*, vol. 6, no. 1, pp. 37–46, 2002.

[34] S. Brown, M. J. Martinez, and L. M. Parsons, "Music and language side by side in the brain: a PET study of the generation of melodies and sentences," *European Journal of Neuroscience*, vol. 23, no. 10, pp. 2791–2803, 2006.

[35] D. E. Callan, V. Tsytsarev, T. Hanakawa et al., "Song and speech: brain regions involved with perception and covert production," *Neuroimage*, vol. 31, no. 3, pp. 1327–1342, 2006.

[36] K. J. Jeffries, J. B. Fritz, and A. R. Braun, "Words in melody: an H215O PET study of brain activation during singing and speaking," *NeuroReport*, vol. 14, no. 5, pp. 749–754, 2003.

[37] A. Riecker, H. Ackermann, D. Wildgruber, G. Dogil, and W. Grodd, "Opposite hemispheric lateralization effects during speaking and singing at motor cortex, insula and cerebellum," *NeuroReport*, vol. 11, no. 9, pp. 1997–2000, 2000.

[38] P. Belin, M. Zilbovicius, P. Remy et al., "Recovery from nonfluent aphasia after melodic intonation therapy: a PET study," *Neurology*, vol. 47, no. 6, pp. 1504–1511, 1996.

[39] J. I. Breier, S. Randle, L. M. Maher, and A. C. Papanicolaou, "Changes in maps of language activity activation following melodic intonation therapy using magnetoencephalography: two case studies," *Journal of Clinical and Experimental Neuropsychology*, vol. 32, no. 3, pp. 309–314, 2010.

[40] M. Jungblut, W. Huber, C. Mais, and R. Schnitker, "Paving the way for speech: voice-training-induced plasticity in chronic aphasia and apraxia of speech—three single cases," *Neural Plasticity*, vol. 2014, Article ID 841982, 14 pages, 2014.

[41] M. van de Sandt-Koenderman, M. Smits, I. van der Meulen, E. Visch-Brink, A. van der Lugt, and G. Ribbers, "A case study of melodic intonation therapy (MIT) in the subacute stage of aphasia: early re-re activation of left hemisphere structures," *Procedia - Social and Behavioral Sciences*, vol. 6, pp. 241–243, 2010.

[42] K.-i. Tabei, M. Satoh, C. Nakano et al., "Improved neural processing efficiency in a chronic aphasia patient following melodic intonation therapy: a neuropsychological and functional MRI study," *Frontiers in Neurology*, vol. 7, p. 148, 2016.

[43] M. W. M. E. van de Sandt-Koenderman, C. P. Mendez Orellana, I. van der Meulen, M. Smits, and G. M. Ribbers, "Language lateralisation after melodic intonation therapy: an fMRI study in subacute and chronic aphasia," *Aphasiology*, pp. 1–19, 2016.

[44] C. Y. Wan, X. Zheng, S. Marchina, A. Norton, and G. Schlaug, "Intensive therapy induces contralateral white matter changes in chronic stroke patients with Broca's aphasia," *Brain and Language*, vol. 136, pp. 1–7, 2014.

[45] M. L. Benjamin, S. Towler, A. Garcia et al., "A behavioral manipulation engages right frontal cortex during aphasia therapy," *Neurorehabilitation and Neural Repair*, vol. 28, no. 6, pp. 545–553, 2014.

[46] B. Crosson, A. B. Moore, K. M. McGregor et al., "Regional changes in word-production laterality after a naming treatment designed to produce a rightward shift in frontal activity," *Brain and Language*, vol. 111, no. 2, pp. 73–85, 2009.

[47] B. W. Vines, A. C. Norton, and G. Schlaug, "Non-invasive brain stimulation enhances the effects of melodic intonation therapy," *Frontiers in Psychology*, vol. 2, p. 230, 2011.

[48] A. M. Muller and M. Meyer, "Language in the brain at rest: new insights from resting state data and graph theoretical analysis," *Frontiers in Human Neuroscience*, vol. 8, p. 228, 2014.

[49] Y. Tie, L. Rigolo, I. H. Norton et al., "Defining language networks from resting-state fMRI for surgical planning—a feasibility study," *Human Brain Mapping*, vol. 35, no. 3, pp. 1018–1030, 2014.

[50] A. U. Turken and N. F. Dronkers, "The neural architecture of the language comprehension network: converging evidence from lesion and connectivity analyses," *Frontiers in Systems Neuroscience*, vol. 5, p. 1, 2011.

[51] H.-D. Xiang, H. M. Fonteijn, D. G. Norris, and P. Hagoort, "Topographical functional connectivity pattern in the perisylvian language networks," *Cerebral Cortex*, vol. 20, no. 3, pp. 549–560, 2010.

[52] L. Zhu, Y. Fan, Q. Zou, J. Wang, J.-H. Gao, and Z. Niu, "Temporal reliability and lateralization of the resting-state language network," *PLoS One*, vol. 9, no. 1, article e85880, 2014.

[53] G. A. James, Z.-L. Lu, J. W. VanMeter, K. Sathian, X. P. Hu, and A. J. Butler, "Changes in resting state effective connectivity in the motor network following rehabilitation of upper extremity poststroke paresis," *Topics in Stroke Rehabilitation*, vol. 16, no. 4, pp. 270–281, 2009.

[54] K. Marcotte, V. Perlbarg, G. Marrelec, H. Benali, and A. I. Ansaldo, "Default-mode network functional connectivity in aphasia: therapy-induced neuroplasticity," *Brain and Language*, vol. 124, no. 1, pp. 45–55, 2013.

[55] S. van Hees, K. McMahon, A. Angwin, G. de Zubicaray, S. Read, and D. A. Copland, "A functional MRI study of the relationship between naming treatment outcomes and resting state functional connectivity in post-stroke aphasia," *Human Brain Mapping*, vol. 35, no. 8, pp. 3919–3931, 2014.

[56] R. Wertz, L. LaPointe, and J. C. Rosenbek, *Apraxia of Speech in Adults: the Disorder and Its Management*, Singular, San Diego, CA, USA, 1984.

[57] H. Goodglass, E. Kaplan, and B. Barresi, *The Assessment of Aphasia and Related Disorders*, Lippincott Williams & Wilkins, Philadelphia, PA, USA, 2001.

[58] D. Howard and K. Patterson, *The Pyramids and Palm Trees Test: a Test of Semantic Access from Words and Pictures*, Thames Valley Test Company, Suffolk, UK, 1992.

[59] M. Coltheart, J. Kay, and R. Lesser, *PALPA: Psycholinguistic Assessments of Language Processing in Aphasia*, Introduction, Auditory Processing, Reading & Spelling, Erlbaum, Hove, UK, 1992.

[60] M. H. Thaut, G. C. McIntosh, and V. Hoemberg, "Neurobiological foundations of neurologic music therapy: rhythmic entrainment and the motor system," *Frontiers in Psychology*, vol. 5, p. 1185, 2015.

[61] N. Helm-Estabrooks, *Helm Elicited Language Program for Syntax Stimulation*, Pro-Ed, Austin, TX, USA, 1981.

[62] C. J. Price, "A review and synthesis of the first 20 years of PET and fMRI studies of heard speech, spoken language and reading," *NeuroImage*, vol. 62, no. 2, pp. 816–847, 2012.

[63] S. Brown, A. R. Laird, P. Q. Pfordresher, S. M. Thelen, P. Turkeltaub, and M. Liotti, "The somatotopy of speech: phonation and articulation in the human motor cortex," *Brain and Cognition*, vol. 70, no. 1, pp. 31–41, 2009.

[64] P. Nachev, C. Kennard, and M. Husain, "Functional role of the supplementary and pre-supplementary motor areas," *Nature Reviews Neuroscience*, vol. 9, no. 11, pp. 856–869, 2008.

[65] L. I. Shuster, "The effect of sublexical and lexical frequency on speech production: an fMRI investigation," *Brain and Language*, vol. 111, no. 1, pp. 66–72, 2009.

[66] N. Tzourio-Mazoyer, B. Landeau, D. Papathanassiou et al., "Automated anatomical labeling of activations in SPM using a macroscopic anatomical parcellation of the MNI MRI single-subject brain," *NeuroImage*, vol. 15, no. 1, pp. 273–289, 2002.

[67] C. W. Sandberg, J. W. Bohland, and S. Kiran, "Changes in functional connectivity related to direct training and generalization effects of a word finding treatment in chronic aphasia," *Brain and Language*, vol. 150, pp. 103–116, 2015.

[68] R. Prakash and S. T. Carmichael, "Blood–brain barrier breakdown and neovascularization processes after stroke and traumatic brain injury," *Current Opinion in Neurology*, vol. 28, no. 6, pp. 556–564, 2015.

[69] S. J. Wilson, K. Parsons, and D. C. Reutens, "Preserved singing in aphasia: a case study of the efficacy of melodic intonation therapy," *Music Perception*, vol. 24, no. 1, pp. 23–36, 2006.

[70] M. S. Hough, "Melodic intonation therapy and aphasia: another variation on a theme," *Aphasiology*, vol. 24, no. 6-8, pp. 775–786, 2010.

[71] B. Bonakdarpour, A. Eftekharzadeh, and H. Ashayeri, "Melodic intonation therapy in Persian aphasic patients," *Aphasiology*, vol. 17, no. 1, pp. 75–95, 2003.

[72] G. Luppino, A. Murata, P. Govoni, and M. Matelli, "Largely segregated parietofrontal connections linking rostral intraparietal cortex (areas AIP and VIP) and the ventral premotor cortex (areas F5 and F4)," *Experimental Brain Research*, vol. 128, no. 1-2, pp. 181–187, 1999.

[73] M. Petrides, *Neuroanatomy of Language Regions of the Human Brain*, Elsevier, London, UK, 2014.

[74] F. X. Alario, H. Chainay, S. Lehericy, and L. Cohen, "The role of the supplementary motor area (SMA) in word production," *Brain Research*, vol. 1076, no. 1, pp. 129–143, 2006.

[75] J. A. Tourville and F. H. Guenther, "The DIVA model: a neural theory of speech acquisition and production," *Language and Cognitive Processes*, vol. 26, no. 7, pp. 952–981, 2011.

[76] H. Ackermann and A. Riecker, "The contribution(s) of the insula to speech production: a review of the clinical and functional imaging literature," *Brain Structure and Function*, vol. 214, no. 5-6, pp. 419–433, 2010.

[77] J. V. Baldo, D. P. Wilkins, J. Ogar, S. Willock, and N. F. Dronkers, "Role of the precentral gyrus of the insula in complex articulation," *Cortex*, vol. 47, no. 7, pp. 800–807, 2011.

Right Hemisphere Grey Matter Volume and Language Functions in Stroke Aphasia

Sladjana Lukic,[1,2] Elena Barbieri,[1,2] Xue Wang,[1,3] David Caplan,[1,4] Swathi Kiran,[1,5] Brenda Rapp,[1,6] Todd B. Parrish,[1,3] and Cynthia K. Thompson[1,2,7]

[1]Center for the Neurobiology of Language Recovery, Northwestern University, Evanston, IL, USA
[2]Department of Communication Sciences and Disorders, School of Communication, Northwestern University, Evanston, IL, USA
[3]Department of Radiology, Feinberg School of Medicine, Northwestern University, Chicago, IL, USA
[4]Department of Neurology, Massachusetts General Hospital, Harvard Medical School, Boston, MA, USA
[5]Department of Speech, Language, and Hearing, College of Health & Rehabilitation, Boston University, Boston, MA, USA
[6]Department of Cognitive Science, Krieger School of Arts & Sciences, Johns Hopkins University, Baltimore, MD, USA
[7]Department of Neurology, Neurology, Feinberg School of Medicine, Northwestern University, Chicago, IL, USA

Correspondence should be addressed to Sladjana Lukic; sladjanalukic2015@u.northwestern.edu

Academic Editor: Anthony J. Hannan

The role of the right hemisphere (RH) in recovery from aphasia is incompletely understood. The present study quantified RH grey matter (GM) volume in individuals with chronic stroke-induced aphasia and cognitively healthy people using voxel-based morphometry. We compared group differences in GM volume in the entire RH and in RH regions-of-interest. Given that lesion site is a critical source of heterogeneity associated with poststroke language ability, we used voxel-based lesion symptom mapping (VLSM) to examine the relation between lesion site and language performance in the aphasic participants. Finally, using results derived from the VLSM as a covariate, we evaluated the relation between GM volume in the RH and language ability across domains, including comprehension and production processes both at the word and sentence levels and across spoken and written modalities. Between-subject comparisons showed that GM volume in the RH SMA was reduced in the aphasic group compared to the healthy controls. We also found that, for the aphasic group, increased RH volume in the MTG and the SMA was associated with better language comprehension and production scores, respectively. These data suggest that the RH may support functions previously performed by LH regions and have important implications for understanding poststroke reorganization.

1. Introduction

Research shows that undamaged tissue in both the contralesional (usually right) and ipsilesional (left) hemispheres of the brain is recruited to support recovery in stroke-induced aphasia (see reviews by [1–7]). Neuroimaging studies show that in early stages of recovery, the right hemisphere (RH) is active during language tasks; however, a shift in activation to the left hemisphere (LH) regions has been found across tasks, including word repetition, rhyme judgment, auditory word/sentence comprehension, semantic association, and reading [8–12]. Functional neuroimaging studies conducted with chronic aphasic individuals also confirm a primary role of ipsilesional tissue in recovery, finding significant correlations between recovery of language function and activation in the LH during confrontation-naming tasks [13, 14].

Other studies, however, have found RH recruitment, even in late stages of recovery [15–23]. Patients studied by Musso and coworkers [18] with lesions in the LH superior temporal gyrus (STG) showed activation in the RH STG during a sentence comprehension task, which positively correlated with off-line performance on a measure of auditory verbal comprehension. Similarly, Perani et al. [20] reported patients with damage to the LH inferior frontal gyrus (IFG) who showed activation of the RH homologue of this region when performing a verbal fluency task. In keeping with these findings, a recent meta-analysis of 12 neuroimaging studies in chronic stroke-induced aphasia [24] showed that, although aphasic individuals evince activation in the LH (i.e., the IFG and middle temporal gyrus (MTG), similar to healthy controls, as well as the left middle frontal gyrus (MFG) and insula), they also show the right hemisphere activation across a variety of language tasks (i.e., in the postcentral gyrus (PCG) and MTG).

Evidence of RH recruitment to support language recovery also comes from studies examining treatment-induced neural plasticity in chronic aphasia, showing increased RH activation associated with treatment gains [17, 25–31]. Recently, Kiran et al. [29] examined neural activation and effective connectivity within the left language network and right homologous regions following language treatment in eight chronic aphasic individuals. The results showed posttreatment increases in neural activity, bilaterally, in picture naming and semantic feature verification tasks. Importantly, effective connectivity maps in individuals with aphasia revealed that the LH IFG and the connection between the RH IFG and the RH MFG, respectively, most consistently modulated as a function of rehabilitation. Several other studies have shown similar patterns of posttreatment increases in the RH regions on picture naming (see [13, 32]) as well as semantic (compared to orthographic and phonological) processing tasks [33, 34]. Thompson et al. [35] also found a bilateral posttreatment upregulation of activation in the temporoparietal region in six chronic aphasic individuals who showed treatment-induced improvement in syntactic processing. These data indicate that the RH regions are engaged in language processing following damage to LH language networks. However, whether or if engagement of the RH is associated with maximally effective language processing has been questioned.

Some research suggests that rather than benefitting language processing, RH recruitment may be maladaptive and reflect inefficient language processing, finding, for example, either no association between increased RH activation and performance on a verb generation task [36] or a correlation between RH frontal activation and production of inaccurate responses on a picture-naming task [37]. An inefficient/maladaptive role of the RH has also been suggested by brain stimulation studies, showing that inhibitory repetitive transcranial magnetic stimulation (rTMS) applied to the RH regions (i.e., the IFG) improves language function ([38–41]; also see [6] for review), putatively secondary to inhibition of the maladaptive RH regions, which thereby facilitates LH processing (but see [42–44] for evidence suggesting that excitatory stimulation directed to the RH positively impacts language performance in chronic aphasic individuals). These and other studies have led to the assertion that recruitment of ipsilesional, rather than contralesional, tissue into the language network may result in greater language gains. Some recent neuroimaging studies also suggest that the contribution of the RH to recovery from aphasia may not reflect restoration of language processes, but rather the engagement of domain-general networks responsible for attention and

cognitive control [45, 46], or processing of perceptual aspects of verbal stimuli [47].

One way to estimate the functionality of cortical tissue is to examine the density of grey matter (GM) tissue, with the assumption that greater GM volume is associated with greater functionality and lesser (i.e., cortical atrophy) associated with decreased function [48, 49]. Studies on the recovery of motor function in chronic stroke have found both increases and decreases in GM volume in motor regions of the brain in patients following recovery (versus healthy controls). Zhang et al. [50] examined 26 hemiparetic individuals (with partial or complete recovery) and 25 age-matched controls on motor tasks before and after physical therapy. They found reduced cortical volume in the ipsilesional motor region for all patients compared to controls with no GM changes in contralesional motor areas. However, in another study, Gauthier et al. [51] found increased GM volume in RH motor regions, homologous to lesioned tissue in the LH, associated with recovery of function in 85 individuals with chronic stroke (also see [52]).

Few studies have examined GM volume in patients with cognitive impairments resulting from stroke. Stebbins et al. [53], using voxel-based morphometry (VBM, [54]), reported significant GM volume reductions (mostly in the thalamus) for stroke patients ($n = 91$) with cognitive impairment (compared to those without). In another study, Xing et al. [55] reported increased GM volume (compared to healthy, unimpaired control participants) in the right temporoparietal cortex (i.e., the supramarginal gyrus (SMG) and STG) in individuals with chronic stroke-induced aphasia. They further showed that GM volume was positively associated with overall aphasia severity as well as performance on production subtests of the *Western Aphasia Battery-Revised* (WAB-R; [56]) (i.e., spontaneous speech, repetition, and naming). Although the study was not longitudinal, the authors interpreted the results as suggesting a compensatory role of the right posterior regions in chronic aphasia. In addition, by partialing out participant variables (e.g., age, gender, level of education, and handedness) as well as the effect of lesion volume on language performance, the authors found the right hypertrophic temporoparietal regions, suggesting that these regions play a role in language recovery.

The present study examined RH GM volume in individuals with chronic stroke-induced aphasia and cognitively healthy people using voxel-based morphometry (VBM; [54]), a voxel-wise neuroimaging technique used for measuring variables associated with brain anatomy (e.g., GM volume). We compared group differences (healthy versus aphasic participants) in GM volume in the entire RH and in RH regions-of-interest (ROIs) where aphasic individuals exhibited a significant relation between GM volume and language performance. Given that lesion site is a critical source of heterogeneity associated with poststroke language ability, we then used voxel-based lesion symptom mapping (VLSM; [55]) to examine the relation between lesion site and language performance in the aphasic participants. Finally, using results derived from the VLSM analysis as a covariate (following Xing et al. [56]), we evaluated the relation between GM volume in the RH and language scores

TABLE 1: Demographic data for aphasic and age-matched healthy participants.

	N	Age (yrs)	Gender	Education (yrs)	Time poststroke (months)
AM controls	40	58.9 (±11.8)	22F; 18M	15.6 (±2.4)	N/A
AM NU	11	54.8 (±8.2)	5F; 6M	16.4 (±1.6)	
AM BU	17	58.2 (±13.4)	8F; 9M	15.4 (±2.8)	
AM JHU	12	63.7 (±11.7)	9F; 3M	15.0 (±2.3)	
All aphasics	40	59.4 (±12.4)	14F; 26M	16.1 (±2.2)	57.2 (±52.3)
NU	11	49.0 (±8.0)	4F; 7M	16.9 (±2.1)	49.3 (±32.5)
BU	17	62.1 (±12.2)	5F; 12M	15.0 (±2.3)	44.3 (±40.7)
JHU	12	65.1 (±10.6)	5F; 7M	16.8 (±1.5)	82.7 (±72.7)

across domains, including comprehension and production processes both at the word and sentence level and across spoken and written modalities.

In line with the aforementioned studies showing structural changes after LH stroke, we expected differences in GM volume in the RH in the aphasic participants compared to healthy controls (i.e., either decreased or increased volumes). We also predicted that if the RH supports language function, then a positive correlation between performance on language tasks and RH GM volume would be observed, independently of differences in lesion volume. Conversely, if the RH does not support language functions, we expected no correlation between language performance and RH GM volume in the group of aphasic participants.

2. Method

2.1. Participants. Forty participants with aphasia (14 female) resulting from a single-left hemisphere stroke and 40 cognitively healthy age-matched (AM) controls (18 female) were recruited for the study from three research sites: Northwestern (NU), Boston (BU and MGH), and Johns Hopkins (JHU) Universities. All were native English speakers, passed a puretone audiometric screening and evinced normal or corrected-to-normal vision (self-reported). All participants were right handed, with the exception of one aphasic speaker who was left handed prior to the stroke that affected his left hemisphere. Participants at each site were recruited as part of a large-scale study examining treatment-induced changes in brain function and, hence, were selected for specific language-deficit patterns: agrammatism (NU), anomia (BU, MGH), and dysgraphia (JHU).

Across sites, the aphasic and control groups were matched for age (t (77.9) = −0.166; $p > 0.05$), ranging from 35 to 81 (59.4 ± 12.4 yrs) and 24–80 (58.9 ± 11.8 yrs) for the two participant groups, respectively, and years of education (aphasic group mean = 16.1 ± 2.2; control group mean = 15.6 ± 2.4 (t (71.5) = −0.936; $p > 0.05$)). Within site, participant groups also did not differ in age (NU: t (20) = 1.678, $p > 0.05$; BU: t (31.7) = −0.882, $p > 0.05$; and JHU: t (21.8) = −0.293, $p > 0.05$), and years of education were matched between participant groups for all sites except JHU, where patients were more highly educated than the control participants (NU: t (19) = −0.571, $p > 0.05$; BU: t (22.7) = 0.398, $p > 0.05$; and JHU: t (18.9) = −2.275, $p = 0.035$). All participants completed

written consent form approved by NU, BU, and JHU Institutional Review Boards (IRB). See Table 1 for demographic data.

Aphasic participants were at least eight months post onset of stroke (57.2 ± 52.3 months) and presented with aphasia based on administration of the *Western Aphasia Battery-Revised* (WAB-R; [57]) and a uniform set of cross-site language measures. The WAB Aphasia Quotient score (WAB-AQ) ranged from 25.2 to 98.4 (70.2 ± 20.5), with no significant differences between participants enrolled at NU and those enrolled at the other sites (NU versus BU: $t = 1.282$, $p > 0.05$; NU versus JHU: $t = −1.536$, $p > 0.05$), while aphasic participants enrolled at BU showed lower WAB-AQ scores than those at JHU ($t = −2.452$, $p = 0.021$). The type and severity of language impairment were characterized using a test battery, which included selected subtests of the *Northwestern Naming Battery* (NNB; [58]), *Psycholinguistic Assessments of Language Processing in Aphasia* (PALPA; [59]); and *Northwestern Assessment of Verbs and Sentences* (NAVS; [60]).

2.2. Language Measures. Language measures selected to examine participants' abilities across domains included the confrontation-naming (CN) and auditory comprehension (AC) subtests from the NNB to quantify single-word naming and comprehension. These subtests use the same sets of nouns and verbs for testing in both domains. From the PALPA, subtests 35, 40, and 51 were selected to evaluate oral reading of words with regular and irregular orthography (PALPA35), spelling-to-dictation of words with high and low frequency (PALPA40), and semantic association between written words (PALPA51), respectively. Finally, the Sentence Production Priming Test (SPPT) and the Sentence Comprehension Test (SCT) from the NAVS were used to evaluate production and comprehension of sentences of different complexity (same sentences tested across domains).

2.3. MRI Image Acquisition. A 3T Trio Siemens scanner at NU, a 3T Skyra at BU, and a Phillips Intera scanner at JHU were used to obtain anatomical T1-weighted scans. Across all sites, standard T1-weighted 3D MPRAGE scans were acquired in the sagittal plane (TR/TE = 2300/2.91 ms, Flip angle = 9°, 1 × 1 × 1 mm), together with a T2-weighted FLAIR sequence (TR/TE = 9000/90 ms, Flip angle = 150°, 0.86 × 0.86 × 5 mm), which was coregistered and resliced for resolution and orientation consistency with T1 images

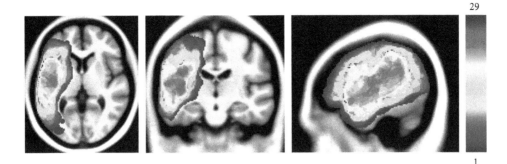

FIGURE 1: Lesion overlap map of 40 participants with aphasia, showing areas of overlap, from no overlap (blue) to maximum overlap (red; $N = 29$ participants).

by participant. Prior to the study, imaging sequences were equated across sites, with the same parameters used for data acquisition across scanners, and quality control was performed to ensure high-quality data from each site.

2.4. MRI Preprocessing (NUNDA Pipeline Description). Anatomical images were corrected for bias field inhomogeneities [61], and lesioned brain regions were masked out before being subjected to a standard voxel-based morphometry workflow using VBM8 toolbox (developed by Christian Gaser). Analysis steps included tissue segmentation, rigid registration, and DARTEL normalization to the template space (Template_1_IXI550_MNI152.nii). The normalized and modulated GM segments were smoothed by 8 mm FWHM Gaussian Kernel and masked using a right hemisphere (RH) GM mask of the T1 brain template.

2.5. Lesion Identification. The chronic stroke lesion mask was manually generated using MRIcron [62] in native space by trained professionals from each site. To delineate the borders of the necrotic tissue for each patient, intensity measures for white and grey matter (WM and GM) in the contralateral right hemisphere were used for each axial slice. The left hemisphere lesioned tissue was drawn on each slice using the pen tool of MRIcron, and then applying the minimum intensity to the outlined area using the intensity filter function. Additional manual correction was applied by visualizing the volume in all three planes simultaneously. All brains and lesions were normalized into Montreal Neurological Institute (MNI) space as part of the anatomical preprocessing pipeline provided by the Northwestern University Neuroimaging Data Archive (NUNDA; [63]) prior to VLSM analysis. Figure 1 displays a lesion overlap map for the aphasic participant group.

2.6. Data Analyses

2.6.1. Analysis 1: Between-Subject (Aphasic Participants, AM Controls) Differences in GM Volume. The group differences (healthy versus aphasic participants) in grey matter volume were examined in the entire RH and in selected region of interest (ROI). The ROIs were derived from the VBM Analysis 3 (see next). Specifically, for any cluster in which grey matter volume was found to be significantly associated with

any of our seven language measures (VBM Analysis 3), we identified the ROI within which the peak voxel for that cluster resided. The so identified ROIs included the right supplementary motor area (SMA), MTG, insula, hippocampus, postcentral, and pallidum areas (see Figure 2). These ROIs were anatomically defined using the AAL atlas within the MarsBaR toolbox in SPM8 [64]. For each ROI, a linear regression analysis was conducted using R 3.2.3 [65], where the mean GM volume was used as a dependent variable, and group (healthy versus aphasic individuals) as an independent variable. Age and total intracranial volume (computed as the sum of grey and white matter and cerebrospinal fluid) were included as covariates in all regression models. Additionally, p values resulting from regression analyses were corrected for the number of ROIs examined using the Benjamini-Hochberg correction [66], with n being the total number of ROIs examined (6). Only Benjamini-Hochberg-corrected results are reported in the Results.

2.6.2. Analysis 2: The Effect of LH Lesion on Language Performance. A voxel-based lesion symptom mapping (VLSM) approach was used to analyze the relationship between lesions in the left hemisphere and language performance [55], using the VLSM toolbox (http://www.crl.ucsd.edu/vlsm) running under Matlab R2014a. (MathWorks Inc., 2014). The participants' lesion images (binary) and language scores (% correct) were entered into a VLSM analysis. For each voxel, aphasic participants were divided into two groups based on the presence (1) or absence (0) of a lesion in that voxel. Only voxels in which more than four (at least 10%) participants had lesions were included in the analysis. VLSM analyses were run with $n = 1000$ permutation tests, resulting in T-maps that reflected critical regions in the LH where lesioned tissue was associated with performance on a given language measure. The total lesion volume was automatically calculated from the lesion masks and served as a covariate in the analysis. Significant results were derived from voxel-wise t-tests using a threshold of $p < 0.05$ with permutation-based correction for multiple comparisons. Cluster level p values then underwent the Benjamini-Hochberg correction [66] for multiple comparisons (with n being the total number of VLSM analyses conducted, that is, seven, one for each language measure). Only corrected p

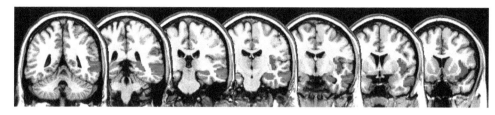

FIGURE 2: Six right hemisphere regions of interest (ROIs), derived from VBM analysis, used to evaluate between-group differences in the grey matter volume. SMA = green, MTG = red, insula = blue, hippocampus = violet, postcentral = yellow, and pallidum = cyan.

TABLE 2: Aphasic participants' scores on language measures.

Language domain		Test	All patients		BU		JHU		NU	
			Mean	SD	Mean	SD	Mean	SD	Mean	SD
Comprehension	*Aphasia severity*	WABAQ	70.2	20.5	62.2	24.3	80.6	16.1	71.3	13.0
	Spoken word comprehension	NNB AC	92.5	14.5	85.5	20.0	98.1	3.8	97.3	4.5
	Word semantic association	PALPA 51	64.0	20.1	54.1	23.7	73.3	16.2	69.7	13.6
	Sentence comprehension	NAVS SCT	71.4	17.3	71.0	19.6	78.9	17.9	63.9	8.5
Production	*Spoken word production*	NNB CN	70.5	29.7	59.6	37.4	76.6	21.6	80.7	17.8
	Oral reading	PALPA 35	65.1	34.3	56.4	41.3	68.5	28.0	76.0	25.9
	Spelling-to-dictation	PALPA 40	37.1	26.8	35.1	32.5	42.8	20.7	33.8	24.2
	Sentence production	NAVS SPPT	39.4	31.5	30.0	34.5	54.0	31.7	40.6	22.2

values are reported in the text. Additionally, effect sizes for significant comparisons were calculated using the following formula, based on the T-statistics (t) and the degrees of freedom (df) $\sqrt[2]{(t^2/(t^2 + \mathrm{df}))}$.

2.6.3. Analysis 3: The Effect of RH GM Volume on Language Performance. The relationship between grey matter volume in the right hemisphere and language performance on the seven language domain measures was analyzed by performing voxel-wise multiple linear regression using the VBM8 toolbox (http://dbm.neuro.uni-jena.de/vbm8) in Statistical Parametric Mapping software (SPM8; http://www.fil.ion.ucl.ac.uk/spm). The segmented, modulated, normalized, and smoothed GM images and language scores (% correct) were entered in each regression model, resulting in T-maps that showed regions where GM volume was significantly associated with language performance. As pointed by Xing et al. [56], when determining the contribution of GM volume in the RH to language performance, it is important to account for the contribution of LH lesioned tissue to the performance on the same language measure, as any correlation found between RH GM volume and language performance may be influenced by the effect of the LH lesion size/site on the participants' performance. In order to account for this, as in Xing et al. [56], the "proportion of critical area of damage" (PCAD) was entered as a covariate together with age and the total intracranial volume (computed as the sum of grey and white matter, and cerebrospinal fluid) in the VBM analysis to partial out their effects on language performance. The PCAD was computed by intersecting the map derived from the group VLSM with each participant's lesion, divided by the VLSM map volume. The PCAD, then, ranged from 0 (when there was no overlap between a patient's lesion and the group map) to 1 (when there was total overlap, with all voxels lesioned in the group map

also lesion for the patient). Group T-maps derived from VBM analyses conducted on language measures were then thresholded by determining the minimum cluster size based on a $p < 0.001$ voxel-level threshold and on an estimate of image smoothness in AFNI [67], following the evidence of a disproportionately high rate of false-positive results yielded by family-wise (FWE) cluster-level correction in SPM [68]. The group residuals derived from the SPM T-maps were run through the 3dfwhmx function in AFNI, which uses the latest version of the autocorrelation function, to derive an estimate of image smoothness, and thresholded at a conservative $p < 0.001$ voxel level using the 3dClustSim function, to determine the appropriate cluster size threshold for each regression analysis. T-maps were also multiplied by a GM mask to ensure significant clusters would be restricted to grey matter and by the Automated Anatomical Labeling (AAL) atlas to obtain MNI coordinates for every peak in every significant cluster. The AAL template was then overlaid onto each binarized T-map using MRIcron [62] to identify the region corresponding to each peak coordinate. Cluster p values were finally corrected for multiple comparisons (with n being the number of regressions performed, that is, seven, one for each language measure) using the Benjamini-Hochberg correction [66]. As for VLSM, effect sizes for each VBM regression analysis were computed as described above, and only corrected p values are reported in the text.

3. Results

3.1. Language Measures. Participant scores derived from administration of language measures across language domains are shown in Table 2. Within the comprehension domain, participants performed well on spoken word comprehension (NNB AC: 92.5 ± 14.5), while scores obtained

TABLE 3: Results of VLSM analyses by language measure.

Language measure	Test	LH regions (AAL)	Cluster size	Peak coordinates px	Peak coordinates py	Peak coordinates pz	t value	df	p (perm) correction	Benjamini-Hochberg correction	Effect size
Spoken word comprehension	NNB AC	*Putamen*	949	−32	−17	0	5.15	35	0.026	0.068	0.656
		IFG									
		STG									
		Rolandic operculum									
Word semantic association	PALPA51	*Putamen*	796	−33	3	−9	4.49	34	0.015	0.068	0.61
		Insula									
		STG/MTG									
		Caudate									
Sentence comprehension	NAVS SCT	*MTG*	1040	−44	−23	0	4.98	35	0.029	0.068	0.644
		STG									

Note. Table 3 summarizes regions where lesion volume was significantly associated with language performance in the comprehension domain. The results are presented at a threshold of $p < 0.05$, based on cluster size and the permutation method. In addition, the permutation-corrected p values were corrected for the total number of language measures examined ($n = 7$) using the Benjamini-Hochberg procedure. Significant peak regions are reported with the corresponding coordinates, T and p values, degrees of freedom, and effect sizes, as well as AAL regions included in the significant cluster; LH: left hemisphere; IFG: inferior frontal gyrus; STG: superior temporal gyrus; MTG: middle temporal gyrus.

on semantic association and sentence comprehension were lower on average and more variable (PALPA51: 64.0 ± 20.1; NAVS SCT: 71.4 ± 17.3). Within the production domain, aphasic participants scored better on spoken word production and oral reading (NNB CN: 70.5 ± 29.7; PALPA 35: 65.1 ± 34.3) than on spelling-to-dictation (PALPA40: 37.1 ± 26.8) and sentence production (NAVS SPPT: 39.4 ± 31.5).

3.2. Between-Subject (Aphasic Participants, AM Controls) Differences in GM Volume.

Between-subject analysis of GM volume for the entire RH showed no significant differences between the aphasic participants and age-matched controls. The results of the ROI analyses revealed between-group differences in the right SMA ($p = 0.054$), where patients showed reduced GM volume compared to healthy participants. To follow up on this result, a median split was used to divide patients into two groups, that is, those with good (>65% correct) ($n = 21$) and poor (<65% correct) ($n = 19$) production ability, based on a composite score (the average percentage correct across the three production measures: spoken word production, oral reading, and sentence production). A between-group (healthy controls, good performers, and poor performers) analysis was run on the mean RH GM volume in the SMA, with age and total intracranial volume included as covariates. The results showed a significant difference between healthy controls and poor performers in GM volume within the RH SMA ($p = 0.004$), while no difference was found between healthy controls and good performers ($p = 0.294$).

3.3. Effect of the LH Lesion on Language Performance (VLSM Results) in Aphasic Participants.

The following results were derived from the VLSM analysis and illustrate the relation between LH lesion and language performance. The results of VLSM analyses are reported in Table 3. Figure 3 displays the relationship between LH lesion site and performance on each language measure.

For measures assessing comprehension, VLSM analysis of *spoken word comprehension* revealed a trend toward a negative relationship between lesions in the left IFG, STG, putamen, and rolandic operculum and spoken word comprehension scores ($p = 0.068$). Similarly, *word semantic association* performance was negatively associated with lesions in the left IFG, STG, and putamen, as well as in two unlabeled clusters spatially contiguous to the insula and caudate ($p = 0.068$). Finally, for *sentence comprehension*, a trend toward a negative relationship was observed with lesions in the left MTG and STG ($p = 0.068$).

VLSM analyses of production measures revealed no significant relationships between lesions and performance on *spoken word production, oral reading, spelling-to-dictation*, or *sentence production* (all corrected ps > 0.1).

3.4. Effect of the RH GM Volume on Language Performance (VBM Results) in Aphasic Participants.

The following results were derived from the VBM regression analysis and illustrate the relation between RH GM volume and language performance where the relations between LH lesioned tissue and language performance (as derived from the VLSM analyses) were taken into account and entered as nuisance variables. VBM maps indicating RH regions in which GM volume was significantly positively associated with language performance are shown in Figure 4. The results of VBM analysis for the aphasic participants are reported in Table 4.

The voxel-wise linear regression of *spoken word comprehension* on GM volume revealed a significant positive relationship between single-word comprehension scores and GM volume in the right MTG and insula. VBM analyses conducted on measures of *word semantic association* and *sentence comprehension* did not yield any significant clusters. For production measures, the voxel-wise linear regression of *spoken word production* on the GM volume revealed a significant positive relationship between word production scores and GM volume in the right SMA and insula.

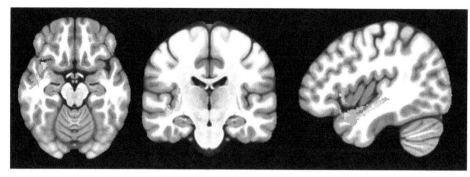

(a) Spoken word comprehension

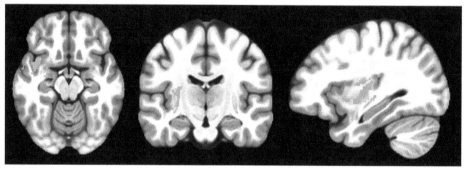

(b) Word semantic association

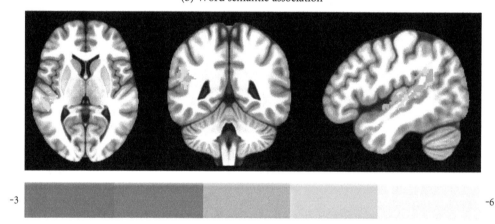

(c) Sentence comprehension

FIGURE 3: VLSM maps showing left hemisphere regions that were significantly associated with language performance. Panels (a–c) display lesions correlated with comprehension measures: (a) spoken word comprehension, (b) word semantic association, and (c) sentence comprehension. All voxels shown in color survived a threshold of $p < 0.05$, based on cluster size and the permutation method. The color bar reflects the range of t values from minimum (red) to maximum (yellow).

Similarly, *oral reading* and *sentence production* performances were positively related with GM volume within the right SMA, whereas *oral reading* performance was also associated with GM volume in the pallidum and hippocampus. Finally, for *spelling-to-dictation,* a positive relationship between GM volume and performance was observed in the right hippocampus and postcentral region.

4. Discussion

This study examined the right hemisphere (RH) grey matter (GM) volume in a group of 40 individuals with stroke-induced chronic aphasia using voxel-based morphometry (VBM). We first compared values derived from the patient group to those derived from 40 age-matched healthy controls, finding reduced GM volume in the RH supplementary motor area (SMA) in aphasic individuals compared to healthy age-matched controls. Follow-up analyses also revealed a significant difference in SMA GM volume only between healthy controls and aphasic individuals with more severe impairment in language production, while no difference emerged between patients with milder language production deficits and healthy individuals. Next, we evaluated the relation between RH GM volume and language performance in the aphasic participant group, controlling for the left hemisphere lesion site, using VBM. The results revealed two findings: (1) better word comprehension was associated with increased RH GM volume in the middle

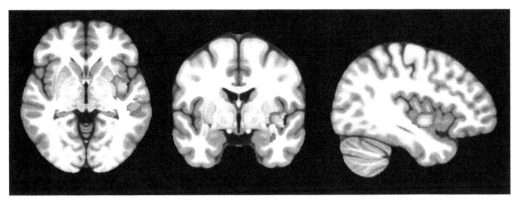

(a) Spoken word comprehension

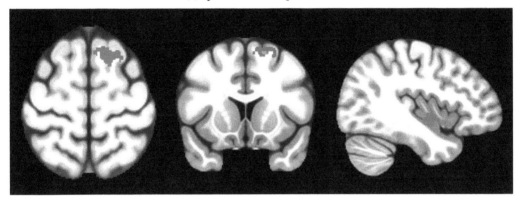

(b) Spoken word production

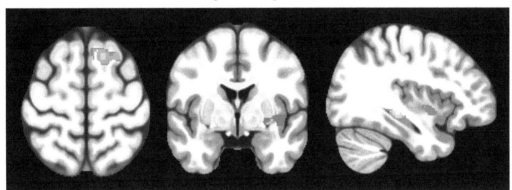

(c) Oral reading

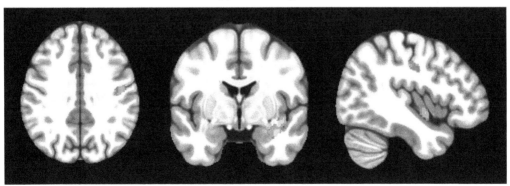

(d) Spelling-to-dictation

FIGURE 4: Continued.

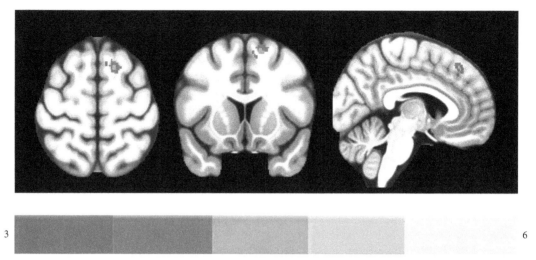

(e) Sentence production

FIGURE 4: VBM maps showing right hemisphere regions where GM volume was significantly associated with language performance. Panel (a) shows the relationship between RH gray matter volume and spoken word comprehension. Panels (b–e) display the relationship between RH gray matter volume and production measures: (b) spoken word production, (c) oral reading, (d) spelling-to-dictation, and (e) sentence production. All voxels shown in color survived a threshold of $p < 0.05$, cluster-level FWE corrected. The color bar reflects the range of t values from minimum (red) to maximum (yellow).

TABLE 4: Results of VBM analyses by language measure.

Language Measure	Test	RH regions (AAL)	Cluster size	Peak coordinates px	py	pz	t value	df	FWE correction	Benjamini-Hochberg correction	Effect size
Spoken word comprehension	NNB AC	Insula	1458	40.5	−4.5	−7.5	5.861	35	0.0000	0.0000	0.70
		MTG	732	55.5	−25.5	−4.5	4.646		0.0000	0.0001	0.62
Word semantic association	PALPA51				No sig. clusters						
Sentence comprehension	NAVS SCT				No sig. clusters						
Spoken word production	NNB CN	SMA	545	13.5	16.5	61.5	4.302	35	0.0001	0.0002	0.59
		Insula	267	40.5	−7.5	−7.5	4.106		0.0002	0.0003	0.57
Oral reading	PALPA35	SMA	502	13.5	15	61.5	4.549	34	0.0001	0.0001	0.62
		Pallidum	430	25.5	−1.5	−4.5	3.861		0.0005	0.0005	0.55
		Hippocampus	294	33	−28.5	−6	5.274		0.0000	0.0001	0.67
Spelling-to-dictation	PALPA40	Hippocampus	503	36	−1.5	−22.5	4.593	35	0.0001	0.0001	0.61
		Postcentral	258	49.5	−12	36	3.981		0.0003	0.0004	0.56
Sentence production	NAVS SPPT	SMA	275	13.5	15	58.5	4.625	34	0.0001	0.0001	0.62

Note. Table 4 summarizes regions where GM volume was significantly associated with language performance in both comprehension and production domains. The results are presented at a threshold of $p < 0.05$, based on $p < 0.001$ voxel-level threshold and a minimum cluster size (665–708 mm^3) determined by an estimate of image smoothness. In addition, cluster p values were corrected for the total number of language measures examined ($n = 7$) using the Benjamini-Hochberg procedure. Significant peak regions are reported with corresponding coordinates, T and p values, degrees of freedom, and effect sizes; RH: right hemisphere; SMA: supplementary motor area; MTG: middle temporal gyrus.

temporal gyrus (MTG) and insula, and (2) better word and sentence production was associated with increased RH GM volume in the SMA.

Language comprehension was evaluated using standardized measures of spoken word comprehension, semantic association, and sentence comprehension. The spoken word comprehension measure examined participants' ability to comprehend single words (nouns and verbs) from an array

of semantically or argument structure-related items, respectively. Accordingly, failure on this task reflects inability to either link spoken words to objects/actions or to access semantic knowledge [58]. The semantic association task also examined word comprehension, although from the visual modality, requiring participants to select semantically related words. To perform the sentence comprehension (i.e., sentence-picture matching) task, individuals needed to access lexical and semantic information stored in long-term memory and integrate it into syntactic structure.

The VBM analysis shows that GM volume in the right MTG and insula was positively associated with performance on *spoken word comprehension,* but no association was found between the RH GM volume and the other two comprehension measures, that is, *semantic association* and *sentence comprehension* in any region. Lesion-deficit patterns derived from VLSM showed that lower performance on both word comprehension and semantic association measures were associated with a lesion in the left IFG and STG, whereas lower sentence comprehension scores were associated with lesions in the left STG and MTG. However, given that VLSM analyses yielded results that were only marginally significant after applying a correction for multiple comparisons, the discussion will focus primarily on the results of the VBM analyses, and VLSM results will be discussed within the context of the explanation of the VBM results.

The finding of an association between performance on spoken word comprehension and GM volume in the right temporal cortex suggests that the RH temporal region may support lexical access during word processing. This finding is in line with neuroimaging studies showing increased RH activation in temporal lobe regions with improved lexical-semantic (compared to orthographic and phonological) processing in aphasic participants [33]. The results are also consistent with studies showing increased posttreatment activation bilaterally in the MTG (in addition to the frontal cortex) on a semantic feature verification task, which also requires access to semantic knowledge [24, 29]. Moreover, when looking at the results of the lesion-deficit analyses for spoken word comprehension and semantic association tasks, within the context of the aforementioned RH results, damage in the left IFG and STG likely affected lexical selection and storage of lexical representations, respectively. This is consistent with studies showing an association between damage to temporal lobe structures and comprehension/semantic deficits in aphasic individuals [69, 70].

In addition to recruitment of the RH temporal lobe, the VBM analysis showed that performance on spoken word comprehension was also associated with GM volume in the insula. Neuroimaging studies have shown activation in the left insula during phonological discrimination tasks [71, 72], although its role in word processing is debated, as several neuroimaging studies have found activation of the insula using a variety of language tasks including naming and word generation ([73–75], see [76] for a review). However, a role for the insula in word comprehension has been suggested in functional connectivity studies, showing significant connections between the insula and the temporal lobe, namely the STG and MTG [76].

Notably, we observed no relationship between GM volumes and sentence comprehension in the right hemisphere. According to most studies with cognitively healthy people, sentence comprehension is supported by a primarily left lateralized temporofrontal network (see [77] for a neurocognitive model of sentence comprehension; also see [5]),

with neuroimaging studies showing increased activation in the left frontal and posterior temporal cortex when comparing sentences with plausible versus implausible meanings [78], grammatical versus ungrammatical sentences [79], or syntactically complex versus simple sentences [31, 80, 81]. These findings suggest that the left temporal and frontal tissue is recruited when strategic, combinatorial, and/or memory processes come into play during sentence processing [82]. In the present study, the absence of a sentence-level comprehension effect in the RH as well as our VLSM lesion-deficit results, revealing a significant negative correlation in the left STG and MTG and sentence comprehension, that is, poorer sentence comprehension was associated with lesions in these regions, consistent with previous findings [31, 70, 83, 84], reflect a reliance on the left hemisphere for sentence comprehension for our patients [1].

Turning to language production, spoken word and sentence production, oral reading, and spelling-to-dictation were tested using standardized measures. Language production engages many of the same processes involved in comprehension, including semantic mediation, phonological processing, and in the case of sentence production, integration of semantic, and syntactic information. However, production also engages motor planning, articulatory, and associated processes.

For *spoken word production, sentence production,* and *oral reading,* we found increased RH GM volume in the right SMA associated with better performance. This finding is in line with the results of several neuroimaging studies, which have found significant SMA activation in production tasks in healthy speakers in both silent (covert) and overt production tasks (see [85] and [3] for review; [86–88]). Although SMA activation often is associated with motor planning and articulatory processes, some authors suggest that this region also is involved in lexical selection and word form encoding [89, 90]. Positive correlations between GM volume in the RH SMA found in the present study across production (but not comprehension) tasks support this, suggesting that the right homologue of the SMA may be recruited to support production processes in individuals with aphasia resulting from stroke.

In addition, the VBM analysis showed that performance on word production was associated with increased GM volume in the insula. Neuroimaging studies examining naming and word generation in healthy speakers have found LH insula activation (see [76] for a review). Previous lesion-deficit correlation analyses also have found an association between lesions in the insula and performance on verbal fluency [54], speech initiation, and motor planning [91, 92]. In addition, the insula has been shown to have strong connections to the LH prefrontal cortex, including the MFG and SMA [76], suggesting that in our patients, lesions affecting the LH insula and its connections with the LH SMA, the RH homologous frontal regions may result in recruitment of the RH insula and SMA for production processes. Alternatively, the RH SMA and insula may support these processes independent of lesioned tissue in the homologue LH regions.

Lastly, performance on the *spelling-to-dictation* measure was associated with GM volume in the right hippocampus and postcentral areas. Associations between performance on this task and GM volume in the RH hippocampal structures are in line with studies indicating a role of the hippocampus in healthy language learning [93–95], as well as with studies showing a positive correlation between treatment outcome and GM volume in the LH [96, 97] or bilateral hippocampus during recovery from stroke. Although—as previously acknowledged—the present study does not directly reflect "recruitment" of RH regions as part of recovery from aphasia, and the findings of a relation between GM volume and structures supporting healthy learning may not be coincidental. Further studies are necessary to investigate the role of the hippocampus as a structure supporting recovery in stroke-induced aphasia. Similarly, recruitment of the RH postcentral area may be implicated in recovery from aphasia. Previous neuroimaging studies in aphasic individuals have found RH postcentral gyrus activation across a variety of language tasks [24, 29].

Overall, our VBM results are inconsistent with those reported by Xing et al. [56]. Whereas Xing et al. found that GM volumes in right temporoparietal areas are related to speech production, but not comprehension, we found the opposite pattern. We found strong correlations between GM volumes in right temporal cortex and comprehension, but not production, and in the domain of production, we found that increased GM volume within the frontal region was associated with better production. It should be noted that the tasks used to test both comprehension and production differed across studies. To evaluate comprehension, Xing et al. [56] used data derived from WAB comprehension subtests and to evaluate production, spontaneous speech data and performance on a repetition task were used, whereas we used linguistically controlled, standardized comprehension and production tasks designed explicitly to elicit both comprehension and production of written and spoken words and sentences. We suggest that controlled tasks designed to measure specific language processes may better reflect neural recruitment patterns associated with recovery from aphasia.

To the extent that GM volume reflects functionality, the positive association between word comprehension and production ability and GM volume in the RH MTG and SMA, respectively, suggests that these regions may play a compensatory role in language recovery in aphasia. Although the precise mechanisms underlying RH GM volume are not completely understood, this finding is in keeping with one theory of language recovery—that RH regions are recruited to perform language functions when the LH is damaged. Notably, however, theories of language recovery suggest that RH compensation occurs in regions homologous to LH damaged regions. For example, in one study, Turkeltaub et al. [24] showed that people with lesions in the left IFG were more likely to recruit the right IFG than those without lesions in that area. Similarly, Buckner et al. [98] reported results of a single-stroke patient who showed activation in the right inferior prefrontal region during a word-stem completion task to compensate for lesioned tissue in the left frontal region, activated by healthy speakers. Also, see studies by Musso et al.

and Perani et al., for similar patterns [18, 20]. However, the present data do not completely support this idea. Whereas, our patients with word comprehension impairments evinced lesions within the LH MTG, perhaps leading to recruitment of RH MTG, and our patients with sentence comprehension impairments evinced LH STG and MTG lesions, but no increases in GM volume were found in any RH regions. Further, our patients with production impairments did not present with LH SMA lesions but nevertheless showed increases in GM volume in the RH SMA, a nonhomologous region. One explanation for this latter finding is that the LH SMA is highly connected to regions within the LH that were damaged in our patients, perhaps leading to recruitment of its RH homologue.

In the absence of longitudinal data, however, we refrain from making strong claims regarding the relation between RH GM volume and recovery. Although RH regions may be recruited to support functions previously performed by LH regions, it is possible that RH recruitment may be maladaptive, as suggested by some repetitive transcranial magnetic stimulation studies (rTMS; see [6] for review). It also is possible that individual differences among participants before (rather than following) stroke may explain the RH GM volume differences we found between aphasic and healthy individuals. Although difficult to accomplish, longitudinal research in which individuals are tested prior to and following stroke could help to address this alternative hypothesis. Research examining GM volume in poststroke patients over time also will provide further insight into the extent to which GM changes are associated with language change. Indeed, the present data are part of a larger longitudinal study examining brain behavior changes associated with treatment (versus no treatment), and the results of which will be informative regarding neural recovery trajectories associated with improved language performance and yield a more comprehensive understanding of both structural and functional plasticity associated with language recovery in stroke aphasia.

5. Conclusion

This study examined the relation between the right hemisphere grey matter volume, left hemisphere lesion site, and both spoken and written comprehension and production of words and sentences in chronic stroke-induced aphasia. To the extent that RH grey matter volume reflects neural shifts associated with recovery from left hemisphere brain damage, our results indicate that right hemisphere regions, both homologous and nonhomologous to the left hemisphere lesioned regions, are recruited to support language, with unique recruitment patterns associated with language domain. Although further research is needed, the present findings have important implications for understanding poststroke neural reorganization.

Acknowledgments

This work was supported by the NIH-NIDCD, Clinical Research Center Grant P50DC012283 (PI: Cynthia K. Thompson). The authors are very grateful to Dr. Ajay Shashikumar Kurani and James Patrick Higgins for their help and assistance with the data analysis and Sarah Dove Chandler for her assistance with the manuscript preparation.

References

[1] G. Gainotti, "Contrasting opinions on the role of the right hemisphere in the recovery of language. A critical survey," *Aphasiology*, vol. 29, no. 9, pp. 1020–1037, 2015.

[2] S. Kiran, "What is the nature of poststroke language recovery and reorganization?" *ISRN Neurology*, vol. 2012, Article ID 786872, 13 pages, 2012.

[3] C. J. Price, "A review and synthesis of the first 20 years of PET and fMRI studies of heard speech, spoken language and reading," *NeuroImage*, vol. 62, no. 2, pp. 816–847, 2012.

[4] C. K. Thompson and D. B. den Ouden, "Neuroimaging and recovery of language in aphasia," *Current Neurology and Neuroscience Reports*, vol. 8, no. 6, pp. 475–483, 2008.

[5] C. K. Thompson and A. Kielar, "Neural bases of sentence processing: evidence from neurolinguistic and neuroimaging studies," in *The Oxford Handbook of Language Production*, M. Goldrick, V. Ferreira and M. Miozzo, Eds., pp. 47–69, Oxford University Press, New York, NY, USA, 2014.

[6] P. Turkeltaub, "Brain stimulation and the role of the right hemisphere in aphasia recovery," *Current Neurology and Neuroscience Reports*, vol. 15, no. 72, pp. 1–9, 2015.

[7] M. M. Watila and S. A. Balarabe, "Factors predicting poststroke aphasia recovery," *Journal of the Neurological Sciences*, vol. 352, no. 1, pp. 12–18, 2015.

[8] B. Fernandez, D. Cardebat, J. Demonet et al., "Functional MRI follow-up study of language processes in healthy subjects and during recovery in a case of aphasia," *Stroke*, vol. 35, no. 9, pp. 2171–2176, 2004.

[9] W. Heiss, A. Thiel, J. Kessler, and K. Herholz, "Disturbance and recovery of language function: correlates in PET activation studies," *NeuroImage*, vol. 20, Supplement 1, pp. S42–S49, 2003.

[10] T. Ino, K. Tokumoto, K. Usami, T. Kimura, Y. Hashimoto, and H. Fukuyama, "Longitudinal fMRI study of reading in a patient with letter-by-letter reading," *Cortex*, vol. 44, no. 7, pp. 773–781, 2008.

[11] H. Karbe, K. Herholz, M. Halber, and W. D. Heiss, "Collateral inhibition of transcallosal activity facilitates functional brain asymmetry," *Journal of Cerebral Blood Flow & Metabolism*, vol. 18, no. 10, pp. 1157–1161, 1998.

[12] D. Saur, R. Lange, A. Baumgaertner et al., "Dynamics of language reorganization after stroke," *Brain*, vol. 129, no. 6, pp. 1371–1384, 2006.

[13] Y. Cao, E. M. Vikingstad, K. P. George, A. F. Johnson, and K. M. A. Welch, "Cortical language activation in stroke patients recovering from aphasia with functional MRI," *Stroke*, vol. 30, no. 11, pp. 2331–2340, 1999.

[14] J. Fridriksson, L. Bonilha, J. Baker, D. Mosen, and C. Rorden, "Activity in preserved left hemisphere regions predicts anomia severity in aphasia," *Cerebral Cortex*, vol. 20, no. 5, pp. 1013–1019, 2010.

[15] V. Blasi, A. C. Young, A. P. Tansy, S. E. Petersen, A. Z. Snyder, and M. Corbetta, "Word retrieval learning modulates right frontal cortex in patients with left frontal damage," *Neuron*, vol. 36, no. 1, pp. 159–170, 2002.

[16] J. Crinion and C. J. Price, "Right anterior superior temporal activation predicts auditory sentence comprehension following aphasic stroke," *Brain*, vol. 128, no. 12, pp. 2858–2871, 2005.

[17] B. Crosson, A. B. Moore, K. M. McGregor et al., "Regional changes in word-production laterality after a naming treatment designed to produce a rightward shift in frontal activity," *Brain and Language*, vol. 111, no. 2, pp. 73–85, 2009.

[18] M. Musso, C. Weiller, S. Kiebel, S. P. Müller, P. Bülau, and M. Rijntjes, "Training-induced brain plasticity in aphasia," *Brain*, vol. 122, no. 9, pp. 1781–1790, 1999.

[19] M. Ohyama, M. Senda, S. Kitamura, K. Ishii, M. Mishina, and A. Terashi, "Role of the nondominant hemisphere and undamaged area during word repetition in poststroke aphasics. A PET activation study," *Stroke*, vol. 27, no. 5, pp. 897–903, 1996.

[20] D. Perani, S. F. Cappa, M. Tettamanti et al., "A fMRI study of word retrieval in aphasia," *Brain and Language*, vol. 85, no. 3, pp. 357–368, 2003.

[21] C. Y. Wan, X. Zheng, S. Marchina, A. Norton, and G. Schlaug, "Intensive therapy induces contralateral white matter changes in chronic stroke patients with Broca's aphasia," *Brain and Language*, vol. 136, pp. 1–7, 2014.

[22] C. Weiller, C. Isensee, M. Rijntjes et al., "Recovery from Wernicke's aphasia: a positron emission tomographic study," *Annals of Neurology*, vol. 37, no. 6, pp. 723–732, 1995.

[23] L. Winhuisin, A. Thiel, B. Schumacher et al., "Role of the contralateral inferior frontal gyrus in recovery of language function in poststroke aphasia: a combined repetitive transcranial magnetic stimulation and positron emission tomography study," *Stroke*, vol. 36, no. 8, pp. 1759–1763, 2005.

[24] P. Turkeltaub, S. Messing, C. Norise, and R. H. Hamilton, "Are networks for residual language function and recovery consistent across aphasic patients?" *Neurology*, vol. 76, no. 20, pp. 1726–1734, 2011.

[25] J. I. Breier, L. M. Maher, B. Novak, and A. C. Papanicolau, "Functional imaging before and after constraint-induced language therapy for aphasia using magnetoencephalography," *Neurocase*, vol. 12, no. 6, pp. 322–331, 2006.

[26] O. Elkana, R. Frost, U. Kramer, D. Ben-Bashat, and A. Schweiger, "Cerebral language reorganization in the chronic stage of recovery: a longitudinal fMRI study," *Cortex*, vol. 49, no. 1, pp. 71–81, 2013.

[27] J. Fridriksson, L. Morrow-Odom, D. Moser, A. Fridriksson, and G. Baylis, "Neural recruitment associated with anomia treatment in aphasia," *NeuroImage*, vol. 32, no. 3, pp. 1402–1412, 2006.

[28] J. Fridriksson, D. Moser, L. Bonilha et al., "Neural correlates of phonological and semantic-based anomia treatment in aphasia," *Neuropsychologia*, vol. 45, no. 8, pp. 1812–1822, 2007.

[29] S. Kiran, E. L. Meier, K. J. Kapse, and P. A. Glynn, "Changes in task-based effective connectivity in language networks following rehabilitation in post-stroke patients with aphasia," *Frontiers in Human Neuroscience*, vol. 9, p. 316, 2015.

[30] M. Meinzer, J. Obleser, T. Flaisch, C. Eulitz, and B. Rockstroh, "Recovery from aphasia as a function of language therapy in an early bilingual patient demonstrated by fMRI," *Neuropsychologia*, vol. 45, no. 6, pp. 1247–1256, 2007.

[31] C. K. Thompson, D. B. den Ouden, B. Bonakdarpour, K. Garibaldi, and T. B. Parrish, "Neural plasticity and treatment-induced recovery of sentence processing in agrammatism," *Neuropsychologia*, vol. 48, no. 11, pp. 3211–3227, 2010.

[32] G. Raboyeau, X. De Boissezon, N. Marie et al., "Right hemisphere activation in recovery from aphasia lesion effect or function recruitment?" *Neurology*, vol. 70, no. 4, pp. 290–298, 2008.

[33] S. Abel, C. Weiller, W. Huber, and K. Willmes, "Neural underpinnings for model-oriented therapy of aphasic word production," *Neuropsychologia*, vol. 57, pp. 154–165, 2014.

[34] B. T. Gold and A. Kertesz, "Right hemisphere semantic processing of visual words in an aphasic patient: an fMRI study," *Brain and Language*, vol. 73, no. 3, pp. 456–465, 2000.

[35] C. K. Thompson, E. A. Riley, D. B. Den Ouden, A. Meltzer-Asscher, and S. Lukic, "Training verb argument structure production in agrammatic aphasia: behavioral and neural recovery patterns," *Cortex*, vol. 49, no. 9, pp. 2358–2376, 2013.

[36] J. B. Allendorfer, B. M. Kissela, S. K. Holland, and J. P. Szaflarski, "Different patterns of language activation in post-stroke aphasia are detected by overt and covert versions of the verb generation task," *Medical Science Monitor: International Medical Journal of Experimental and Clinical Research*, vol. 18, no. 3, pp. CR135–CR137, 2012.

[37] W. Postman-Caucheteux, R. Birn, R. Pursley et al., "Single-trial fMRI shows contralesional activity linked to overt naming errors in chronic aphasic patients," *Journal of Cognitive Neuroscience*, vol. 22, no. 6, pp. 1299–1318, 2010.

[38] C. Barwood, B. Murdoch, B. Whelan et al., "Improved language performance subsequent to low-frequency rTMS in patients with chronic non-fluent aphasia post-stroke," *European Journal of Neurology*, vol. 18, no. 7, pp. 935–943, 2010.

[39] R. Hamilton, E. Chrysikou, and H. B. Coslett, "Mechanisms of aphasia recovery after stroke and the role of noninvasive brain stimulation," *Brain and Language*, vol. 118, no. 1-2, pp. 40–50, 2011.

[40] P. I. Martin, M. A. Naeser, M. Ho et al., "Overt naming fMRI pre- and post-TMS: two nonfluent aphasia patients, with and without improved naming post-TMS," *Brain and Language*, vol. 111, no. 1, pp. 20–35, 2009.

[41] M. Naeser, P. Martin, M. Nicholas et al., "Improved picture naming in chronic aphasia after TMS to part of right Broca's area: an open-protocol study," *Brain and Language*, vol. 93, no. 1, pp. 95–105, 2005.

[42] R. Chieffo, F. Ferrari, P. Battista et al., "Excitatory deep transcranial magnetic stimulation with H-coil over the right homologous Broca's region improves naming in chronic post-stroke aphasia," *Neurorehabilitation and Neural Repair*, vol. 28, no. 3, pp. 291–298, 2014.

[43] G. Hartwigsen, D. Saur, C. J. Price, S. Ulmer, A. Baumgaertner, and H. R. Siebner, "Perturbation of the left inferior frontal gyrus triggers adaptive plasticity in the right homologous area during speech production," *PNAS*, vol. 110, no. 41, pp. 16402–16407, 2013.

[44] W. Kakuda, M. Abo, N. Kaito, M. Watanabe, and A. Senoo, "Functional MRI-based therapeutic rTMS strategy for aphasic stroke patients: a case series pilot study," *International Journal of Neuroscience*, vol. 120, no. 1, pp. 60–66, 2010.

[45] F. Geranmayeh, S. L. Brownsett, and R. J. Wise, "Task-induced brain activity in aphasic stroke patients: what is driving recovery?" *Brain*, vol. 137, no. 10, pp. 2632–2648, 2014.

[46] C. A. van Oers, M. Vink, M. J. van Zandvoort et al., "Contribution of the left and right inferior frontal gyrus in recovery from aphasia. A functional MRI study in stroke patients with preserved hemodynamic responsiveness," *NeuroImage*, vol. 49, no. 1, pp. 885–893, 2010.

[47] A. Baumgaertner, G. Hartwigsen, and H. R. Siebner, "Right-hemispheric processing of non-linguistic word features: implications for mapping language recovery after stroke," *Human Brain Mapping*, vol. 34, no. 6, pp. 1293–1305, 2013.

[48] G. Fein, S. McGillivray, and P. Finn, "Older adults make less advantageous decisions than younger adults: cognitive and psychological correlates," *Journal of the International Neuropsychological Society*, vol. 13, no. 3, pp. 480–489, 2007.

[49] D. Mungas, B. R. Reed, W. J. Jagust et al., "Volumetric MRI predicts rate of cognitive decline related to AD and cerebrovascular disease," *Neurology*, vol. 59, no. 6, pp. 867–873, 2002.

[50] J. Zhang, L. Meng, W. Qin, N. Liu, F. D. Shi, and C. Yu, "Structural damage and functional reorganization in ipsilesional m1 in well-recovered patients with subcortical stroke," *Stroke*, vol. 45, no. 3, pp. 788–793, 2014.

[51] L. V. Gauthier, E. Taub, V. W. Mark, A. Barghi, and G. Uswatte, "Atrophy of spared gray matter tissue predicts poorer motor recovery and rehabilitation response in chronic stroke," *Stroke*, vol. 43, no. 2, pp. 453–457, 2012.

[52] J. D. Schaechter, C. I. Moore, B. D. Connell, B. R. Rosen, and R. N. Dijkhuizen, "Structural and functional plasticity in the somatosensory cortex of chronic stroke patients," *Brain*, vol. 129, no. 10, pp. 2722–2733, 2006.

[53] G. T. Stebbins, D. L. Nyenhuis, C. Wang et al., "Gray matter atrophy in patients with ischemic stroke with cognitive impairment," *Stroke*, vol. 39, no. 3, pp. 785–793, 2008.

[54] J. Ashburner and K. J. Friston, "Voxel-based morphometry—the methods," *NeuroImage*, vol. 11, no. 6 Pt 1, pp. 805–821, 2000.

[55] E. Bates, S. M. Wilson, A. P. Saygin et al., "Voxel-based lesion–symptom mapping," *Nature Neuroscience*, vol. 6, no. 5, pp. 448–450, 2003.

[56] S. Xing, E. H. Lacey, L. M. Skipper-Kallal et al., "Right hemisphere grey matter structure and language outcomes in chronic left hemisphere stroke," *Brain*, vol. 139, no. 1, pp. 227–241, 2016.

[57] A. Kertesz, *Western Aphasia Battery (Revised)*, PsychCorp, San Antonio, 2007.

[58] C. K. Thompson and S. Weintraub, *Northwestern Naming Battery (NNB)*, Northwestern University, Evanston, IL, 2014, http://northwestern.flintbox.com/public/project/22014/.

[59] J. Kay, R. Lesser, and M. Coltheart, "Psycholinguistic assessments of language processing in aphasia (PALPA): an introduction," *Aphasiology*, vol. 10, no. 2, pp. 159–180, 1996.

[60] C. K. Thompson, *Northwestern Assessment of Verbs and Sentences (NAVS)*, Northwestern University, Evanston, IL, 2012, http://northwestern.flintbox.com/public/project/9299/.

[61] N. J. Tustison, B. B. Avants, P. A. Cook et al., "N4ITK: improved N3 bias correction," *IEEE Transactions on Medical Imaging*, vol. 29, no. 6, pp. 1310–1320, 2010.

[62] C. Rorden and M. Brett, "Stereotaxic display of brain lesions," *Behavioural Neurology*, vol. 12, no. 4, pp. 191–200, 2000.

[63] K. Alpert, A. Kogan, T. Parrish, D. Marcus, and L. Wang, "The Northwestern University Neuroimaging Data Archive (NUNDA)," *NeuroImage*, vol. 124, part B, pp. 1131–1136, 2016.

[64] M. Brett, J. L. Anton, R. Valabregue, and J. B. Poline, "Region of interest analysis using the MarsBar toolbox for SPM 99," *NeuroImage*, vol. 16, no. 2, p. S497, 2002.

[65] R Core Team, *R: A Language and Environment for Statistical Computing*, R Foundation for Statistical Computing, Vienna, Austria, 2015, URL https://www.R-project.org/.

[66] Y. Benjamini and Y. Hochberg, "Controlling the false discovery rate: a practical and powerful approach to multiple testing," *Journal of the Royal Statistical Society. Series B (Methodological)*, vol. 57, no. 1, pp. 289–300, 1995.

[67] R. W. Cox, "AFNI: software for analysis and visualization of functional magnetic resonance neuroimages," *Computers and Biomedical Research*, vol. 29, no. 3, pp. 162–173, 1996.

[68] A. Eklund, T. E. Nichols, and H. Knutsson, "Cluster failure: why fMRI inferences for spatial extent have inflated false-positive rates," *Proceedings of the National Academy of Sciences*, vol. 113, no. 28, pp. 7900–7905, 2016.

[69] J. Hart and B. Gordon, "Delineation of single-word semantic comprehension deficits in aphasia, with anatomical correlation," *Annals of Neurology*, vol. 27, no. 3, pp. 226–231, 1990.

[70] N. F. Dronkers, D. P. Wilkins, R. D. Van Valin, B. B. Redfern, and J. J. Jaeger, "Lesion analysis of the brain areas involved in language comprehension," *Cognition*, vol. 92, no. 1, pp. 145–177, 2004.

[71] J. R. Booth, D. D. Burman, J. R. Meyer, D. R. Gitelman, T. B. Parrish, and M. M. Mesulam, "Modality independence of word comprehension," *Human Brain Mapping*, vol. 16, no. 4, pp. 251–261, 2002.

[72] L. K. Tyler, W. D. Marslen-Wilson, and E. A. Stamatakis, "Differentiating lexical form, meaning, and structure in the neural language system," *Proceedings of the National Academy of Sciences of the United States of America*, vol. 102, no. 23, pp. 8375–8380, 2005.

[73] S. C. Baker, C. D. Frith, and R. J. Dolan, "The interaction between mood and cognitive function studied with PET," *Psychological Medicine*, vol. 27, no. 3, pp. 565–578, 1997.

[74] M. Berlingeri, D. Crepaldi, R. Roberti, G. Scialfa, C. Luzzatti, and E. Paulesu, "Nouns and verbs in the brain: grammatical class and task specific effects as revealed by fMRI," *Cognitive Neuropsychology*, vol. 25, no. 4, pp. 528–558, 2008.

[75] S. Kemeny, F. Q. Ye, R. Birn, and A. R. Braun, "Comparison of continuous overt speech fMRI using BOLD and arterial spin labeling," *Human Brain Mapping*, vol. 24, no. 3, pp. 173–183, 2005.

[76] A. Ardila, B. Bernal, and M. Rosselli, "Participation of the insula in language revisited: a meta-analytic connectivity study," *Journal of Neurolinguistics*, vol. 29, pp. 31–41, 2014.

[77] A. D. Friederici, "Towards a neural basis of auditory sentence processing," *Trends in Cognitive Sciences*, vol. 6, no. 2, pp. 78–84, 2002.

[78] C. Rogalsky and G. Hickok, "Selective attention to semantic and syntactic features modulates sentence processing networks in anterior temporal cortex," *Cerebral Cortex*, vol. 19, no. 4, pp. 786–796, 2009.

[79] A. D. Friederici, S. A. Kotz, S. K. Scott, and J. Obleser, "Disentangling syntax and intelligibility in auditory language comprehension," *Human Brain Mapping*, vol. 31, no. 3, pp. 448–457, 2010.

[80] A. D. Friederici, M. Makuuchi, and J. Bahlmann, "The role of the posterior superior temporal cortex in sentence comprehension," *Neuroreport*, vol. 20, no. 6, pp. 563–568, 2009.

[81] J. E. Mack, A. Meltzer-Asscher, E. Barbieri, and C. K. Thompson, "Neural correlates of processing passive sentences," *Brain Sciences*, vol. 3, no. 3, pp. 1198–1214, 2013.

[82] C. J. Price, "The anatomy of language: a review of 100 fMRI studies published in 2009," *Annals of the new York Academy of Sciences*, vol. 119, no. 1, pp. 62–88, 2010.

[83] D. Caplan, J. Michaud, and R. Hufford, "Mechanisms underlying syntactic comprehension deficits in vascular aphasia: new evidence from self-paced listening," *Cognitive Neuropsychology*, vol. 32, no. 5, pp. 283–313, 2015.

[84] S. Lukic, B. Bonakdarpour, D. B. den Ouden, C. Price, and C. K. Thompson, "Neural mechanisms of verb and sentence production: a lesion-deficit study," *Procedia - Social and Behavioral Sciences*, vol. 94, pp. 34–35, 2013.

[85] P. Indefrey and W. J. Levelt, "The spatial and temporal signatures of word production components," *Cognition*, vol. 92, no. 1, pp. 101–144, 2004.

[86] R. Kawashima, J. Okuda, A. Umetsu et al., "Human cerebellum plays an important role in memory-timed finger movement: an fMRI study," *Journal of Neurophysiology*, vol. 83, no. 2, pp. 1079–1087, 2000.

[87] J. W. Bohland and F. H. Guenther, "An fMRI investigation of syllable sequence production," *NeuroImage*, vol. 32, no. 2, pp. 821–841, 2006.

[88] T. M. Loucks, C. J. Poletto, K. Simonyan, C. L. Reynolds, and C. L. Ludlow, "Human brain activation during phonation and exhalation: common volitional control for two upper airway functions," *NeuroImage*, vol. 36, no. 1, pp. 131–143, 2007.

[89] F. X. Alario, H. Chainay, S. Lehericy, and L. Cohen, "The role of the supplementary motor area (SMA) in word production," *Brain Research*, vol. 1076, no. 1, pp. 129–143, 2006.

[90] B. Crosson, J. R. Sadek, L. Maron et al., "Relative shift in activity from medial to lateral frontal cortex during internally versus externally guided word generation," *Journal of Cognitive Neuroscience*, vol. 13, no. 2, pp. 272–283, 2001.

[91] N. F. Dronkers, "A new brain region for coordinating speech articulation," *Nature*, vol. 384, no. 6605, pp. 159–161, 1996.

[92] J. Shuren, "Insula and aphasia," *Journal of Neurology*, vol. 240, no. 4, pp. 216–218, 1993.

[93] C. Breitenstein, A. Jansen, M. Deppe et al., "Hippocampus activity differentiates good from poor learners of a novel lexicon," *NeuroImage*, vol. 25, no. 3, pp. 958–968, 2005.

[94] E. A. Maguire and C. D. Frith, "The brain network associated with acquiring semantic knowledge," *NeuroImage*, vol. 22, no. 1, pp. 171–178, 2004.

[95] B. Opitz and A. D. Friederici, "Interactions of the hippocampal system and the prefrontal cortex in learning language-like rules," *NeuroImage*, vol. 19, no. 4, pp. 1730–1737, 2003.

[96] M. Meinzer, S. Mohammadi, H. Kugel et al., "Integrity of the hippocampus and surrounding white matter is correlated with language training success in aphasia," *NeuroImage*, vol. 53, no. 1, pp. 283–290, 2010.

[97] R. A. Menke, J. Scholz, K. L. Miller et al., "MRI characteristics of the substantia nigra in Parkinson's disease: a combined quantitative T1 and DTI study," *NeuroImage*, vol. 47, no. 2, pp. 435–441, 2009.

[98] R. L. Buckner, M. E. Raichle, F. M. Miezin, and S. E. Petersen, "Functional-anatomic studies of the recall of pictures and words from memory," *The Journal of Neuroscience*, vol. 16, no. 19, pp. 6219–6235, 1996.

3

The Effect of rTMS over the Different Targets on Language Recovery in Stroke Patients with Global Aphasia

Caili Ren ⓘ,[1,2] Guofu Zhang,[2] Xinlei Xu,[1] Jianfeng Hao,[1] Hui Fang,[1] Ping Chen,[1] Zhaohui Li,[1] Yunyun Ji,[1] Qingjie Cai,[1] and Fei Gao[1]

[1]*Department of Neurological Rehabilitation, Wuxi Tongren Rehabilitation Hospital of Nanjing Medical University, Wuxi, Jiangsu Province, China*
[2]*Department of Psychiatry, The Affiliated Wuxi Mental Health Center of Nanjing Medical University, Wuxi, Jiangsu Province, China*

Correspondence should be addressed to Caili Ren; sally7226@163.com

Academic Editor: Alfredo Conti

Objective. To evaluate and compare the effects of repetitive transcranial magnetic stimulation (rTMS) over the right pars triangularis of the posterior inferior frontal gyrus (pIFG) and the right posterior superior temporal gyrus (pSMG) in global aphasia following subacute stroke. *Methods.* Fifty-four patients with subacute poststroke global aphasia were randomized to 15-day protocols of 20-minute inhibitory 1 Hz rTMS over either the right triangular part of the pIFG (the rTMS-b group) or the right pSTG (the rTMS-w group) or to sham stimulation, followed by 30 minutes of speech and language therapy. Language outcomes were assessed by aphasia quotient (AQ) scores obtained from the Chinese version of the Western Aphasia Battery (WAB) at baseline and immediately after 3 weeks (15 days) of experimental treatment. *Results.* Forty-five patients completed the entire study. The primary outcome measures include the changes in WAB-AQ score, spontaneous speech, auditory comprehension, and repetition. These measures indicated significant main effect between the baseline of the rTMS-w, rTMS-b, and sham groups and immediately after stimulation ($P<0.05$). Compared with the sham group, the increases were significant for auditory comprehension, repetition, and AQ in the rTMS-w group ($P<0.05$), whereas the changes in repetition, spontaneous speech, and AQ tended to be higher in the rTMS-b group ($P<0.05$). *Conclusions.* Inhibitory rTMS targeting the right pIFG and pSTG can be an effective treatment for subacute stroke patients with global aphasia. The effect of rTMS may depend on the stimulation site. Low-frequency rTMS inhibited the right pSTG and significantly improved language recovery in terms of auditory comprehension and repetition, whereas LF-rTMS inhibited the right pIFG, leading to apparent changes in spontaneous speech and repetition.

1. Introduction

Stroke-related aphasia is one of the most common consequences of cerebrovascular diseases and occurs in one-third of acute or subacute stroke patients [1]. Global aphasia is one of the most serious and common aphasia types in acute and subacute stroke patients. This type is usually caused by infarction of the left middle cerebral artery. Patients with global aphasia have difficulties with communication, which is affected gravely and comprehensively in the domains of spontaneous speech, auditory comprehension, naming, and repetition. The most important period of language recovery usually occurs in the first to the third month after stroke, which is the key time for neurophysiological restoration and reorganization of the language cortex [2].

Mounting studies have demonstrated that inhibitory low-frequency repetitive transcranial magnetic stimulation (LF-rTMS) (≤ 1 Hz) over the unaffected hemisphere can improve language function in poststroke aphasic patients with left-hemispheric lesions [3–6]. Language functional recovery occurs because of compensatory facilitation of the left hemisphere following the reduction of interhemispheric inhibition by suppressive LF-rTMS. Ideally, when used therapeutically for aphasia to reduce interhemispheric inhibition and facilitate the neural activity of the compensatory areas, LF-rTMS should be applied to an area homologous to the compensatory areas with impaired language function [7]. Our previous work [8] identified seven randomized controlled trials involving 160 stroke patients for a meta-analysis that investigated the positive effect of low-frequency rTMS targeting the pars triangularis of the right posterior inferior frontal gyrus (pIFG) [9–12]. Abo et al. [13] reported that low-frequency rTMS over the superior temporal gyrus (STG) of the temporal lobe improved language function in patients with fluent aphasia. A positron emission tomographic study found right hemisphere activation in STG in patients with Wernicke's aphasia [14]. The right posterior part of the superior temporal gyrus (pSTG), homotopic to the left Wernicke's area, is the other optimal target of rTMS stimulation.

The right pars triangularis (BA45) was selected as a stimulation site because previous imaging studies have shown that activation occurs in all patients in whom the perisylvian language cortex of the dominant hemisphere is damaged, and 1 Hz inhibitory TMS over the right pars triangularis but not the pars opercularis can improve anomia in patients with aphasia [15]. The rationale for the utilization of the right pSTG as the other stimulation site was that it is an important area of the language network and a key point of the ventral stream, which is involved in mapping sound onto meaning [16]. Therefore, this suggests that LF-rTMS over the right pSTG in global aphasia may improve auditory comprehension significantly by promoting a recovery semantic language network.

However, little is known about the effects of LF-rTMS over the right pSTG combined with speech and language therapy (SLT) in the treatment of subacute global aphasia poststroke. The present randomized sham-stimulation-controlled study aimed to investigate the efficacy of LF-rTMS over the right pSTG or the right pIFG in global aphasic patients with subacute stroke.

2. Materials and Methods

2.1. Subjects. A total of 45 right-handed (assessed by the Edinburgh Handedness Inventory; Oldfield, 1971) subjects suffering from subacute stroke with global aphasia participated in this experiment. All subjects were native Chinese speakers aged 45 to 75 years. Table 1 provides the detailed demographic and clinical information of the participants. The inclusion criteria were as follows: (1) a first-ever left-sided middle cerebral artery (MCA) stroke with the lesion site verified by magnetic resonance imaging (MRI); (2) the time between 4 and 12 weeks after suffering from the stroke; (3) global aphasia defined by WAB-AQ scores; and (4) written informed consent from all subjects who participated in the study.

The exclusion criteria were as follows: (1) vision and hearing disabilities that might interfere with diagnostic and therapeutic treatment; (2) medications altering the level of cortical excitability (e.g., antiepileptics, neuroleptics or benzodiazepines); (3) a history of substance abuse, premorbid dementia or any neuropsychiatric diseases; and

(4) contraindications for rTMS according to the safety guidelines [17, 18].

The Ethics Committee of the Medical University of Nanjing approved the study protocol. We registered the protocol of the present randomized controlled study in the Chinese Clinical Trial Registry (no. ChiCTR-IPR-15007382).

2.2. Procedure. This study was randomized, double-blinded, and sham controlled. A completely randomized digital table was used to generate the random allocation sequence. The patients were randomly assigned to three groups: those receiving real inhibiting rTMS on the right pars triangularis of the pIFG, which is the homolog of the left Broca's area (the rTMS-b group); those receiving real inhibiting rTMS on the right pSTG, which is the homolog of the left Wernicke's area (the rTMS-w group); and those receiving sham rTMS (the sham group), all in combination with SLT. The allocations were stored in sealed, numbered envelopes. The subjects did not know whether they were receiving real or sham rTMS. The language therapist assessed speech and language abilities and was blinded to the patients' group assignments. All subjects, investigators (except the investigator responsible for rTMS application), clinicians, speech, and language therapists were blinded to patient assignment to real or sham rTMS.

The therapeutic procedure consisted of rTMS sessions and SLT. Subjects in all three groups underwent SLT sessions for 30 minutes immediately after finishing rTMS treatment from Monday to Friday for 3 weeks. The speech and language training mainly focused on the comprehension and expression of spoken language. The rehabilitation program focused on specific training to stimulate various aspects of the language system (e.g., semantic, phonological, syntactic or motor).

A language assessment was performed at baseline and immediately after 3 weeks of real or sham rTMS treatment using the Western Aphasia Battery (WAB), which evaluated the capabilities of spontaneous speech, auditory comprehension, repetition and naming. The AQ was obtained after the examination. This measure reflects the severity of aphasia and can be used as an index for evaluating the improvement and deterioration of aphasia. The highest AQ score is 100, and the normal range is 98.4-99.6. AQ<93.8 is classified as aphasia. When the measure results of patients reach the score of spontaneous speech 0~4, auditory comprehension 0~3.9, repetition 0~4.9, and naming 0-6, they are defined as the patients of global aphasia.

2.3. Transcranial Magnetic Stimulation. rTMS was performed with a MagPro® (MagVenture Company, Farum, Denmark) equipped with an air-cooled figure-of-eight coil (each loop was 70 mm in diameter). The subjects were seated in a chair that allowed their head to lean on the headrest to ensure that it was immobile during the rTMS procedure. The coil was placed tangentially to the scalp over the right pIFG (F4 site on a standard EEG-10/20) or the pSTG (CP6 site on a standard EEG-10/20). Each LF-rTMS session consisted of 1,200 pulses and lasted 20 minutes. Magnetic stimulation was

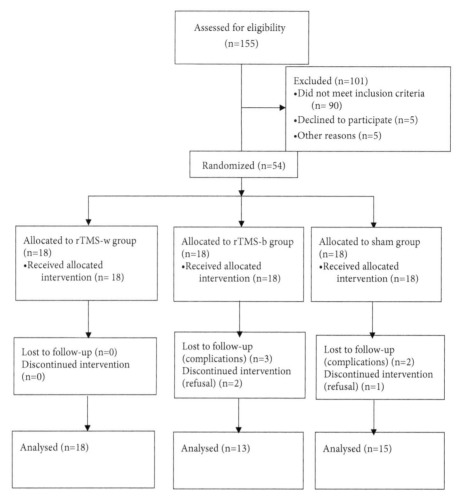

FIGURE 1: CONSORT diagram of patient flow throughout the study.

applied at 80% of the resting motor threshold (RMT) at a 1-Hz frequency. RMT was determined in each subject once before treatment and was defined as the minimum stimulus intensity able to elicit a motor evoked potential of at least 50 mV in 5 or more of 10 consecutive stimulations. MEP was recorded from the first dorsal interosseus muscle of the unaffected hand. The stimulation parameters were chosen according to current safety guidelines for rTMS [19]. The sham stimulation used the same coil and was placed vertically over the vertex with the same stimulation parameters used for the real rTMS procedure.

2.4. Sample Size Calculation. Based on previous studies [9, 20], we expected an effect size of 0.5, with an α of 0.05 and a power of 0.8. The minimum sample size in each group was n=14. If the dropout rate is less than 20%, we need at least 18 participants in each group.

2.5. Statistical Analysis. The necessary sample size was estimated by referring to the previous randomized controlled study [9]. The data analyses were performed with SPSS version 22.0 for Windows statistical software. Differences in categorical data were analyzed using the Chi-square test.

Descriptive data were reported as the mean±SD for normally distributed data or as the median (interquartile range) for discrete variables of baseline characteristics and the language function scores of each group. A 2-factor repeated measures ANOVA was performed to test for differential treatment effects on WAB-AQ and WAB subtests. Post hoc analyses were applied to multiple comparisons. Differences were considered statistically significant when *P*<0.05.

3. Results

3.1. Participant Characteristics. A total of 54 patients participated in the study based on the inclusion and exclusion criteria. Three patients refused to participate in the study after signing informed consent and allocation (2 from the rTMS-b group and 1 from the sham group). Five patients dropped out because of complications (3 from the rTMS-b group and 2 from the sham group). Finally, 45 participants completed the study (rTMS-w group, n=18; rTMS-b group, n=13; sham group, n=15) (Figure 1). All three groups were balanced at baseline with respect to the severity of aphasia, time since onset, participant age, gender and concomitant diseases (*P*>0.05) (Table 1).

TABLE 1: Summary of patients' characteristics.

	rTMS-W group (n=18)	rTMS-b group (n=13)	Sham group (n=15)	Statistics	P
Gender, M/F	12/6	7/6	9/6	$\chi^2=0.528$	0.768
Mean age, years (SD)	65.95 (8.53)	62.46 (10.95)	63.60 (16.71)	$F=-0.561$	0.574
Time of onset, days (SD)	55.90 (19.41)	50.58 (23.80)	61.20 (22.66)	$F=-0.917$	0.407
Hypertension (n)	14	11	12	$\chi^2=0.528$	0.768
Diabetes (n)	5	5	7	$\chi^2=0.152$	0.697
Coronary artery disease (n)	2	3	3	$\chi^2=0.073$	0.787
Atrial fibrillation (n)	4	3	3	$\chi^2=0.167$	0.682
WAB-AQ scores (SD)	9.07 (7.12)	10.48 (12.49)	7.05 (10.67)	$F=-0.427$	0.655

TABLE 2: WAB-AQ and subtest performances of the rTMS-w group, rTMS-b group, and sham group at pre- and posttreatment.

Test	Baseline Pre-rTMS			Post rTMS			F	ANOVA Group *Time (P)
	rTMS-w (n=18)	rTMS-b (n=13)	Sham (n=15)	rTMS-w (n=18)	rTMS-b (n=13)	Sham (n=15)		
Spontaneous speech	1.70±1.59	1.08±1.75	1.07±2.19	2.83±1.58	5.00±3.08	1.93±2.69	17.512	0.001
Auditory comprehension	1.58±0.98	2.02±1.86	1.21±1.57	3.64±1.11	3.68±1.85	2.17±1.92	6.099	0.005
Repetition	1.35±1.78	1.63±2.12	1.09±1.89	2.80±2.22	4.03±2.34	1.37±1.87	9.331	0.001
Naming	0.04±0.18	0.54±1.19	0.03±0.10	0.61±0.85	1.45±2.31	0.60±0.98	0.428	0.655
AQ	9.06±7.12	10.48±12.49	7.05±10.67	19.79±7.53	27.59±18.06	12.37±14.26	11.977	0.001

3.2. Treatment Effects. A comparison of performance between the rTMS-w, rTMS-b and sham groups across baseline and posttreatment is shown in Figure 2 and Table 2. A series of two-way repeated measures analysis of variances (ANOVA) were conducted. Significant differences in the interactions between group and time were found on the following WAB-AQ and the WAB subtests: WAB-AQ scores ($P<0.001$), WAB spontaneous speech scores ($P<0.001$), WAB auditory comprehension scores ($P=0.005$) and WAB repetition scores ($P<0.001$). Post Hoc analyses were conducted between the three groups at baseline and posttreatment (repeated measured t-test). There was no significant difference in WAB scores for spontaneous speech, auditory comprehension, naming, repetition or AQ at baseline among the three groups ($P>0.05$). A significant change in auditory comprehension differences was found only between the rTMS-w group and the sham group ($P=0.001$, 95% CI (-1.73, -0.46)). The change in spontaneous speech remained significantly different between the rTMS-b group and the sham group ($P\leq0.001$, 95% CI (-0.564, -0.235)). No significant difference was found for the changes in WAB scores for AQ ($P=0.083$, 95% CI (-0.413, 0.026)) and auditory comprehension ($P=0.240$, 95% CI (-0.270, 1.051)) between the rTMS-b group and the rTMS-w group.

4. Discussion

The present randomized sham-controlled study investigates the effect of inhibitory rTMS over the right pIFG or the right pSTG combined with SLT on language recovery from subacute global aphasia. A relatively short treatment period of rTMS combined with SLT promoted language recovery for rTMS over the right pIFG and pSTG as opposed to the sham group. LF-rTMS inhibited the right pSTG and led to significantly higher gains in auditory comprehension and repetition, whereas LF-rTMS inhibited the right pIFG and caused changes in spontaneous speech and repetition. These results provide evidence that rTMS may be an effective treatment tool for subacute stroke with global aphasia.

The present study suggested that the efficacy of rTMS on language recovery may be based on the stimulation sites. This study is the first to compare two stimulation sites in a randomized study. We chose global aphasia because these patients have difficulty involved in SLT due to their severely impaired auditory comprehension. Meanwhile, patients with global aphasia displayed little effect from SLT, whose therapeutic effects are quite variable and usually modest (Brady et al., 2012). Previous research has elucidated increased right hemisphere activation in individuals with left hemisphere lesions [21]. Such activation suggests that the brain may be employing a compensatory strategy which could potentially be maladaptive. Low-frequency rTMS provides an opportunity to normalize language function by inhibiting maladaptive brain activation and increasing adaptive activation. The underlying mechanisms for the LF-rTMS over the right two stimulations in patients with global aphasia were needed further study.

The results suggested that LF-rTMS inhibited the right pSTG and significantly improved language performance in WAB-AQ scores, auditory comprehension, and repetition.

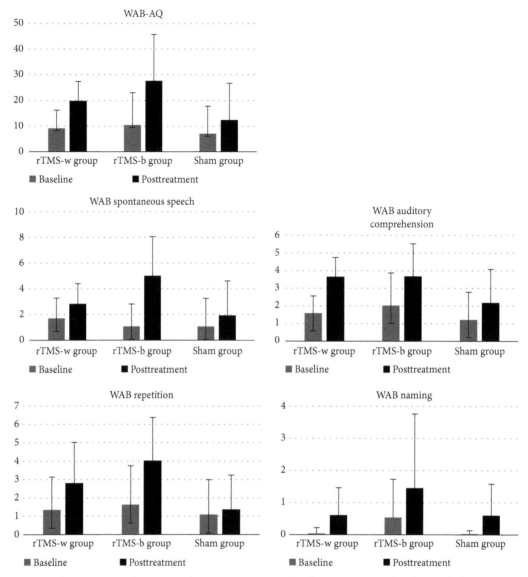

FIGURE 2: Language performance regarding pre- and posttreatment. Graphs showing means at baseline and after treatment for the three groups across WAB-AQ scores and WAB subtests.

These results suggest that the related areas on the right hemisphere may contribute to recovery from aphasia when stimulated. These findings also corroborate a small pilot study by Abo et al. [13], who reported that low-frequency rTMS improved language function over the STG of the temporal lobe in patients with fluent aphasia. We also found that the application of LF-rTMS to the right pIFG displayed apparently beneficial changes in WAB-AQ, spontaneous speech, and repetition. This result is consistent with previous studies that showed that LF-rTMS over the right prIFG exhibited superior performance in spontaneous speech, comprehension, repetition, naming, and AQ in nonfluent aphasia [3, 8, 22, 23]. However, in our study, only small changes were observed in the recovery of naming ability between pre- and posttreatment with rTMS for global aphasia. The reason may be that there is a severe degree of speech injury in poststroke patients with global aphasia. The therapeutic effect

of LF-rTMS over the right pSTG or prIFG may be mediated by increased inhibition of the contra-lesional hemisphere, thus restoring balance that enables the undamaged parts of the language area to function properly. The left anterior temporal lobe is not included in the MCA territory [24]. Furthermore, recovery of auditory comprehension in aphasia after left MCA infarction depends on the reorganization of the remaining language cortex of the left anterior temporal lobe [25]. These studies may provide a theoretical basis for the recovery of auditory comprehension in aphasic patients.

4.1. Study Limitations. The present study also has some limitations. Long-term effects have not been observed, and we did not have functional MRI available to investigate the change in activation of the language cortex before and after rTMS treatment.

5. Conclusions

Many studies have reported that low-frequency rTMS is beneficial for rehabilitating patients with aphasia, but the ideal stimulation sites for rTMS are not known. Low-frequency rTMS applied to the right pIFG and pSTG can be assumed to be an effective treatment for global aphasia following subacute stroke. Even immediately after the 15-day treatment, LF-rTMS inhibited the right pSTG and promoted significantly increased gains in auditory comprehension and repetition, whereas LF-rTMS inhibited the right pIFG and apparently caused changes in spontaneous speech and repetition. Further investigations are necessary to explore the neural mechanisms that underlie the differences in functional recovery observed between the different stimulation sites in this study.

Acknowledgments

The authors thank all those who participated in the trial. This work was supported by the National Natural Science Foundation of China [Grant number 81501949]. Contributor Shuyuan Wu participated in the treatment of participants.

References

[1] P. M. Pedersen, H. S. Jorgensen, H. Nakayama, H. O. Raaschou, and T. S. Olsen, "Aphasia in acute stroke: incidence, determinants, and recovery," *Annals of Neurology*, vol. 38, no. 4, pp. 659–666, 1995.

[2] R. M. Lazar, A. E. Speizer, J. R. Festa, J. W. Krakauer, and R. S. Marshall, "Variability in language recovery after first-time stroke," *Journal of Neurology, Neurosurgery & Psychiatry*, vol. 79, no. 5, pp. 530–534, 2008.

[3] X. Y. Hu, T. Zhang, G. B. Rajah et al., "Effects of different frequencies of repetitive transcranial magnetic stimulation in stroke patients with non-fluent aphasia: a randomized, sham-controlled study," *Neurological Research*, vol. 40, no. 6, pp. 459–465, 2018.

[4] H. Zhang, Y. Chen, R. Hu et al., "rTMS treatments combined with speech training for a conduction aphasia patient: a case report with mri study," *Medicine*, vol. 96, no. 32, article e7399, 2017.

[5] L. Sebastianelli, V. Versace, S. Martignago et al., "Low-frequency rTMS of the unaffected hemisphere in stroke patients: a systematic review," *Acta Neurologica Scandinavica*, vol. 136, no. 6, pp. 585–605, 2017.

[6] M. Ilkhani, H. S. Baghini, G. Kiamarzi, A. Meysamie, and P. Ebrahimi, "The effect of low-frequency repetitive transcranial magnetic stimulation (rTMS) on the treatment of aphasia caused by cerebrovascular accident (CVA)," *Medical Journal of The Islamic Republic of Iran*, vol. 31, no. 1, article 137, 2017.

[7] B. Otal, M. C. Olma, A. Flöel, and I. Wellwood, "Inhibitory non-invasive brain stimulation to homologous language regions as an adjunct to speech and language therapy in post-stroke aphasia: a meta-analysis," *Frontiers in Human Neuroscience*, vol. 9, article 236, 2015.

[8] C.-L. Ren, G.-F. Zhang, N. Xia et al., "Effect of low-frequency rTMS on aphasia in stroke patients: a meta-analysis of randomized controlled trials," *PLoS ONE*, vol. 9, no. 7, Article ID e102557, 2014.

[9] A. Thiel, A. Hartmann, I. Rubi-Fessen et al., "Effects of noninvasive brain stimulation on language networks and recovery in early poststroke aphasia," *Stroke*, vol. 44, no. 8, pp. 2240–2246, 2013.

[10] J. Seniów, K. Waldowski, M. Leśniak, S. Iwański, W. Czepiel, and A. Członkowska, "Transcranial magnetic stimulation combined with speech and language training in early aphasia rehabilitation: a randomized double-blind controlled pilot study," *Topics in Stroke Rehabilitation*, vol. 20, no. 3, pp. 250–261, 2015.

[11] C. H. S. Barwood, B. E. Murdoch, S. Riek et al., "Long term language recovery subsequent to low frequency rTMS in chronic non-fluent aphasia," *NeuroRehabilitation*, vol. 32, no. 4, pp. 915–928, 2013.

[12] K. Waldowski, J. Seniow, M. Lesniak, S. Iwanski, and A. Czlonkowska, "Effect of low-frequency repetitive transcranial magnetic stimulation on naming abilities in early-stroke aphasic patients: a prospective, randomized, double-blind sham-controlled study," *Scientific World Journal*, vol. 2012, Article ID 518568, 8 pages, 2012.

[13] M. Abo, W. Kakuda, M. Watanabe, A. Morooka, K. Kawakami, and A. Senoo, "Effectiveness of low-frequency rtms and intensive speech therapy in poststroke patients with aphasia: a pilot study based on evaluation by fmri in relation to type of aphasia," *European Neurology*, vol. 68, no. 4, pp. 199–208, 2012.

[14] C. Weiller, C. Isensee, M. Rijntjes et al., "Recovery from wernicke's aphasia: a positron emission tomographic study," *Annals of Neurology*, vol. 37, no. 6, pp. 723–732, 1995.

[15] M. A. Naeser, P. I. Martin, H. Theoret et al., "TMS suppression of right pars triangularis, but not pars opercularis, improves naming in aphasia," *Brain and Language*, vol. 119, no. 3, pp. 206–213, 2011.

[16] D. Saura, B. W. Kreher, S. Schnell et al., "Ventral and dorsal pathways for language," *Proceedings of the National Acadamy of Sciences of the United States of America*, vol. 105, no. 46, pp. 18035–18040, 2008.

[17] E. M. Wassermann, "Risk and safety of repetitive transcranial magnetic stimulation: report and suggested guidelines from the international workshop on the safety of repetitive transcranial magnetic stimulation," *Electroencephalography and Clinical Neurophysiology—Evoked Potentials*, vol. 108, no. 1, pp. 1–16, 1998.

[18] S. Anand and J. Hotson, "Transcranial magnetic stimulation: Neurophysiological applications and safety," *Brain and Cognition*, vol. 50, no. 3, pp. 366–386, 2002.

[19] C. Tranulis, B. Guéguen, A. Pham-Scottez et al., "Motor threshold in transcranial magnetic stimulation: comparison of three estimation methods," *Neurophysiologie Clinique/Clinical Neurophysiology*, vol. 36, no. 1, pp. 1–7, 2006.

[20] W.-D. Heiss, A. Hartmann, I. Rubi-Fessen et al., "Noninvasive brain stimulation for treatment of right- and left-handed post-stroke aphasics," *Cerebrovascular Disease*, vol. 36, no. 5-6, pp. 363–372, 2013.

[21] W.-D. Heiss, "Imaging effects related to language improvements by rTMS," *Restorative Neurology and Neuroscience*, vol. 34, no. 4, pp. 531–536, 2016.

[22] T. H. Yoon, S. J. Han, T. S. Yoon, J. S. Kim, and T. I. Yi, "Therapeutic effect of repetitive magnetic stimulation combined with speech and language therapy in post-stroke non-fluent aphasia," *NeuroRehabilitation*, vol. 36, no. 1, pp. 107–114, 2015.

[23] A. Thiel, S. E. Black, E. A. Rochon et al., "Non-invasive repeated therapeutic stimulation for aphasia recovery: a multilingual, multicenter aphasia trial," *Journal of Stroke and Cerebrovascular Diseases*, vol. 24, no. 4, pp. 751–758, 2015.

[24] T. G. Phan, G. A. Donnan, P. M. Wright, and D. C. Reutens, "A digital map of middle cerebral artery infarcts associated with middle cerebral artery trunk and branch occlusion," *Stroke*, vol. 36, no. 5, pp. 986–991, 2005.

[25] H. Robson, R. Zahn, J. L. Keidel, R. J. Binney, K. Sage, and M. A. Lambon Ralph, "The anterior temporal lobes support residual comprehension in Wernicke's aphasia," *Brain*, vol. 137, no. 3, pp. 931–943, 2014.

4

A Middle-Aged Woman with Logopenic Progressive Aphasia as a Precursor of Alzheimer's Disease

Stephanie M. Awad[1] and Amer M. Awad[1,2]

[1] Family Medicine Residency Program, Baton Rouge General Medical Center, Baton Rouge, LA 70806, USA
[2] Baton Rouge Neurology Associates, Baton Rouge General Medical Center, 3600 Florida Boulevard, Baton Rouge, LA 70806, USA

Correspondence should be addressed to Amer M. Awad, ameraldo@gmail.com

Academic Editors: Ö. Ateş and M. Swash

Primary progressive aphasia is a neurodegenerative disorder that was recently classified into three types: fluent (semantic), nonfluent, and logopenic. The logopenic variant is the least common one and is closely related to Alzheimer's disease in comparison to the other two variants that are closely related to frontotemporal dementia. We report the case of a middle-aged woman who presented to our center with progressive aphasia that was undiagnosed for two years. The patient's neurological evaluation including positron emission tomography is consistent with a logopenic variant of primary progressive aphasia.

1. Introduction

Primary progressive aphasia (PPA) is a spectrum of heterogeneous disorders that are characterized by slowly progressive neurodegeneration affecting mainly the language function [1].

The first description of isolated language deteriorations was probably made by Serieux in the late nineteenth century [2]. Comprehensive epidemiological studies are so far lacking to define the exact demographics of PPA. However, PPA is still considered a rare disease with variable progression rates, variable ages of onset and without remarkable gender preponderance.

There has been dramatic progress in our understanding of PPA in the last few decades thanks to the progress in neuropathology, neurogenetics, and neuropsychology. PPA was recently subclassified into three distinct types [3, 4]: progressive nonfluent aphasia (PNFA), semantic dementia (SD), and the recently described logopenic variant (LPA). The logopenic variant accounts for one-third of PPA cases [3]. In this paper we will discuss the case of a patient with LPA that has early Alzheimer's disease features as well.

2. Case Report

The patient is a 54-year-old left-handed Caucasian lady who was referred to our center for evaluation of speech difficulties. The patient noted a gradually progressing speech problem about two years prior to her presentation. Her main difficulties were related to word finding and inability to express herself very well with frequent pauses. Her comprehension was also affected, but much less than her fluency. In addition, she noted that her reading abilities were declining and her writing skills seemed to be deteriorating. The patient denied any history of weakness, trouble swallowing, trouble breathing, numbness, loss of vision, hearing, or balance. Her husband had thought that her short-term memory was also impaired. The patient's family history was significant for Alzheimer's disease that affected her aunt in her 80s. The patient denied any history of strokes, seizures, or head injury. No behavioral abnormalities were reported. Her medical exam was normal, except for high cortical abnormalities. Her cranial nerves, motor system, sensory system, and coordination system exams were normal. The patient scored 23/30 on the Montreal Cognitive Assessment

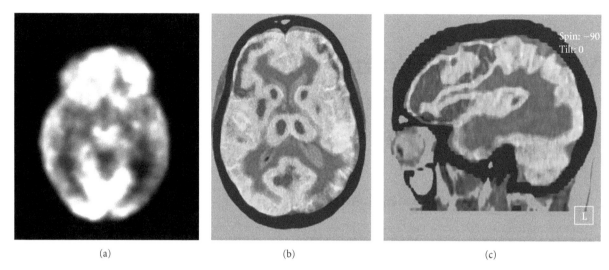

(a)   (b)   (c)

FIGURE 1: (a)–(c) show brain PET scan of the patient showing bilateral, predominantly left-sided, parietotemporal hypometabolism in different orientations.

Exam (MOCA). There was evidence of aphasia on detailed language examination that can be classified as global aphasia. The patient's fluency was decreased with word finding difficulties without agrammatism. Comprehension of isolated words was intact, whereas comprehension of complex sentences was impaired. Repetition and digit span was impaired as well. Naming was mildly affected. Short-term memory including episodic memory was impaired. Cues did not seem to help improve recall. Interestingly, visuospatial function was impaired in a very subtle way. The patient was able to copy a cube but only after several unsuccessful attempts.

Prior to being evaluated by us the patient underwent numerous tests that were reported to be normal including brain magnetic resonance imaging (MRI), comprehensive autoimmune panel, electroencephalography (EEG) and vitamin B12, folic acid, thyroid stimulating hormone (TSH), and rapid plasma reagin (RPR) tests. We evaluated the patient with positron emission tomography (PET) scan which showed hypometabolism in the bilateral parietal as well as temporal lobes (Figures 1(a), 1(b), and 1(c)).

The clinical findings along with the radiological findings are highly suggestive of logopenic primary progressive aphasia (LPA).

3. Discussion

Our patient's neurocognitive assessment is highly suggestive of LPA.

LPA was first described by Gorno-Tempini and his co-workers in 2004 [3]. The disorder typically presents with word finding difficulty with no agrammatism, impaired repetition, impaired comprehension of complex sentences with retained comprehension of isolated words [3, 4].

LPA typically involves an abnormality in the parietotemporal lobes, predominantly, the dominant side [3–6]. Our patient's PET scan revealed bilateral parietotemporal

pathology, predominantly in the left side. This was consistent with the neuroimaging findings.

The majority of LPA cases show AD cerebrospinal fluid (CSF) biomarkers [7, 8]. CSF biomarkers were not yet available at the time of case reporting.

The histopathology of LPA is variable, but pathology of Alzheimer's disease is the most common finding. In the series reported in 2008 by Josephs and coinvestigators, all PPA patients whose pathology showed changes consistent with AD pathology belonged to the LPA group [9]. Other series found AD pathology in the majority of cases, including frontotemporal lobar dementia (FTLD) pathology, in about one-fifth of LPA phenotype [7, 8, 10, 11].

Our patient had very subtle findings that suggest very early AD-like mild visuospatial dysfunction and subtle cortical memory deficits. These findings predict AD-type pathology.

4. Conclusion

LPA is a rare neurodegenerative disorder that is closely related to Alzheimer's disease. The early symptoms are very subtle and require a high index of suspicion. Healthcare providers need to be aware of this entity and other entities that present with subtle cognitive abnormalities. Despite the lack of effective treatment, recruiting these patients to research is invaluable to help improve our understanding of the pathophysiology of the disease that should guide us one day to an effective treatment.

References

[1] M. M. Mesulam, "Slowly progressive aphasia without generalized dementia," *Annals of Neurology*, vol. 11, no. 6, pp. 592–598, 1982.

[2] P. Serieux, "On a case of pure verbal deafness," *Revue Medicale*, vol. 13, pp. 733–750, 1893.

[3] M. L. Gorno-Tempini, N. F. Dronkers, K. P. Rankin et al., "Cognition and amatomy in three variants of primary progressive aphasia," *Annals of Neurology*, vol. 55, no. 3, pp. 335–346, 2004.

[4] M. L. Gorno-Tempini, S. M. Brambati, V. Ginex et al., "The logopenic/phonological variant of primary progressive aphasia," *Neurology*, vol. 71, no. 16, pp. 1227–1234, 2008.

[5] M. Awad, J. E. Warren, S. K. Scott, F. E. Turkheimer, and R. J. S. Wise, "A common system for the comprehension and production of narrative speech," *Journal of Neuroscience*, vol. 27, no. 43, pp. 11455–11464, 2007.

[6] P. C.M. Wong, J. X. Jin, G. M. Gunasekera, R. Abel, E. R. Lee, and S. Dhar, "Aging and cortical mechanisms of speech perception in noise," *Neuropsychologia*, vol. 47, no. 3, pp. 693–703, 2009.

[7] M. Mesulam, A. Wicklund, N. Johnson et al., "Alzheimer and frontotemporal pathology in subsets of primary progressive aphasia," *Annals of Neurology*, vol. 63, no. 6, pp. 709–719, 2008.

[8] J. D. Rohrer, G. R. Ridgway, S. J. Crutch et al., "Progressive logopenic/phonological aphasia: erosion of the language network," *NeuroImage*, vol. 49, no. 1, pp. 984–993, 2010.

[9] K. A. Josephs, J. L. Whitwell, J. R. Duffy et al., "Progressive aphasia secondary to Alzheimer disease vs FTLD pathology," *Neurology*, vol. 70, no. 1, pp. 25–34, 2008.

[10] M. Grossman, S. X. Xie, D. J. Libon et al., "Longitudinal decline in autopsy-defined frontotemporal lobar degeneration," *Neurology*, vol. 70, no. 22, pp. 2036–2045, 2008.

[11] G. D. Rabinovici, W. J. Jagust, A. J. Furst et al., "Aβ amyloid and glucose metabolism in three variants of primary progressive aphasia," *Annals of Neurology*, vol. 64, no. 4, pp. 388–401, 2008.

5

Acute Onset of Hypersomnolence and Aphasia Secondary to an Artery of Percheron Infarct and a Proposed Emergency Room Evaluation

Tamra Ranasinghe ⓘ,[1] **SoHyun Boo,**[2] **and Amelia Adcock** ⓘ[1]

[1]Neurology Department, West Virginia University, USA
[2]Radiology Department, West Virginia University, USA

Correspondence should be addressed to Tamra Ranasinghe; tamrar@gmail.com

Academic Editor: Aristomenis K. Exadaktylos

Artery of Percheron (AOP) is a rare anatomical variant, which supplies bilateral paramedian thalami and the rostral mesencephalon via a single dominant thalamic perforating artery arising from the P1 segment of a posterior cerebral artery. AOP infarcts can present with a plethora of neurological symptoms: altered mental status, memory impairment, hypersomnolence, coma, aphasia, and vertical gaze palsy. Given the lack of classic stroke signs, majority of AOP infarcts are not diagnosed in the emergency setting. Timely diagnosis of an acute bilateral thalamic infarct can be challenging, and this case report highlights the uncommon neurological presentation of AOP infarction. The therapeutic time window to administer IV tPA can be missed due to this delay in diagnosis, resulting in poor clinical outcomes. To initiate appropriate acute ischemic stroke management, we propose a comprehensive radiological evaluation in the emergency room for patients with a high suspicion of an AOP infarction.

1. Introduction

Artery of Percheron (AOP) is a rare anatomical variant, which supplies bilateral paramedian thalami and the rostral mesencephalon via a single dominant thalamic perforating artery arising from the P1 segment of a Posterior Cerebral Artery (PCA) [1]. Percheron described three anatomic variations of the arterial supply to the paramedian thalamic-mesencephalic region [2]. Exact prevalence of AOP is unknown; it is estimated to be seen in 0.6% of cases of all ischemic strokes in an ischemic stroke registry of 2,750 [3]. Bilateral thalamic infarcts can present with a plethora of neurological symptom: altered mental status, memory impairment, hypersomnolence, coma, aphasia, and vertical gaze palsy [4–7].

Given the lack of classic stroke signs, majority of AOP infarcts are not diagnosed in the emergency setting. The diagnosis is usually made following a MRI brain scan, which is usually obtained outside the therapeutic window for IV tissue plasminogen activator (tPA) administration.

Timely diagnosis of an acute bilateral thalamic infarct can be challenging, and this case report highlights the noncommon neurological presentation of AOP infarction. We propose a comprehensive evaluation pathway which includes an extensive diagnostic radiological approach for patients with a high suspicion of an AOP infarction. The proposed evaluation pathway needs to conclude in the emergency department in a time sensitive manner.

2. Case Presentation

69-year-old female with no significant past medical history with the exception of anxiety presented as a transfer from an outside hospital with acute onset of hypersomnolence and aphasia. She was last seen normal the night before by her family. Her vitals on arrival were within normal limits; blood pressure was 134/64 mmHg, heart rate was 88 per minute, respiratory rate was of 22 breaths per minutes, and she was afebrile. On exam she appeared drowsy, nonverbal, and intermittently following one-step commands. Her cranial nerves

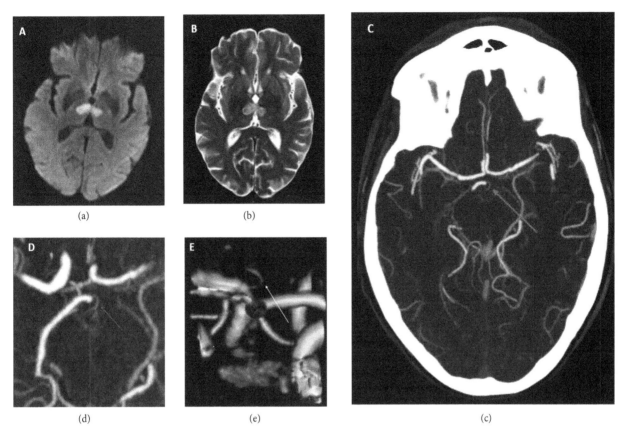

FIGURE 1: MRI brain diffusion weighted imaging series (a) and T2 (b) demonstrating bilateral paramedian thalamic infarcts. CTA vessel study. (c) Axial-Maximum Intensity Projection (MIP); (d) axial-3D-MIP; and (e) reconstructed 3D image demonstrates an Artery of Percheron (arrow) arising from the right Posterior Cerebral Artery P1 segment.

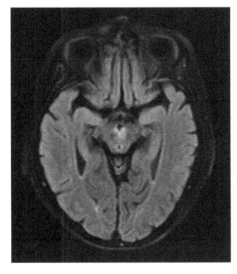

FIGURE 2: MRI brain with fluid attenuated inversion recovery (FLAIR) series demonstrating the "V sign" hyperintensity along the pial surface of the interpeduncular fossa in the midbrain.

were intact and on motor exam she had mild generalized weakness but was able to move all extremities against gravity. Sensory exam was confounded by her decreased mental status. Bilateral plantar reflexes were equivocal. National Institute of Health Stroke Scale (NIHSS) was 10. She was out of the 4.5-hour time window to consider IV thrombolysis therapy and on exam her presenting symptoms did not localize to one cerebral vascular territory.

Initial diagnostic work-up: serum white blood cell count 11000/uL, hemoglobin 14.2g/dL, platelets 190000/uL, sodium 143mmol/L, potassium 5.7mmol/ (repeat 4.4mmol/L), blood urea nitrogen 34mg/dL, creatinine 1.05mg/dL, glucose 323mg/dL, troponins <7ng/L, aspartate aminotransferase 46 U/L, and alanine aminotransferase 45 U/L. Urinary analysis was positive for moderate leukocytes and negative nitrites, and her toxicology screen was negative.

Noncontrasted CT brain demonstrated bilateral thalamic hypodensities. A CT angiogram (CTA) demonstrated focal areas of basilar artery narrowing, an Artery of Percheron (AOP) arising from the right PCA (Figures 1(c), 1(d), and 1(e)) and no large vessel occlusions. MRI brain demonstrated bilateral paramedian thalamic infarcts (Figures 1(a) and 1(b)) extending into the midbrain on diffusion weighted imaging (DWI). Her ejection fraction was 65% with no atrial septum shunt on transthoracic echocardiogram.

Her serum low density lipoprotein was 130mg/dL and her glycosylated hemoglobin was 13.8%. She was diagnosed with diabetes mellitus type 2. Her stroke etiology was thought to be secondary to small vessel disease given the arterial

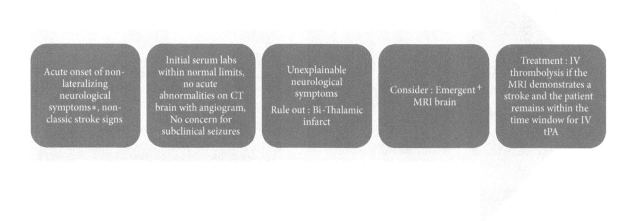

FIGURE 3: Proposed comprehensive radiological evaluation pathway to be completed in the Emergency Department. *Acute onset of any of the following symptoms: altered mental status, memory impairment, hypersomnolence, coma, aphasia, and vertical gaze palsy. +Emergent MRI brain without contrast with limited series of images to be done only if the patient is within the therapeutic window for thrombolysis (<4.5hrs since symptom onset).

bed involved and her uncovered lipohyalinosis risk factors. Patient was discharged on atorvastatin 40 mg, aspirin 81 mg, and an insulin regimen. On discharge to rehab her NIHSS improved to four.

3. Discussion

Vascular supply to the thalamus is described as anterior territory supplied by tuberothalamic (polar) artery, the paramedian territory supplied by the thalamosubthalamic (paramedian) artery, inferolateral territory supplied by thalamogeniculate (inferolateral) artery, and the posterior territory supplied by the posterior choroidal artery [8]. The exact supply to each territory can vary due to anatomical differences and the size of the adjacent vascular territories [9]. AOP is a rare anatomical variant, which supplies bilateral paramedian thalami and the rostral mesencephalon via a single dominant thalamic perforating artery arising from the P1 segment of a PCA.

Lazzaro N.A. et al. described four distinct patterns of AOP infarctions in their retrospective analysis of 37 patients with AOP infarcts [10]. They reported 43% with bilateral paramedian thalami with rostral midbrain, 38% with bilateral paramedian thalami without midbrain, 14% with bilateral paramedian and anterior thalami with midbrain, and 5% with bilateral paramedian and anterior thalami without midbrain infarctions. Further they described a "V-shaped hyperintensity" along the pial surface of the midbrain in the interpeduncular fossa on the axial fluid attenuated inversion recovery (FLAIR) and DWI images. The sensitivity of the "V sign" in their study group was 67% in patients with midbrain involvement. In our patient with the AOP infarction, bilateral paramedian thalami with rostral midbrain was affected with a positive "V sign" (Figure 2) seen on MRI brain FLAIR series.

The AOP is rarely visualized with conventional cerebral angiogram and only four authors have successfully demonstrated this variant on conventional cerebral angiogram [10]. Therefore conventional cerebral angiograms should not be used routinely to diagnose Percheron artery occlusion. AOP is thought to be too small to be visualized on computed tomography (CT) angiogram. However, we report a very rare instance where AOP was visualized on CT angiogram (Figures 1(c), 1(d), and 1(e)).

It is vital to consider bilateral thalamic infarctions in the differential diagnosis when evaluating patients with acute onset of vague nonlateralizing neurological symptoms such as altered mental status, memory impairments, hypersomnolence, coma, aphasia, and oculomotor disturbances. A basilar tip occlusion, venous occlusion, intracranial hemorrhage, expanding subdural hematomas, subclinical seizures, Wernicke encephalopathy, neoplasms, infections, and toxic, metabolic, and inflammatory causes should be also considered in the differential diagnosis.

When a patient with nonlateralizing acute neurological symptoms presents to the emergency department, a CT brain and a CTA with perfusions should be considered with the initial blood and urine test. If the severity of the clinical features does not correlate with the CT brain findings (no acute intracranial abnormalities including hemorrhage) and the initial metabolic, toxic, and infectious work-up is negative, a bithalamic infarction should be high on the differential diagnosis. AOP infarcts are often missed on the initial CT brain scan.

In such patients, we propose a comprehensive evaluation pathway (Figure 3) to be completed in emergency room. This includes a CTA with perfusions and an emergent MRI brain scan if the patient is within the therapeutic time window for thrombolysis (<4.5 hours of from symptom onset). The emergent noncontrasted MRI brain scan should be limited to DWI, apparent diffusion coefficient (ADC) and gradient echo sequences (GRE) series. Given the limited series, MRI brain scan should be completed in a time sensitive manner ~15-20 minutes. If the MRI brain is positive, implying acute ischemia and the patient remains within the therapeutic window for thrombolysis, IV tPA should be administered. Maintaining a high suspicion for thalamic infarct, with AOP occlusion as one etiology, and a low threshold for MRI in patients presenting acutely with otherwise unexplainable neurological symptoms may facilitate diagnosis and decrease morbidity [9].

However, it is essential to keep in mind the low risk of complications including symptomatic intracranial hemorrhage in stroke mimics receiving IV tPA [11, 12]. Hence, if there is a high suspicion of an acute ischemic stroke, CT brain is negative for hemorrhage, and the initial work-up is not suggestive of an alternate diagnosis, thrombolysis with IV tPA should not be delayed to conduct further imaging.

4. Conclusion

Thalamic pathology should be considered in patients with vague nonlateralizing neurological symptoms. Diagnosis of Percheron artery infarction is challenging and often made later in presentation due to lack of clinical awareness and the nonclassic stroke signs/symptoms on presentation. The therapeutic time window to administer IV tPA can be missed due to this delay in diagnosis, resulting in poor clinical outcomes. To initiate appropriate acute ischemic stroke management, we propose a comprehensive radiological evaluation in the emergency room for patients with a high suspicion of an AOP infarction.

References

[1] G. Percheron, "The anatomy of the arterial supply of the human thalamus and its use for the interpretation of the thalamic vascular pathology," *Zeitschrift für Neurologie*, vol. 205, no. 1, pp. 1–13, 1973.

[2] Percheron G., "Les artères du thalamus humain. II. Artères et territoires thalamiques paramédians de l'artère basilaire communicante," *Revue Neurologique*, vol. 132, pp. 309–324, 1976.

[3] E. Kumral, D. Evyapan, K. Balkir, and S. Kutluhan, "Bilateral thalamic infarction. Clinical, etiological and MRI correlates," *Acta Neurologica Scandinavica*, vol. 103, no. 1, pp. 35–42, 2001.

[4] J. Bogousslavsky, F. Regli, and A. Uske, "Thalamic infarcts: clinical syndromes, etiology, and prognosis," *Neurology*, vol. 38, no. 6, pp. 837–848, 1988.

[5] X. Y. Chen, Q. Wang, X. Wang, and K. S. Wong, "Clinical Features of Thalamic Stroke," *Current Treatment Options in Neurology*, vol. 19, no. 2, 2017.

[6] N. Zappella, S. Merceron, C. Nifle et al., "Artery of percheron infarction as an unusual cause of coma: three cases and literature review," *Neurocritical Care*, vol. 20, no. 3, pp. 494–501, 2014.

[7] N. Morparia, G. Miller, A. Rabinstein, G. Lanzino, and N. Kumar, "Cognitive decline and hypersomnolence: Thalamic manifestations of a tentorial dural arteriovenous fistula (dAVF)," *Neurocritical Care*, vol. 17, no. 3, pp. 429–433, 2012.

[8] E. Carrera, P. Michel, and J. Bogousslavsky, "Anteromedian, central, and posterolateral infarcts of the thalamus: three variant types," *Stroke*, vol. 35, no. 12, pp. 2826–2831, 2004.

[9] J. L. Khanni, J. A. Casale, A. Y. Koek, P. H. Espinosa del Pozo, and P. S. Espinosa, "Artery of percheron infarct: an acute diagnostic challenge with a spectrum of clinical presentations," *Cureus*, vol. 10, no. 9, article no e3276, 2018.

[10] N. A. Lazzaro, B. Wright, M. Castillo et al., "Artery of percheron infarction: imaging patterns and clinical spectrum," *American Journal of Neuroradiology*, vol. 31, no. 7, pp. 1283–1289, 2010.

[11] G. Tsivgoulis, R. Zand, A. H. Katsanos et al., "Safety of intravenous thrombolysis in stroke mimics: prospective 5-year study and comprehensive meta-analysis," *Stroke*, vol. 46, no. 5, pp. 1281–1287, 2015.

[12] S. M. Zinkstok, S. T. Engelter, H. Gensicke et al., "Safety of Thrombolysis in Stroke Mimics," *Stroke*, vol. 44, no. 4, pp. 1080–1084, 2013.

6

Regional Alteration within the Cerebellum and the Reorganization of the Cerebrocerebellar System following Poststroke Aphasia

Xiaotong Zhang ⓘ,[1] Zhaocong Chen ⓘ,[1] Na Li,[1] Jingfeng Liang,[1] Yan Zou,[2] Huixiang Wu,[1] Zhuang Kang,[2] Zulin Dou,[1] and Weihong Qiu ⓘ[1]

[1]Department of Rehabilitation Medicine, The Third Affiliated Hospital of Sun Yat-sen University, Guangzhou, Guangdong Province, China
[2]Department of Radiology, The Third Affiliated Hospital of Sun Yat-sen University, Guangzhou, Guangdong Province, China

Correspondence should be addressed to Weihong Qiu; q-weihong@163.com

Xiaotong Zhang and Zhaocong Chen contributed equally to this work.

Academic Editor: Carlo Cavaliere

Recently, an increasing number of studies have highlighted the role of the cerebellum in language processing. However, the role of neural reorganization within the cerebellum as well as within the cerebrocerebellar system caused by poststroke aphasia remains unknown. To solve this problem, in the present study, we investigated regional alterations of the cerebellum as well as the functional reorganization of the cerebrocerebellar circuit by combining structural and resting-state functional magnetic resonance imaging (fMRI) techniques. Twenty patients diagnosed with aphasia following left-hemispheric stroke and 20 age-matched healthy controls (HCs) were recruited in this study. The Western Aphasia Battery (WAB) test was used to assess the participants' language ability. Gray matter volume, spontaneous brain activity, functional connectivity, and effective connectivity were examined in each participant. We discovered that gray matter volumes in right cerebellar lobule VI and right Crus I were significantly lower in the patient group, and the brain activity within these regions was significantly correlated with WAB scores. We also discovered decreased functional connectivity within the crossed cerebrocerebellar circuit, which was significantly correlated with WAB scores. Moreover, altered information flow between the cerebellum and the contralateral cerebrum was found. Together, our findings provide evidence for regional alterations within the cerebellum and the reorganization of the cerebrocerebellar system following poststroke aphasia and highlight the important role of the cerebellum in language processing within aphasic individuals after stroke.

1. Introduction

Aphasia is one of the common complications among individuals after left-hemispheric stroke, and it has been reported that approximately 40% of survivors from left-hemispheric stroke are diagnosed with aphasia [1]. Patients with poststroke aphasia (PSA) have multiple aspects of language impairments, including naming, comprehension, and spontaneous speaking. Because patients with PSA mainly have difficulty communicating with others, it is difficult for them to function in society, thus decreasing the quality of life of patients and financially burdening society [2, 3]. For such reasons, investigating the disease-specific mechanism following PSA is important because it helps improve the present understanding of the language process after stroke and refine the therapeutic strategy for aphasia treatment. Although reorganization of the language network within the cerebral cortex after PSA has been widely studied in recent years [4, 5], few studies currently focus on the reorganization of the cerebrocerebellar system within aphasic individuals, while accumulating evidence hints at the potential role of the cerebellum in language processing.

The concept of a "linguistic cerebellum" is currently drawing attention. On the one hand, patients with cerebellar impairments have shown different aspects of cognitive impairments, including language processing. It has been discovered that patients with resected right cerebellar tumors and individuals who survive right cerebellar infractions tend to show linguistic problems [6]. Among adolescents diagnosed with autism spectrum disorder, decreased activations within the cerebellum during language tasks were found. Also, these patients exhibited reduced functional connectivity between right Crus I and distributed supratentorial language areas [7, 8]. Jeong et al. also found that microstructural impairment of the cerebrocerebellar circuit may be relative to communication problems [9]. On the other hand, studies based on task-based functional magnetic resonance imaging (fMRI) revealed that the cerebellum participated in different aspects of language processing [10–13], and the activation areas during language tasks were mainly located in right Crus I/Crus II, lobule VI, and midline lobule VIIAt, which are characteristic areas of right lateralization [14]. Diffusion imaging analysis also found structural connections linking the supratentorial language areas and the cerebellum [15, 16], and the structural frontal-cerebellar loop might contribute to verbal working memory [17]. Such findings indicated that the cerebellum plays a role in language processing via informative interaction through the cerebrocerebellar circuits, and it is believed that considering the cerebellum when constructing the language network will make the network more accurate [18]. However, whether regional alterations within the cerebellum and functional reorganization of cerebrocerebellar circuits occur within aphasic individuals after stroke remains unknown.

Motivated by the evidence and the limitations mentioned above, in this study, we used structural and resting-state functional magnetic resonance imaging (fMRI) to investigate the structural and functional alterations within the cerebellum and to explore the functional reorganization of the cerebrocerebellar system among patients with aphasia after left-hemispheric stroke. First, voxel-based morphometry (VBM) analysis was used to explore the structural alterations of gray matter volume (GMV) within the cerebellum, accompanied by the calculation of regional spontaneous brain activity by using the amplitude of low-frequency fluctuation (ALFF) as an indicator. Second, regions with significant differences in the VBM analysis were used as regions of interest (ROIs) in the following functional connectivity (FC) analysis with the goal of exploring aberrant FC in the cerebrocerebellar system. Additionally, the Granger causality analysis (GCA) was used to study alterations in effective connectivity (EC) within the cerebrocerebellar circuit. We considered that GCA could be used to recognize changes in the directionality of information flow [19] and thus provide comprehensive evidence for functional reorganization of the cerebrocerebellar system following PSA. We hypothe-

sized that PSA would not only cause changes in regional structure and neural activity in cerebellar language-related areas but also result in functional reorganization within the cerebrocerebellar language system.

2. Methods

2.1. Subjects. Patients who were diagnosed with aphasia after left-hemispheric stroke at the rehabilitation department of the 3rd Affiliated Hospital of Sun Yat-sen University Guangzhou city, China, as well as age- and sex-matched healthy controls (HCs), were recruited for this study. The diagnosis of aphasia was based on the language test criteria from the Chinese version of the Western Aphasia Battery (WAB); patients recruited in this study were native Chinese speakers and had normal language function before stroke. To eliminate heterogeneity, patients with bilateral hemispheric stroke or who had a history of other cerebrovascular or mental diseases were excluded from this study. To ensure the safety of MRI scanning, participants with MRI contraindications were also excluded.

2.2. Language Assessment. Before undergoing MRI scans, each patient's language severity was assessed by the same professional language therapist using the WAB. WAB scores include aphasia quotient (AQ), representing the overall severity of language impairment, and four subtypes, including naming, repetition, comprehension, and spontaneous speech.

2.3. MRI Acquisition. All the participants recruited in the present study underwent MRI scanning with a GE 3.0-Tesla scanner (General Electric Company, USA) in the radiology department of the 3rd Affiliated Hospital of Sun Yat-sen University. rs-fMRI data were first acquired with the gradient-echo EPI sequence: repetition time (TR) = 2000 ms, echo time (TE) = 35 ms, flip angle = 90°, thickness = 4 mm, slice number = 35, field of view = 240 × 240 mm^2, 3.75 mm × 3.75 mm in-plane resolution, and 243 time points for a total of 486 s. During scanning, participants were informed to fixate on the black cross presented on the screen against a white background and avoid thinking of anything. Structural MRI data were acquired with a high-resolution, axial magnetization-prepared rapid gradient echo (MPRAGE) T1-weighted sequence: TR = 8200 ms, TE = 3.2 ms, flip angle = 90°, field of view (FOV) = 256 × 256 mm, slice thickness = 1.2 mm, and voxel size = 1 × 1 × 1 mm^3. Foam paddings were placed inside the head coil to reduce head motion, and earplugs were also used for noise reduction.

2.4. Data Preprocessing. For VBM processing, structural images were processed with the use of the CAT12 toolbox (CAT12 Version 12.6; http://dbm.neuro.uni-jena.de/cat/), which was implemented in SPM12 (SPM12; http://www.fil.ion.ucl.ac.uk/spm/software/spm12/) running in the MATLAB 2020a environment. All T1 images were first manually quality checked by the researchers followed by bias-field inhomogeneities correction. Then, the individual T1 images were segmented into three tissue components, including gray matter (GM), white matter (WM), and cerebrospinal fluid (CSF), using tissue probability maps (TPMs). Total intracranial volume (TIV) was also calculated by adding total GM, WM, and CSF volumes. Afterward, native-space tissue segments were registered to the standard Montreal Neurological Institute (MNI) template by using the DARTEL algorithm. The normalized GM images were subsequently modulated to preserve the original tissue volumes in each voxel and then smoothed with a 6 mm Gaussian kernel with a full width at half maximum (FWHM).

rs-fMRI images were processed with the use of the RESTplus toolbox (RESTplus v1.24; http://restfmri.net/forum/restplus) and SPM12 within the MATLAB 2020a environment. The first 10 time points were excluded to eliminate the influence of participants' adaptation to the scanning noise, followed by slice timing and realignment for the correction of head motion. Before the following spatial normalization, any participant who had maximum translation larger than 3.0 mm or maximum rotation larger than 3.0 degrees was excluded from the rs-fMRI analysis. Spatial normalization was then performed so that the individual images would be standardized into MNI space. After these procedures, functional images were then smoothed with a 6 mm FWHM Gaussian kernel. The linear trend of the time series was removed, and the nuisance signal (Friston's 24 head motion) was regressed out.

2.5. GMV Analysis. To explore the alteration of GMV within the cerebellum, an independent two-sample *t* test was used for voxelwise group comparisons with the use of the spatially unbiased infratentorial template (SUIT, http://www.diedrichsenlab.org/imaging/suit_download.htm), which is a spatially unbiased template of the human cerebellum [20], and age and TIV were used as covariates. The Gaussian random-field (GRF) correction (voxel level: $p < 0.001$, cluster level: $p < 0.05$) was used for multiple comparison correction, and we considered $p < 0.05$ statistically significant. The MNI coordinates of the peak *t*-value from regions with significant differences between groups were then extracted as the center of ROI for the following analysis. The radius of each ROI was 6 mm.

2.6. rs-fMRI Analysis

2.6.1. Cerebellar ALFF Analysis. Regional ALFF was analyzed to study the regional spontaneous neural activity within the regions with significant GMV differences in participants in the patient group. The whole-brain ALFF map of each individual was first calculated. To improve the normality of the data, each individual mean ALFF (mALFF) map was calculated by dividing the ALFF of each voxel by the global average value. The regional mALFF value of each participant was then extracted within each spherical ROI.

2.6.2. Cerebrocerebellar FC Analysis. A seed-based FC analysis was used to analyze FC alterations in the cerebrocerebellar circuit. The average time series of each ROI was extracted, followed by the calculation of the Pearson correlation coefficients between the time series of the ROI and every other voxel within the whole brain. The FC map of each subject was then standardized to a zFC map with Fisher's *r*-to-*z* transformation to improve normality.

2.6.3. GCA. GCA has been thought to be a useful method to investigate EC among discrete regions without prior knowledge [21]. In the theory of GCA, if the past time series of *X* and *Y* predict the current time series of *X* more accurately than the past *X* time series itself, then *Y* has a "causal influence" on *X*, and vice versa [22]. In the present study, we defined the time series of the ROI as the time series of *X* and the time series of each other voxel within the whole brain as the time series of *Y*. The definition of ROIs was the same as the FC analysis. Voxelwise, coefficient-based GCA was performed with the use of the RESTplus toolbox, and the EC map of each individual was created, followed by Fisher's *z* transformation (zGC) to improve normality.

2.7. Statistical Analysis. We used the RESTplus package, mentioned previously, for the statistical analysis of GMV, zFC, and zGC data. For the zFC and zGC data, an independent two-sample *t* test was used for voxelwise group comparisons within the whole brain. We used the GRF correction (voxel level: $p < 0.001$, cluster level: $p < 0.05$) for multiple comparison correction, and $p < 0.05$ was considered statistically significant.

Demographic and regional mALFF data analysis was performed with the IBM SPSS statistics 26. The Shapiro-Wilk test was used to evaluate the normality. For continuous variables, if the data were normally distributed, an independent two-sample test was used to evaluate the difference between groups; otherwise, the Mann–Whitney *U* test was used. For the classified variables, Fisher's precision probability test was used to assess between-group differences. Spearman's correlation analysis was also used to explore the correlation between WAB scores and values of mALFF values, between WAB scores and zFC values, and between WAB scores and zGC values. We considered $p < 0.05$ to indicate statistical significance.

3. Results

3.1. Demographic Data and Language Performance. We finally recruited 20 PSA patients and 20 HCs in the present study. There was no significant difference between age, sex, or education years, and detailed information is shown in Table 1. The lesion overlap of the recruited patients is shown in Figure 1.

3.2. Cerebellar GMV Alteration. The VBM analysis showed that the GMV of two clusters in the right cerebellum, centering at right cerebellum Crus I (rCrus I) and lobule VI (rLobule VI), of patients was significantly lower than that of HCs. (Table 2, Figure 2). The MNI coordinates of the peak *t*-value from regions with significant differences between groups were then extracted as the center of ROI for the following analysis. The radius of each ROI was 6 mm (Figure 3).

3.3. The Results of rs-fMRI Analysis. Two patients were excluded from the rs-fMRI study for head motion, leaving 18 patients in the following re-fMRI analysis.

TABLE 1: Demographic data and language performance.

	Patient group (n = 20)	Control group (n = 20)	p
Age	49.60 ± 9.30	52.05 ± 5.98	0.328
Sex (male/female)	18/2	16/4	0.661
Education (years)	12.10 ± 1.62	12.30 ± 1.84	0.717
Time from stroke (days)	65.25 ± 37.17	NA	NA
AQ	31.20 (31.95)	NA	NA
Naming	11.00 (20.75)	NA	NA
Repetition	37.00 (51.75)	NA	NA
Comprehension	98.00 (49.50)	NA	NA
Spontaneous speech	4.00 (6.50)	NA	NA

Data are presented as the mean ± standard deviation if the variables were normally distributed or presented as the median value (interquartile range) if the variables were the non-normally distributed. NA: not available. AQ: aphasia quotient.

3.3.1. ALFF Result. There was no significant difference in ALFF values within ROIs between participants in the two groups. Correlative analysis revealed that the ALFF value in rCrus I was negatively correlated with comprehension scores in individuals in the patient group (Table 3, Figure 4).

3.3.2. Results of Seed-Based FC Analysis. Aphasic individuals showed significantly lower FC between rCrus I and the left precentral gyrus (lPreCG) as well as between rLobule VI and the lPreCG than participants in the HC group (Table 4, Figure 5). Correlation analysis revealed that reduced FC between rCrus I and the lPreCG was significantly correlated with AQ ($r = -0.480$, $p = 0.044$) and comprehension ($r = -0.677$, $p = 0.002$) scores. In addition, a negative correlation between comprehension scores and FC between rLobule VI and the lPreCG was observed ($r = -0.520$, $p = 0.027$) (see Figure 6).

3.3.3. The Results of GCA. The results of voxelwise GCA are shown in Table 5 and Figure 7. Compared with participants in the HC group, patients with PSA demonstrated decreased EC from rCrus I to the left postcentral gyrus (lPostCG) and from rLobule VI to the left supramarginal gyrus (lSMG). Additionally, the left inferior frontal gyrus pars triangularis (lIFGtri) illustrated a higher causal influence on the rCrus I; also, the lSMG demonstrated an increased causal influence on rLobuleVI among aphasic individuals.

4. Discussion

In the present study, we investigated structural and functional alterations within the cerebellum, as well as functional reorganization of the cerebrocerebellar system following aphasia caused by left-hemispheric stroke. Our results demonstrated that among aphasia patients after stroke, GMVs in rCrus I and rLobule VI were significantly lower than those in HCs, while there was no significant difference in ALFF values of those two regions between individuals in the two groups. FC analysis revealed reduced FC between rCrus I

and the lPreCG as well as between rLobule VI and the lPreCG. In addition, there was enhanced EC from rCrus I to the lPostCG as well as from the lSMG to rLobule VI, whereas EC from the lIFGtri to rCrus I and from rLobuleVI to the lSMG was decreased. Moreover, FC and ALFF values are negatively correlated with WAB scores. To our knowledge, this is the first study to explore structural and functional reorganization of the cerebellum in addition to the reorganization of functional cerebrocerebellar circuits following PSA.

4.1. Structural and Functional Alterations within the Cerebellum. Changes in regional GMVs were demonstrated subsequent to aphasia after stroke. This phenomenon may be the result of the extension of anatomical lesions from the supratentorial area, as previous studies indicated that regions distant from the anatomical lesion tend to show structural alterations if these regions were in the same network [23, 24]. An increasing number of studies have confirmed that rLobule VI and rCrus I are activated during variations in language performance, suggesting that these two regions are part of the language network and play an important role in normal language processing. Accompanied by correlation findings from the present study, demonstrating that the value of ALFF in rCrus I were negatively correlated with language performance, we verified the participation of the cerebellum in language processing in aphasic individuals. Another explanation of the structural damage in the cerebellum may be caused by crossed cerebellar diaschisis (CCD). CCD is the phenomenon of decreased blood flow and metabolism within the contralateral cerebellum after supratentorial structural impairment and can be commonly recognized [25–27]. It has been reported that patients diagnosed with CCD often show cerebellar hypofunction with an intact cortical structure [24, 28], but some patients in the chronic stage may further experience cerebellar atrophy [29, 30]. However, although cerebellar atrophy was demonstrated in participants in the patient group, we did not find a decrease in ALFF values, which is one of the indicators of regional spontaneous neural activity, in these atrophic regions compared with HCs. Considering that the calculation of the ALFF value of each ROI is the average value within the region, the significant difference may be offset by the decreased GMV in the resulting regions. Moreover, the patients recruited in our study were mainly subacute aphasic patients whose GMV of the cerebellar cortex might be more likely to decrease after long-term hypometabolism; thus, we assumed that regional ALFF reductions in rCrus I and rLobule VI might be recognized if the aphasic individuals were in the acute stage after stroke.

4.2. Changes of Cerebrocerebellar FC. Reduced FC between rCrus I and the lPreCG, as well as between rLobule VI and the lPreCG, was observed in our study. The precentral gyrus, which is part of the dorsal stream in the language network, plays a role in mapping sound to meaning in the language process [31] and is thought to be related to phonological processing. It has been reported that patients with impairment of the precentral gyrus show inability in phonological

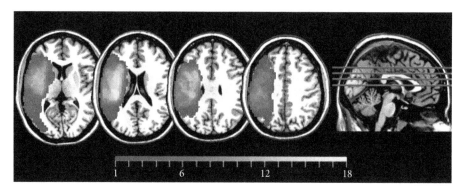

FIGURE 1: Lesion overlap of 20 PSA patients. The color bar represents the number of patients with a lesion in a specific voxel (maximum 18 out of 20).

TABLE 2: Between-group differences in VBM analysis (patient>control).

Area	Peak MNI coordinates			Voxel size	Peak t-value
	x	y	z		
rCrus I	36	-67.5	-36	813	-4.890
rLobule VI	22.5	-69	-22.5	1213	-5.195

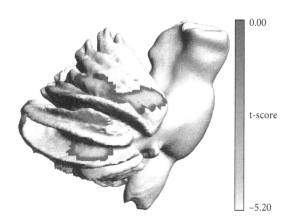

FIGURE 2: Resulting clusters of VBM analysis.

judgment [32]; in addition, activation of the precentral gyrus during phonological tasks is well recognized among healthy individuals [33, 34]. Moreover, elderly individuals with hearing loss showed activation of several areas, including the precentral gyrus, when encountering complex sentences [35], suggesting that functional activity of the precentral gyrus is important in language processing when individuals already have impaired language ability. Combining accumulating evidence of the precentral gyrus in phonology and the notion that the frontal-cerebellar circuit is crucial in language processing, we assumed that the cerebrocerebellar circuits of rCrus I-lPreCG and rLobule VI-lPreCG are parts of the phonological network and influence language performance in aphasic individuals. Phonological processing is the procedure that understands spoken words by using language sounds [34, 36]. Our correlation analysis results showed that the FC between rCrus I and the lPreCG was

negatively correlated with comprehension scores in the patient group, further verifying our assumption.

4.3. GCA. In the present study, aberrant EC between the cerebellum and language-related areas was also found, indicating the alteration of information flow within the cerebrocerebellar system following stroke. The inferior frontal gyrus (IFG) is considered the hub of the language network as it has a role in both phonologic and semantic processes. Studies based on lesion-symptom mapping (LSM) revealed that damage to the supramarginal gyrus and the postcentral gyrus among poststroke individuals is related to phonological deficits in single-word production [37–39]. A task-based fMRI study revealed that both regions participate in picture naming tasks among healthy individuals [40]. In general, these two areas together are thought to contribute to fluent speech production by phonetic-articulatory planning [41]. The postcentral gyrus, as a part of the sensorimotor system, also contributes to semantic processing, particularly action-related words [42]. In addition, an impaired structural connection between the postcentral gyrus and language-related areas due to the influence of a stroke on language performance [43] indicated the potential role of the postcentral gyrus in language processing.

Previous studies discovered that the severity of speech apraxia among patients was related to the degree of impairment of the supramarginal gyrus and the postcentral gyrus. Interestingly, in some cases, patients with only cerebellar damage showed similar symptoms of apraxia, suggesting that the disruption of the cerebrocerebellar circuit may cause the same outcome. Associative diffusion MRI analyses revealed that there are contralateral interconnections between the cerebellum and the cerebral cortex via the thalamus [16], and the dentate nucleus is structurally connected to various areas in the contralateral frontal lobe [15]. Such evidence may be the basis of information interplay between the cerebrum and the cerebellum in language processing. In the theory of cerebellar internal models, the cerebellum plays a role in motor speech planning by transmitting predictions on coming linguistic information and modifying speech execution if needed [44]. Through the dense structural connectivity between the cerebrum and the cerebellum, the linguistic cerebellum receives information from the

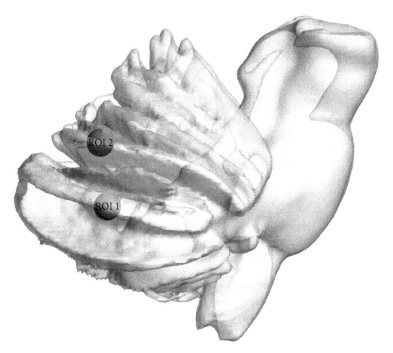

FIGURE 3: The MNI coordinates of the peak t-value from regions with significant between-group differences in VBM analysis were extracted as the center of ROI. ROI 1 (36, -67.5, and -36): rCrus I; ROI 2 (22.5, -69, and -22.5): rLobule VI.

TABLE 3: Between-group differences in ALFF within ROI 1 (rCrus I) and ROI 2 (rLobule VI).

	Patient group ($n = 18$)	Control group ($n = 20$)	p
ROI 1: rCrus I	0.760 ± 0.195	0.773 ± 0.127	0.805
ROI 2: rLobule VI	1.150 ± 0.385	1.226 ± 0.295	0.493

Data are presented as the mean ± standard deviation.

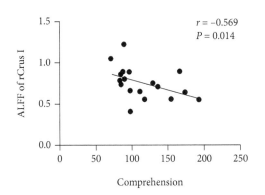

FIGURE 4: Correlation analysis between ALFF values of rCrus I and comprehension scores ($r = -0.569$, $p = 0.014$).

frontotemporal area during speech production [45] and conveys predictive information to the prefrontal cortex to ensure accurate actual expression [46]. DCM is an alternative way to analyze the EC between regions; with the use of DCM, Sobczak found that the EC from lIFG to the pons and subsequently to the right superior cerebellum (rLobule VI/ rCrus I) might contribute to verbal working tasks among healthy individuals [17]. They assumed that the right superior cerebellum might serve a role in the predictive mechanism [17]. Here, in the GCA results, we discovered that patients with aphasia had alterations in information flow both in the input and output stages within the internal model. We assumed that the decreased EC from the supratentorial area to the cerebellum might reflect the specific disease mechanism following PSA. When language-related areas, such as the IFG and supramarginal gyrus (SMG), are damaged, the information flow to the contralateral cerebellum might be subsequently reduced and might affect the information input to the cerebellar internal model and thus affect the expression of patients with aphasia. Furthermore, the increased EC from the cerebellum to the supratentorial areas might indicate compensation for the decreased informative interplay caused by a stroke and help individuals with language recovery. Consistent with our hypothesis, a study of the cerebellum as a neuromodulation target demonstrated that anodal tDCS to rCrus I helps language performance and increases FC between the cerebellum and the language hub [18, 47]. However, we noticed that cathodal tDCS to the right cerebellum also helped language recovery in some studies. The exact effect of tDCS intervention on the right cerebellum on the recovery of language in individuals with aphasia after stroke and the underlying mechanism of this effect are still worth exploring.

4.4. Limitation. There were limitations in the present study. First, this was an observational study with a relatively small sample, and it might be helpful to fully understand the specific mechanism within the cerebrocerebellar system after PSA with an enlarged sample size. Second, although the

TABLE 4: Regions with significant between-group differences in seed-based FC analysis (patient>control).

Seed	Region	Voxel size	Peak MNI			Peak t-value
			x	y	z	
ROI 1: rCrus I	lPreCG	75	-51	9	33	-5.295
ROI 2: rLobule VI	lPreCG	317	-54	0	27	-5.723

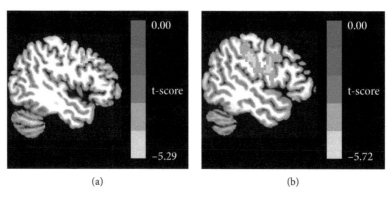

(a)   (b)

FIGURE 5: With the use of ROI 1 and ROI 2 as the seed in seed-based FC analysis separately, the result showed decreased FC (a) between the rCrus I and the lPreCG, as well as (b) between the rLobule VI and the lPreCG.

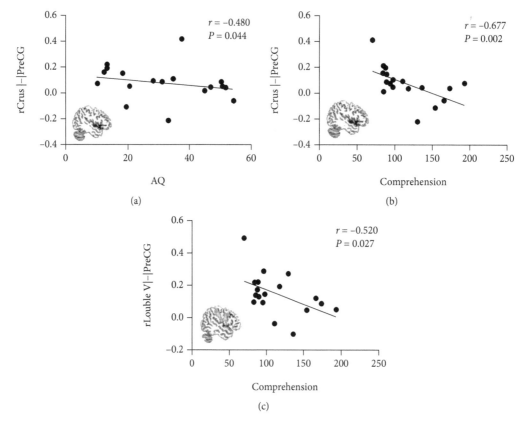

FIGURE 6: (a) Negative correlation between rCrus I-lPreCG and AQ scores ($r = -0.480$, $p = 0.044$). (b) Negative correlation between rCrus I-lPreCG and comprehension scores ($r = -0.677$, $p = 0.002$). (c) Negative correlation between rLobule VI-lPreCG and comprehension scores ($r = -0.520$, $p = 0.027$).

results of the study presented here showed functional reorganization within the cerebrocerebellar system after PSA, we did not explore the microstructural integrity of WM fibers between these areas. Notably, diffusion MRI is a useful technique that could be used to solve this problem and could be employed in future studies.

TABLE 5: Regions with significant between-group differences in GCA (patient>control).

		Region	Voxel size	Peak MNI x	y	z	Peak t-value
ROI 1: rCrus I	X2Y	lPostCG	1579	-63	-6	21	6.193
	Y2X	lIFGtri	646	-42	30	9	-7.387
ROI 2: rLobuleVI	X2Y	lSMG	204	-60	-24	15	5.692
	Y2X	lSMG	81	-54	-24	24	-5.185

X2Y: the causal outflow from the ROI (X) to the rest of the whole brain (Y); Y2X: the causal inflow to the ROI (X) from the rest of the whole brain (Y).

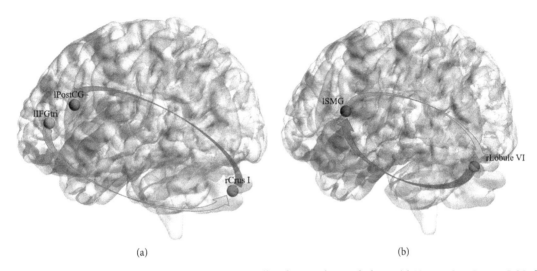

(a)   (b)

FIGURE 7: Aberrant effective connectivity from and to rCrus I as well as from and to rLobule VI. (a) Using rCrus I as an ROI, decreased EC from the lIFGtri to rCrus I and increased EC from rCrus I to the lPostCG were found. (b) Using rLobule VI as an ROI, decreased EC from the lSMG to rLobule and increased EC from rLobule VI to the lSMG were found.

5. Conclusion

To our knowledge, this is the first article to explore neural reorganization within the cerebellum subsequent to PSA both from regional and integrative viewpoints. We discovered that PSA not only causes reduced matter volumes in right cerebellar lobule VI and Crus I but also induces aberrant functional connectivity as well as effective connectivity between the cerebellum and the supratentorial language-related areas. Together, this study may provide a new perspective to understand the reorganization of the cerebellum following aphasia caused by supratentorial lesion.

Acknowledgments

This study was supported by grants from the National Natural Science Foundation of China (No. 81401869), the National Key Research and Development Program (No. 2020YFC2004201), and the Natural Science Foundation of Guangdong Province (No. 2016A030313327).

References

[1] S. T. Engelter, M. Gostynski, S. Papa et al., "Epidemiology of aphasia attributable to first ischemic stroke: incidence, severity, fluency, etiology, and thrombolysis," *Stroke*, vol. 37, no. 6, pp. 1379–1384, 2006.

[2] R. H. Hamilton, "Neuroplasticity in the language system: reorganization in post-stroke aphasia and in neuromodulation interventions," *Restorative Neurology and Neuroscience*, vol. 34, no. 4, pp. 467–471, 2016.

[3] W. H. Qiu, H. X. Wu, Q. L. Yang et al., "Evidence of cortical reorganization of language networks after stroke with subacute Broca's aphasia: a blood oxygenation level dependent-functional magnetic resonance imaging study," *Neural Regeneration Research*, vol. 12, no. 1, pp. 109–117, 2017.

[4] S. Xing, E. H. Lacey, L. M. Skipper-Kallal et al., "Right hemisphere grey matter structure and language outcomes in chronic left hemisphere stroke," *Brain*, vol. 139, Part 1, pp. 227–241, 2016.

[5] J. D. Stefaniak, A. D. Halai, and M. A. Lambon Ralph, "The neural and neurocomputational bases of recovery from post-stroke aphasia," *Nature Reviews. Neurology*, vol. 16, no. 1, pp. 43–55, 2020.

[6] D. Riva and C. Giorgi, "The cerebellum contributes to higher functions during development: evidence from a series of children surgically treated for posterior fossa tumours," *Brain*, vol. 123, no. 5, pp. 1051–1061, 2000.

[7] S. M. Hodge, N. Makris, D. N. Kennedy et al., "Cerebellum, language, and cognition in autism and specific language impairment," *Journal of Autism and Developmental Disorders*, vol. 40, no. 3, pp. 300–316, 2010.

[8] A. M. D'Mello and C. J. Stoodley, "Cerebro-cerebellar circuits in autism spectrum disorder," *Frontiers in Neuroscience*, vol. 9, p. 408, 2015.

[9] J. W. Jeong, D. C. Chugani, M. E. Behen, V. N. Tiwari, and H. T. Chugani, "Altered white matter structure of the dentatorubrothalamic pathway in children with autistic spectrum disorders," *Cerebellum*, vol. 11, no. 4, pp. 957–971, 2012.

[10] M. Frings, A. Dimitrova, C. F. Schorn et al., "Cerebellar involvement in verb generation: an fMRI study," *Neuroscience Letters*, vol. 409, no. 1, pp. 19–23, 2006.

[11] J. G. Ojemann, R. L. Buckner, E. Akbudak et al., "Functional MRI studies of word-stem completion: reliability across laboratories and comparison to blood flow imaging with PET," *Human Brain Mapping*, vol. 6, no. 4, pp. 203–215, 1998.

[12] C. J. Stoodley, E. M. Valera, and J. D. Schmahmann, "Functional topography of the cerebellum for motor and cognitive tasks: an fMRI study," *NeuroImage*, vol. 59, no. 2, pp. 1560–1570, 2012.

[13] V. van de Ven, L. Waldorp, and I. Christoffels, "Hippocampus plays a role in speech feedback processing," *NeuroImage*, vol. 223, article 117319, 2020.

[14] C. J. Stoodley and J. D. Schmahmann, "Functional topography in the human cerebellum: a meta-analysis of neuroimaging studies," *NeuroImage*, vol. 44, no. 2, pp. 489–501, 2009.

[15] Q. Ji, A. Edwards, J. O. Glass, T. M. Brinkman, Z. Patay, and W. E. Reddick, "Measurement of projections between dentate nucleus and contralateral frontal cortex in human brain via diffusion tensor tractography," *Cerebellum*, vol. 18, no. 4, pp. 761–769, 2019.

[16] F. Palesi, J. D. Tournier, F. Calamante et al., "Contralateral cerebello-thalamo-cortical pathways with prominent involvement of associative areas in humans in vivo," *Brain Structure & Function*, vol. 220, no. 6, pp. 3369–3384, 2015.

[17] M. Sobczak-Edmans, Y. C. Lo, Y. C. Hsu et al., "Cerebro-cerebellar pathways for verbal working memory," *Frontiers in Human Neuroscience*, vol. 12, p. 530, 2018.

[18] C. Vias and A. S. Dick, "Cerebellar contributions to language in typical and atypical development: a review," *Developmental Neuropsychology*, vol. 42, no. 6, pp. 404–421, 2017.

[19] Y. Shi, W. Liu, R. Liu et al., "Investigation of the emotional network in depression after stroke: a study of multivariate Granger causality analysis of fMRI data," *Journal of Affective Disorders*, vol. 249, pp. 35–44, 2019.

[20] J. Diedrichsen, "A spatially unbiased atlas template of the human cerebellum," *NeuroImage*, vol. 33, no. 1, pp. 127–138, 2006.

[21] Z. Zhang, X. Zhou, J. Liu, L. Qin, W. Ye, and J. Zheng, "Aberrant executive control networks and default mode network in patients with right-sided temporal lobe epilepsy: a functional and effective connectivity study," *The International Journal of Neuroscience*, vol. 130, no. 7, pp. 683–693, 2020.

[22] A. K. Seth, A. B. Barrett, and L. Barnett, "Granger causality analysis in neuroscience and neuroimaging," *The Journal of Neuroscience*, vol. 35, no. 8, pp. 3293–3297, 2015.

[23] E. Carrera and G. Tononi, "Diaschisis: past, present, future," *Brain*, vol. 137, Part 9, pp. 2408–2422, 2014.

[24] N. Zhang, M. Xia, T. Qiu et al., "Reorganization of cerebrocerebellar circuit in patients with left hemispheric gliomas involving language network: a combined structural and resting-state functional MRI study," *Human Brain Mapping*, vol. 39, no. 12, pp. 4802–4819, 2018.

[25] M. Reivich, "Crossed cerebellar diaschisis," *AJNR. American Journal of Neuroradiology*, vol. 13, no. 1, pp. 62–64, 1992.

[26] Z. Patay, C. Parra, H. Hawk et al., "Quantitative longitudinal evaluation of diaschisis-related cerebellar perfusion and diffusion parameters in patients with supratentorial hemispheric high-grade gliomas after surgery," *Cerebellum*, vol. 13, no. 5, pp. 580–587, 2014.

[27] H. Yamauchi, H. Fukuyama, and J. Kimura, "Hemodynamic and metabolic changes in crossed cerebellar hypoperfusion," *Stroke*, vol. 23, no. 6, pp. 855–860, 1992.

[28] A. Boyer, J. Deverdun, H. Duffau et al., "Longitudinal changes in cerebellar and thalamic spontaneous neuronal activity after wide-awake surgery of brain tumors: a resting-state fMRI study," *Cerebellum*, vol. 15, no. 4, pp. 451–465, 2016.

[29] E. Le Strange, N. Saeed, F. M. Cowan, A. D. Edwards, and M. A. Rutherford, "MR imaging quantification of cerebellar growth following hypoxic-ischemic injury to the neonatal brain," *AJNR. American Journal of Neuroradiology*, vol. 25, no. 3, pp. 463–468, 2004.

[30] R. D. Tien and B. C. Ashdown, "Crossed cerebellar diaschisis and crossed cerebellar atrophy: correlation of MR findings, clinical symptoms, and supratentorial diseases in 26 patients," *AJR. American Journal of Roentgenology*, vol. 158, no. 5, pp. 1155–1159, 1992.

[31] G. Hickok and D. Poeppel, "The cortical organization of speech processing," *Nature Reviews. Neuroscience*, vol. 8, no. 5, pp. 393–402, 2007.

[32] G. Vallar, A. M. Di Betta, and M. C. Silveri, "The phonological short-term store-rehearsal system: patterns of impairment and neural correlates," *Neuropsychologia*, vol. 35, no. 6, pp. 795–812, 1997.

[33] M. Yen, A. T. DeMarco, and S. M. Wilson, "Adaptive paradigms for mapping phonological regions in individual participants," *NeuroImage*, vol. 189, pp. 368–379, 2019.

[34] V. J. Hodgson, M. A. Lambon Ralph, and R. L. Jackson, "Multiple dimensions underlying the functional organization of the language network," *NeuroImage*, vol. 241, article 118444, 2021.

[35] M. Vogelzang, C. M. Thiel, S. Rosemann, J. W. Rieger, and E. Ruigendijk, "Effects of age-related hearing loss and hearing aid experience on sentence processing," *Scientific Reports*, vol. 11, no. 1, p. 5994, 2021.

[36] R. A. Poldrack, A. D. Wagner, M. W. Prull, J. E. Desmond, G. H. Glover, and J. D. Gabrieli, "Functional specialization for semantic and phonological processing in the left inferior prefrontal cortex," *NeuroImage*, vol. 10, no. 1, pp. 15–35, 1999.

[37] G. S. Dell, M. F. Schwartz, N. Nozari, O. Faseyitan, and C. H. Branch, "Voxel-based lesion-parameter mapping: identifying the neural correlates of a computational model of word production," *Cognition*, vol. 128, no. 3, pp. 380–396, 2013.

[38] D. Mirman, Q. Chen, Y. Zhang et al., "Neural organization of spoken language revealed by lesion-symptom mapping," *Nature Communications*, vol. 6, p. 6762, 2015.

[39] M. F. Schwartz, O. Faseyitan, J. Kim, and H. B. Coslett, "The dorsal stream contribution to phonological retrieval in object naming," *Brain*, vol. 135, Part 12, pp. 3799–3814, 2012.

[40] H. Zhang, A. Eppes, A. Beatty-Martínez, C. Navarro-Torres, and M. T. Diaz, "Task difficulty modulates brain-behavior correlations in language production and cognitive control: behavioral and fMRI evidence from a phonological go/no-go picture-naming paradigm," *Cognitive, Affective, & Behavioral Neuroscience*, vol. 18, no. 5, pp. 964–981, 2018.

[41] D. Mirman, A. E. Kraft, D. Y. Harvey, A. R. Brecher, and M. F. Schwartz, "Mapping articulatory and grammatical subcomponents of fluency deficits in post-stroke aphasia," *Cognitive, Affective, & Behavioral Neuroscience*, vol. 19, no. 5, pp. 1286–1298, 2019.

[42] F. R. Dreyer, T. Picht, D. Frey, P. Vajkoczy, and F. Pulvermüller, "The functional relevance of dorsal motor systems for processing tool nouns- evidence from patients with focal lesions," *Neuropsychologia*, vol. 141, article 107384, 2020.

[43] R. M. Besseling, J. F. Jansen, G. M. Overvliet et al., "Reduced structural connectivity between sensorimotor and language areas in rolandic epilepsy," *PLoS One*, vol. 8, no. 12, article e83568, 2013.

[44] H. Zhang, Y. Bao, Y. Feng, H. Hu, and Y. Wang, "Evidence for reciprocal structural network interactions between bilateral crus lobes and Broca's complex," *Frontiers in Neuroanatomy*, vol. 14, p. 27, 2020.

[45] M. J. Pickering and S. Garrod, "Do people use language production to make predictions during comprehension?," *Trends in Cognitive Sciences*, vol. 11, no. 3, pp. 105–110, 2007.

[46] G. P. Argyropoulos, "The cerebellum, internal models and prediction in 'non-motor' aspects of language: a critical review," *Brain and Language*, vol. 161, pp. 4–17, 2016.

[47] A. M. D'Mello, P. E. Turkeltaub, and C. J. Stoodley, "Cerebellar tDCS modulates neural circuits during semantic prediction: a combined tDCS-fMRI study," *The Journal of Neuroscience*, vol. 37, no. 6, pp. 1604–1613, 2017.

7

The Nature of Lexical-Semantic Access in Bilingual Aphasia

Swathi Kiran, Isabel Balachandran, and Jason Lucas

Department of Speech Language and Hearing Sciences, Boston University Sargent College, 635 Commonwealth Avenue, Boston, MA 02215, USA

Correspondence should be addressed to Swathi Kiran; kirans@bu.edu

Academic Editor: Jubin Abutalebi

Background. Despite a growing clinical need, there are no clear guidelines on assessment of lexical access in the two languages in individuals with bilingual aphasia. *Objective.* In this study, we examined the influence of language proficiency on three tasks requiring lexical access in English and Spanish bilingual normal controls and in bilingual individuals with aphasia. *Methods.* 12 neurologically healthy Spanish-English bilinguals and 10 Spanish-English bilinguals with aphasia participated in the study. All participants completed three lexical retrieval tasks: two picture-naming tasks (BNT, BPNT) and a category generation (CG) task. *Results.* This study found that across all tasks, the greatest predictors for performance were the effect of group and language ability rating (LAR). Bilingual controls had a greater score or produced more correct responses than participants with bilingual aphasia across all tasks. The results of our study also indicate that normal controls and bilinguals with aphasia make similar types of errors in both English and Spanish and develop similar clustering strategies despite significant performance differences between the groups. *Conclusions.* Differences between bilingual patients and controls demonstrate a fundamental lexical retrieval deficit in bilingual individuals with aphasia, but one that is further influenced by language proficiency in the two languages.

1. Introduction

Naming deficits are a commonly acquired disorder, manifesting in all types of aphasia [1, 2]; however, we are still unclear about the nature and mechanisms underlying lexical processing deficits in monolingual and bilingual individuals with aphasia. Theories of normal bilingual language processing indicate variable degrees of overlap between the two languages. For instance, the *revised hierarchical model* (RHM; [3–5]) allows for language proficiency differences by proposing connections between both L1 and L2 and the semantic system; these connections differ in their strengths as a function of fluency in L1 relative to L2. In bilingual individuals with a dominant language, the lexicon of L1 is generally assumed to be larger than that of L2 because more words are known in the dominant language. Also, lexical associations from L2 to L1 are assumed to be stronger than those from L1 to L2. Conversely, the links between the semantic system and L1 are assumed to be stronger than from the semantic system to L2. With regards to activation of phonological representations from the semantic system, the prevailing theory suggests that activation flows from the semantic system to the phonological system of both languages simultaneously, indicating that lexical access is target language-nonspecific [6, 7]. Thus, targets in both languages are potentially active subsequent to semantic activation, but through a process of competitive selection, the target in the accurate language is ultimately produced. An alternate, but not necessarily contradictory hypothesis, is the fact that in order for bilinguals to access the target language, the nontarget language must be inhibited [8–10]. In other words, a speaker activates target language lemmas while simultaneously inhibiting the lemmas of the nontarget language.

There are several methods to examine lexical access in bilingual individuals. The most common approach has been confrontation picture naming. In general, performance on picture naming tasks is constrained by the images presented and influenced by word frequency and imageability. One such picture naming task that has been used extensively as a measure of lexical access in monolinguals and bilinguals is the Boston Naming Test (BNT, [11]). For instance, Kohnert et al.

[12] showed that normal young bilinguals performed better in English than Spanish on the BNT and that naming accuracy significantly correlated with self-ratings of language skills. Similarly, Roberts et al. [13] examined naming on the BNT in French/English and Spanish/English bilinguals and found that both bilingual groups scored significantly below the monolingual English group on the BNT.

Another approach to examining lexical access includes category generation verbal fluency tasks [14–17]. Verbal fluency has been found to be dependent on a multitude of factors, including two qualitative features, clustering and switching ability. These strategic processes are mediated by executive functioning and verbal memory storage and have therefore been a successful predictor of lexical access ability [18, 19]. Performance on the task is highly contingent on the success of the generation of semantically related words in a subcategory, or clustering, which utilizes an individual's language stores. There is also an equally essential component of switching between subordinate categories in the verbal fluency task, which relies on an efficient cognitive flexibility [20–22]. Therefore, simply examining the number of correct words is not sufficient to understand the performance on the task [16].

The nature of semantic organization in the two languages of a bilingual individual affects influences their performance on verbal fluency tasks. For instance, Roberts and Le Dorze [23] examined category generation in French-English participants and found that there was no language effect on the number of correct responses across languages. However, for *animals*, French-English bilinguals recalled more subcategories (*birds, insects, etc.*) in French than English. The authors suggested that some semantic fields may have similar type of semantic organization across languages, whereas others may differ between languages even in balanced bilinguals. The authors suggested that childhood experiences and the cultural environment play an important role in determining the nature of semantic system.

In another set of studies, Rosselli et al. [24] first compared Spanish-English bilinguals with English monolinguals and Spanish monolinguals on word fluency task using either phoneme letter cues or semantic categories. Results showed a lower performance in the bilingual participants compared to their monolingual counterparts on the semantic category cued task but not on the phoneme letter cue task. They indicated that the shared elements of concrete nouns across languages may further the interference between the two languages. There may also be a greater conflict between the languages while the individual is searching through their verbal stores for semantically related words [24]. Interestingly, age of acquisition of L2 did interact with language, bilinguals who learned English earlier in life as L2 performed significantly higher than later learners on English versions of the tests. In a follow-up study, Rosselli et al. [25] examined the use of grammatical words versus content words for phonemic word generation and analyzed the relationship between productivity and semantic association for the responses in category generation. Results for generation of words within phonemic categories were similar to the previous study [24] in which bilinguals produced almost an identical number

of words as both English and Spanish monolinguals. There are other studies that have examined verbal fluency as a measure of lexical-semantic access in bilingual individuals in other language combinations (e.g., Zulu/English, [26]; Finnish/English, [27]) and found differences in the degree of performance across the two languages of the bilingual. To summarize, most studies examining category fluency in bilingual individuals have demonstrated that participants tend to produce more items in one language relative to another and to task set (e.g., semantic or phonological cues), but no study has systematically examined the nature of category fluency in bilingual individuals across a set of semantic categories by taking into account language proficiency.

Both lexical access tasks described above, picture naming and verbal fluency, test lexical access but in slightly different ways. In both tasks, the measure of lexical access theoretically involves parallel activation of both languages with highly interactive phonological and semantic representations that spread through the levels of language representation [6]. However, sufficient crucial differences in the theoretical basis between the tasks exist to investigate different properties of lexical access. Performance on picture naming tasks is constrained by the images presented, making nonlinguistic strategies like clustering and switching ineffective. Performance on the picture naming tasks is driven mainly by word frequency and imageability. Also, categories in the category generation task have a certain degree of flexibility with regard to items that belong to a given category which is not present in a picture naming task. On the verbal fluency task, however, nonlinguistic and semantically unrelated phonological strategies are effective means of performing the task. Grouping clusters is dependent on the way semantically related words are organized in the brain. Clustering and switching abilities on the verbal fluency task are dependent on individual language exposure. The relative freedom of the category generation task (to semantically organize the categories) also aids in the performance of the task by facilitating the individual language abilities of the participants.

In contrast to studies on lexical access in nonbrain damaged bilingual individuals, examination of lexical access in bilingual aphasia is relatively sparse and most studies are case studies of individuals with interesting but atypical language impairment profiles [11, 28–33]. In one group study, Tschirren et al. [34] examined the interaction of late age of acquisition (AoA) on L2 syntactic deficits in bilingual aphasia. A total of 12 late bilingual patients with aphasia (six with anterior lesions and six with posterior lesions) were examined. The authors found that, as a group, the L1 and L2 aphasia severity scores did not differ; however, four patients with lesions in the prerolandic area did exhibit lower scores in L2 syntactic processing compared to L1 syntactic processing.

A few studies have specifically examined lexical access in bilingual aphasia. For instance, Roberts and Deslauriers [35] examined the relationship between the mental representation of the two languages and how effectively individuals switched between languages. During naming performance on cognate nouns, the study found that bilingual individuals with aphasia produced cognate nouns with higher accuracy than noncognates in both languages. In another study, Muñoz and Marquardt [36] compared language history and language proficiency self-ratings with poststroke picture naming and identification ability in four Spanish-English patients with bilingual aphasia with 20 neurologically healthy Spanish-English adults who were gender, ethnicity, and age matched and completed the same experiment diagnostics. The bilingual nonbrain damaged individuals showed that more frequent use of the English language is consistent with between-language differences in proficiency and literacy. The four patients fell into three patterns. For two patients differences in naming and identification scores in Spanish and English were correlated with varying degrees of skill between two languages instead of a differential impairment. For a third patient, it was predicted that his performance in English would outperform Spanish based on the language history; however, this trend was not observed and the authors identified a differential impairment. Finally, the fourth patient presented with a language profile that predicted similar impairments across languages; however, the English picture naming task was less impaired than the Spanish whereas the opposite trend in results was observed for the picture identification task. For this patient, the authors speculate that higher English picture naming scores may be attributed to strategies learned in years of English therapy that did not transfer to Spanish. Overall, the experiment results strongly suggest that an in-depth premorbid language history is a vital piece to the evaluation and identification of deficits and language pattern impairments in bilingual aphasia.

These studies highlight the fact that lexical retrieval is influenced by proficiency and the nature of brain damage, but these results are not necessarily generalizable to the larger population of bilingual aphasia. A systematic examination of a larger group of patients on different language tasks while accounting for language proficiency will help better understand the nature of lexical access in individuals with bilingual aphasia and guide better diagnosis and treatment of lexical impairment in these individuals.

The present study examines lexical access in English and Spanish with respect to both premorbid proficiency and the effect of stroke on language ability in ten patients with bilingual aphasia and their nonbrain damaged controls. We compared picture naming on the BNT with a separate normed naming task to examine any differences (or similarities) between these two tasks. While the BNT is used often in the assessment of lexical impairment in individuals with bilingual aphasia, it has clear limitations as a valid measure of lexical access due to the relatively low frequency of certain items in the task [27]. Therefore, in the present study, we directly compared performance on the BNT with another naming task that developed to examine lexical retrieval in bilingual individuals [37, 38] and that has items that are generally frequent in both English and Spanish cultures. Additionally, we compared confrontation naming on these two tasks with category generation across three categories for the reasons described above. In addition to examining accuracy on the confrontation naming task, we also systematically examined the nature of target and nontarget language errors that were produced by patients and controls. Likewise, in addition to examining the number of correct words generated on the category generation task, we also examined strategies in verbal fluency including semantic clusters and switches between subclusters across three semantic categories.

In addition to comparing the three lexical access tasks across two languages (English, Spanish), the main goal of this paper was to examine the effect of language proficiency on differences in bilingual lexical access in normal bilingual controls as well as in individuals with bilingual aphasia. To this end, we obtained detailed measures of language background, use, and proficiency in both bilingual controls and in patients with bilingual aphasia. We predicted that bilingual controls would outperform the patients on all three measures of lexical access, but both groups would demonstrate a variance in the nature of strategies employed in lexical retrieval. As such, we expected bilingual controls to produce different semantic clusters and switches and fewer semantic errors compared to bilingual individuals with aphasia. In addition, we predicted language proficiency measures such as language exposure, self-rating of language proficiency, and other parameters to positively correlate with the extent to which participants successfully retrieved words in the two languages.

2. Methods

2.1. Participants. Twelve Spanish-English bilingual nonbrain damaged individuals between the ages of 18 and 70 (mean age = 34.92 years, standard deviation = 18.89, see Table 1 for a complete description of demographic information). Control subjects were paid $10 each for their participation. Ten Spanish/English bilingual speakers with aphasia participated in the study (see Table 2 for a complete description of demographic information). All participants experienced a single, unilateral cerebral vascular event (CVA, or stroke) in the distribution of the left middle cerebral artery at least 6 months prior to initiation of the experiment with the exception of BA04 who experienced a gunshot wound in the left hemisphere. Participants with apraxia were excluded from the study because the motor complexity can impact oral naming, which was the main task in the study.

2.1.1. Assessment of Language Proficiency Levels. All participants received extensive background language assessments and a comprehensive LUQ [39]. This questionnaire obtained information about the period of *age of language acquisition* (AoA). Next, participants were required to *self-rate their proficiency* (prestroke for bilinguals with aphasia) in each language in terms of their ability to speak and understand the language in formal and informal situations and read and write in each language. Again, an average proportion score in each language reflected participants' perception of their own *language ability rating* (LAR). Additionally, a proportion of language exposure in hearing, speaking, and reading domains during the entire lifetime for each individual was obtained. A weighted average of the proportion of language exposure in the three domains was obtained for each language; for the participants, this information primarily reflected their prestroke *lifetime language exposure*.

TABLE 1: Demographic information for bilingual normal controls.

Control	Age	Sex	AoA		Lifetime exposure %		Confidence %		Current exposure %		Family proficiency %		Education history %		Language ability rating %	
			Eng.	Sp.	Eng.	Sp.	Eng.	Sp.	Eng.	Sp.	Eng.	Sp.	Eng.	Sp.	Eng.	Sp.
BC01	18	F	5	0	40.83	59.17	48.33	75.83	79.35	20.65	58.33	91.67	55.56	44.44	97.14	85.71
BC02	19	F	8	0	53.89	46.11	87.50	98.61	93.33	6.67	58.33	91.67	61.11	38.89	100.00	91.43
BC03	21	F	0	9	82.94	17.06	100.00	31.25	58.14	41.86	100.00	33.33	72.22	27.78	100.00	91.43
BC05	42	M	0	0	54.63	45.37	88.10	100.00	75.21	24.79	91.67	100.00	11.11	88.89	100.00	100.00
BC06	20	F	2	0	57.34	42.66	88.33	89.44	63.79	36.21	75.00	100.00	72.22	27.78	100.00	100.00
BC07	60	M	30	0	45.13	54.87	55.00	100.00	88.95	11.05	8.33	100.00	33.33	66.67	62.86	100.00
BC08	20	M	0	0	38.10	61.90	95.56	95.56	50.00	50.00	91.67	100.00	50.00	50.00	80.00	100.00
BC09	20	F	3	0	50.00	50.00	86.94	85.56	57.50	42.50	37.50	100.00	72.22	27.78	100.00	94.29
BC10	58	F	48	0	20.46	79.20	24.14	75.86	45.58	54.42	0.00	100.00	0.00	100.00	48.57	100.00
BC11	34	F	14	0	88.07	11.93	100.00	40.63	91.07	8.93	100.00	0.00	100.00	0.00	100.00	71.43
BC12	62	M	12	0	42.47	57.53	61.54	100.00	82.77	17.23	50.00	100.00	16.67	83.33	94.29	100.00
BC14	61	F	10	0	43.90	56.10	37.91	100.00	40.91	59.09	0.00	100.00	25.00	75.00	45.71	100.00

Note: AoA: Age of acquisition, Eng.: English, Sp.: Spanish.

TABLE 2: Demographic information for bilingual individuals with aphasia.

Patient	Age	Sex	AoA Eng.	AoA Sp.	Lifetime exposure % Eng.	Lifetime exposure % Sp.	Confidence % Eng.	Confidence % Sp.	Current exposure % Eng.	Current exposure % Sp.	Family proficiency % Eng.	Family proficiency % Sp.	Education history % Eng.	Education history % Sp.	Language ability rating % Eng.	Language ability rating % Sp.
BA01	43	M	19	0	28.00	72.00	42.00	94.00	22.00	78.00	33.00	100.00	0.00	100.00	89.00	89.00
BA04	36	M	0	0	74.00	26.00	81.00	100.00	66.00	34.00	67.00	100.00	100.00	0.00	100.00	89.00
BA07	65	F	45	0	10.00	90.00	5.00	100.00	2.00	98.00	0.00	100.00	0.00	100.00	32.00	100.00
BA10	76	M	40	0	4.00	96.00	15.00	100.00	0.00	100.00	0.00	100.00	0.00	100.00	47.00	100.00
BA17	53	M	6	0	66.00	34.00	96.00	98.00	55.00	45.00	75.00	100.00	58.00	42.00	100.00	100.00
BA18	73	F	17	0	40.00	60.00	80.00	100.00	0.00	100.00	58.00	100.00	25.00	75.00	100.00	100.00
BA19	75	M	27	0	16.00	84.00	13.00	76.00	15.00	85.00	0.00	100.00	0.00	100.00	20.00	100.00
BA21	88	F	5	0	72.00	28.00	100.00	100.00	99.00	1.00	100.00	100.00	100.00	0.00	31.00	23.00
BA22	42	M	18	0	10.00	90.00	11.00	92.00	38.00	63.00	17.00	100.00	0.00	100.00	34.00	94.00
BA23	42	F	9	0	33.00	67.00	42.00	100.00	29.00	71.00	33.00	100.00	22.00	78.00	66.00	94.00

Note: AoA: Age of acquisition, Eng: English, Sp: Spanish.

TABLE 3: Average scores for bilinguals with aphasia and bilingual normal controls on BAT-Comprehension, BAT-Semantics, BNT, and BPNT in English and Spanish. Scores for bilingual normal controls are provided for BNT and BPNT (standard deviations are in parenthesis).

Group	BAT Comp %		BAT Sem %		Boston naming test %		Bilingual picture naming task %	
	English	Spanish	English	Spanish	English	Spanish	English	Spanish
Controls					75.00 (21.66)	61.81 (15.33)	85.52 (19.45)	80.73 (12.41)
Patients	47.96 (28.33)	69.26 (20.72)	45.71 (14.90)	51.67 (13.54)	18.83 (22.91)	24.51 (19.44)	34.73 (34.72)	46.05 (29.95)

A similar set of questions obtained a proportion of confidence in hearing, speaking, and reading domains during the entire lifetime for each individual. A weighted average of the proportion of confidence in language use in the three domains was obtained for each language; for the participants, this piece of information primarily reflected their prestroke *language confidence use*. Participants estimated the time spent conversing in each language hour by hour during a typical weekday and typical weekend. A weighted average of this score reflected the proportion of language use in the two languages; for the participants with aphasia this piece of information reflected their *current (poststroke) language* use. Participants were also asked to rate their *family proficiency* (estimates of parent/sibling proficiency) in each of the two languages. Finally, participants also filled out a detailed *educational history* form in which they were asked to provide the language of instruction and the predominant language used during educational interactions.

2.1.2. Assessment of Language Impairment for Participants with Aphasia. Because there is inadequate evidence to guide a priori hypotheses about lexical-semantic impairments, no explicit criteria other than the ability to perform the experimental task were set for inclusion in the experiment. The three pictures subtest of *Pyramids and Palm Trees (PAPT)* [20], the *Bilingual Aphasia Test (BAT)* [40], and the *Boston Naming Test* [12, 41] were administered in both languages (English/Spanish) on separate days by separate examiners (see Table 3 for score information). The BNT was administered in its entirety (all sixty items) according to the protocol including the guidelines for basal and ceiling scoring as indicated in the manual. Scoring for the Spanish items was done according to the procedures reviewed by Kohnert et al. [12]. With the exception of the BNT which was analyzed further for differences, results from the remaining tests are reported as patient demographic information to provide additional information about the nature of language impairment.

2.2. Materials. In addition to the BNT, a second picture naming task that included primarily high frequency concrete nouns obtained from specific categories (Bilingual Picture Naming Task, BPNT) was administered. Stimuli for this task were chosen from our previous work that included a corpus of 200 words that varied across semantic categories [37, 38]. In both language pairs, cognates (e.g., *elephant* and *elefante*) and words with at least 50% phonetic similarity (e.g., *cat* and *gato*) were eliminated from the set. The picture stimuli were chosen from Art Explosion Software (NOVA Inc.) and modified to

approximately 4×6 inches. The picture naming task consisted of 108 pictures. Stimuli were presented in language blocks with the order of stimuli pseudorandomized within each block to ensure that items from the same category were not presented sequentially. Prior to presentation of stimuli in each language, the bilingual clinician verbally conversed with the participant for a minimum of five minutes (i.e., general everyday conversation) to ensure that participants were aware of the target language and to facilitate lexical access of the target language.

All participants were also administered a Category Generation (CG) task as a measure of verbal fluency. Three categories were selected: *animals, clothing,* and *food* in English and Spanish. Participants were asked to produce as many semantically related words in two minutes in each of the assigned categories. Again, the order of presentation of languages and categories for the task was counterbalanced across sessions for each participant.

2.3. Data Scoring

2.3.1. Picture Naming Scoring. For both naming tests, bilingual controls were shown the target stimuli and given up to thirty seconds to generate a response. Responses were counted as correct if they matched the target response. All other responses were coded on a 20-point error scale that included the following error codes: no response; neologism; perseveration; unrelated word; circumlocution; semantic error; mixed error; phonemic error; correct in nontarget language; accent influence in target language (see Table 6 for descriptions and examples). Target language indicates the language in which testing was taking place at the time. Nontarget language denotes responses that were given in the language not being tested.

The same scoring procedure was used for patients and controls, with minor differences made to compensate for the participants' deficits. In particular, responses were counted as correct if they matched the target response, or contained one phonemic substitution, omission, or addition to the target response; however, for controls, responses had to be accurate productions of the target. Additionally, participants with aphasia were given up to one minute to generate a response to the stimuli pictures.

2.3.2. Category Generation Scoring. For the CG task, the responses of all participants were transcribed and tabulated. This was performed separately for each category and each language. Three measures were obtained from this data: (a) the total number words produced, (b) total correct words produced, (c) mean semantic cluster size, and (d) mean semantic switching in each subcategory for each language, Spanish and English [22, 34]. Outlined below is the scoring procedure for the four categories analyzed.

(a) Total Words. The number of responses, either intelligible or unintelligible, was calculated for each category and language.

(b) Total Correct Words. The accuracy of the words produced in the task was determined through a 20-point error analysis procedure outlined in Table 6. Only intelligible and appropriate words for each category and language were deemed correct. Incorrect responses and any cross linguistic errors, perseverations, two or more repetitions of the same item, were considered as incorrect items.

(c) Mean Semantic Cluster Score. In order to calculate clusters produced within each category, several constraints were utilized based on previously published work. For the category of *animals*, the method of analysis was taken directly from Tschirren et al. [34]. The coding system for *clothing* was guided by work done by Rosselli et al. [25]. A coding system for *food items* was developed by applying the methods stated in [21]. The average of all of the semantic clusters in one category and one language was then determined for each subject to produce a final score. (The individual categories are listed in Appendix A.)

(d) Mean Semantic Switching Score. The scoring for the mean semantic cluster score was consistent between each category and each language [34]. This score was calculated as the total amount of changes between clusters (Appendix A).

We did not collect formal measures of reliability. The transcription of oral responses was completed by the testing clinician and the error coding was performed by a research assistant who checked all transcribed responses against the targets prior to coding the errors.

3. Results

3.1. Analysis of Language History and Proficiency. Tables 1 and 2 reveal that there were differences between the two groups in terms of language history and proficiency. Simple factorial ANOVAs were performed on the various variables (e.g., language ability rating, lifetime language exposure) with group (patient, control) and language (English, Spanish) as independent variables. Results showed a significant main effect of group ($F(1, 42) = 6.9$, $P < 0.01$) and language ($F(1, 42) = 4.3$, $P < 0.05$) indicating that language ability ratings were generally higher for the controls relative to the patients ($P < 0.05$) and in Spanish relative to English ($P < 0.05$). For lifetime language exposure, a significant interaction effect of group and language was observed ($F(1, 42) = 6.8$, $P < 0.01$) indicating that lifetime exposure in Spanish was higher than English for patients ($P < 0.01$) but no significant differences were observed for controls. Similarly, for current language use, a significant interaction of group and language was observed ($F(1, 42) = 25.7$, $P < 0.0001$) indicating that

current language use was higher in English than in Spanish ($P < 0.01$) for controls, whereas current language use was higher in Spanish than in English ($P < 0.001$) for patients. Interestingly, current use of Spanish in the patients was higher than controls ($P < 0.01$). Analysis of language confidence revealed a significant effect of language ($F(1, 42) = 5.7$, $P < 0.02$) with the overall confidence in Spanish being higher than in English. Analysis of family proficiency revealed significant main effects of language ($F(1, 42) = 19.5$, $P < 0.0001$) and interaction effects of group and language ($F(1, 42) = 4.8$, $P < 0.03$) essentially indicating higher family proficiency in Spanish relative to English in patients ($P < 0.0001$), however, the differences were not significant for controls. Analysis on education history was not significant for patients or controls. In summary, these results indicate that both groups demonstrated greater language history and proficiency in Spanish than in English, with the difference between the two languages being larger for the patient group than the control group. Notably, controls demonstrated an interesting split between language history (where values were generally higher in Spanish than English) and current language use (where current use was higher in English than in Spanish).

3.2. Picture Naming. Separate regression analyses were used to analyze the dependent variables (performance on the BNT and BPNT) to investigate the factors most responsible for the performance of the groups. The categorical predictors were group (patient, controls) and language (English, Spanish), and the continuous predictors were the variables of the LUQ: LAR, Confidence, Lifetime Exposure, Current Exposure, Family Proficiency, and Education History. For BNT, the overall regression equation was significant ($R^2 = 0.834$, $F(1, 38) = 21.14$, $P < 0.00001$). The significant predictors were group ($\beta = 0.68$, $t(38) = 9.31$, $P < 0.0001$), LAR ($\beta = 0.29$, $t(38) = 3.01$, $P < 0.001$) and language ($\beta = 0.25$, $t(38) = 2.74$, $P < 0.01$). For the *BPNT*, which was also significant ($R^2 = 0.765$, $F(1, 36) = 13.03$, $P < 0.0001$) significant predictors of performance were group ($\beta = 0.52$, $t(34) = 5.91$, $P < 0.0001$) and LAR ($\beta = 0.46$, $t(34) = 4.00$, $P < 0.001$).

Since the regression equations revealed group and at least one aspect of language proficiency to be major predictors for both the BNT and BPNT, the data for the patients and bilingual controls were separated andanalyzed to examine if differences in language performance was observed once language proficiency measures were controlled within each participant group. Also, since the regression analysis for both picture naming tasks revealed LAR as the only significant LUQ predictor, only this variable was entered into a subsequent ANCOVA analysis, with language as the independent variable. For the BNT, there was a significant effect of language even after controlling for LAR ($F(1, 21) = 16.68$, $P < 0.001$). Post hoc tests indicated that naming accuracy on the BNT was higher in English than Spanish ($P < 0.005$). For the BPNT, there was also a significant effect of language after controlling for LAR ($F(1, 21) = 8.87$, $P < 0.05$). However, the post hoc analysis was not significant ($P > 0.20$) with trends indicating that naming performance in English was slightly

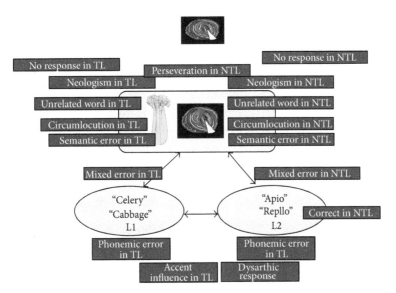

FIGURE 1: Schematic explaining the hypothesized locus of naming errors that is based on a two-step model of naming that includes semantic access and phonological access in the two languages. All error types may occur in the target language (TL) or nontarget language (NTL). No responses, perseverations, and neologisms are presumed to occur prior to semantic access of the target lemma. Unrelated word, circumlocutions, and semantic errors may occur due to varying degrees of incomplete access at the semantic representation level. Mixed errors (combinations of semantic and phonological errors) may occur due to impaired connections between semantic and language specific phonological levels. Phonemic errors, accent influences, and dysarthric responses are all presumed to occur after language specific phonological access has occurred. Cross-language translations are coded as correct responses in the nontarget language.

higher than in Spanish. Results for the bilinguals with aphasia were not significant on the ANCOVA analysis for either BNT or BPNT.

3.3. *Error Analysis.* Responses on the BPNT were further analyzed for the nature of errors produced (providing stimulus cues during BNT makes it difficult to interpret the nature of semantic errors on the task) and interpreted within a framework of lexical access (see Figure 1). Analysis of responses for the BPNT showed that despite the significant differences in accuracy and distribution of error types, no significant differences were observed between bilingual controls and participants with aphasia on English error types ($t(20) = 0.32$; $P = 0.06$). As seen in Figure 2, bilingual controls performed with 84.3% accuracy on English targets. Error types greater than 1% were (a) Circumlocution in target language (4.9%), (b) Semantic error in target language (4.9%), (c) No response/idk in target language (3.8%), and (d) Correct in nontarget language (1.3%). The remaining error types were produced either less than 1% of the time or were not produced at all by bilingual controls in English. Participants with aphasia produced a greater variety of error types, evidenced by their average accuracy of 27.5% in English. The main error types were No response/idk in target language (30%), Correct in nontarget language (9.4%), Circumlocution in nontarget language (10.9%), Neologism in target language (4.8%), Semantic error in target language (3.9%), Neologism in nontarget language (2.4%), Semantic error in nontarget language (2.4%), Unrelated word in nontarget language (2.1%), Unrelated word in target language (1.7%), and Circumlocution in target language (1.1%).

The Spanish data in Figure 2 show even greater similarity between the bilingual controls and participants with aphasia in terms of types of errors produced than the English data ($t(20) = 0.33$, $P = 0.20$). Bilingual controls performed with 79.5% accuracy. Error types greater than 1% included (a) No response/idk in target language (9.3%), (b) Semantic error in target language (6.2%), (c) Circumlocution in target language (2.1%), and (d) Correct in nontarget language (1.07%). Other error types were produced either below 1% or not produced at all by this group. Participants with aphasia performed with 38.1% accuracy in Spanish. The main error types were No response/idk in target language (27%), Circumlocution in target language (17%), Semantic error in target language (9.2%), Neologism in target language (7.8%), Unrelated word in target language (1.5%), and Correct in nontarget language (1.3%).

3.4. *Category Generation Task.* As in the picture naming tasks, a regression analysis was performed on the number of correct words (across the three categories), mean semantic cluster scores, and mean semantic switching scores on the CG task, the categorical predictors were group (patient, bilingual controls) and language (English, Spanish), and the continuous predictors were the variables of the LUQ: LAR, Confidence, Lifetime Exposure, Current Exposure, Family Proficiency, and Education History.

(a) Correct Words. A regression analysis for total correct words was significant ($R^2 = 0.922$, $F(1, 36) = 22.58$, $P = 0.00$), the strongest predictor on the task was group ($\beta = 0.764, t(36) = 10.56$, $P = 0.00$), followed by language of the task ($\beta = 0.273$, $t(36) = 3.09$, $P < 0.001$). Thus, controls

TABLE 4: Mean correct words on the category generation task, mean semantic cluster scores, and mean semantic switching scores for bilingual normal controls and bilinguals with aphasia (standard deviations are in parenthesis).

Group	Correct words		Mean semantic cluster score		Mean semantic switching score		Mean ratio of correct words to semantic switches	
	English	Spanish	English	Spanish	English	Spanish	English	Spanish
Controls	29.70 (9.10)	24.36 (6.18)	2.07 (0.86)	1.47 (0.50)	8.94 (2.53)	9.75 (2.89)	3.36 (0.81)	2.55 (0.41)
Patients	4.60 (5.90)	5.87 (4.24)	0.36 (0.41)	0.41 (0.36)	5.10 (3.84)	3.93 (2.54)	1.06 (0.84)	1.58 (0.65)

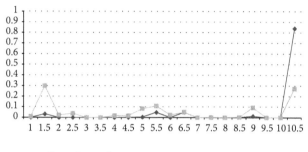

— Normal controls

(a)

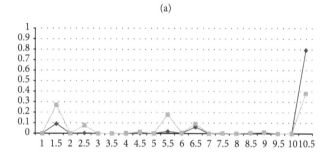

— Normal controls
— Bilinguals with Aphasia

(b)

FIGURE 2: (a) Comparison between accurate production and errors on BPNT for normal controls and bilinguals with aphasia on English targets. (b) Comparison between accurate production and errors on BPNT for normal controls and participants with aphasia on Spanish targets. Correct responses are scored 10.5 (Correct responses in TL). The greatest errors made being No response/idk in TL (1.5), Circumlocution in TL (5.5), Correct response in NTL (9). Error Percentages Spanish (across patients): (1) No response/idk NTL. (1.5) No response/idk TL. (2) Neologism in NTL. (2.5) Neologism in TL. (3) Perseveration to a nonprobe. (3.5) Perseveration to a probe in session. (4) Unrelated word in NTL. (4.5) Unrelated word in TL. (5) Circumlocution in NTL. (5.5) Circumlocution in TL. (6) Semantic error in NTL. (6.5) Semantic error in TL. (7) Mixed error in NTL. (7.5) Mixed error in TL. (8) Phonemic error in NTL. (8.5) Phonemic error in TL. (9) Correct in NTL. (9.5) Dysarthric/apractic intelligible response. (10) Accent Influence in TL. (10.5) Correct in TL.

produced more words than patients, and words generated in English were higher than in Spanish ($P < 0.05$). Also, of the variables assessed with the LUQ, LAR was the only significant predictor ($\beta = 0.226$, $t(36) = 2.65$, $P < 0.01$).

(b) Mean Semantic Cluster Score. The regression analysis for the mean semantic cluster scores was significant ($R^2 = 0.753$, $F(1, 36) = 12.89$, $P < 0.0001$), and the strongest predictor of performance on the task was group ($\beta = 0.677$, $t(36) = 5.30$, $P < 0.0001$). Bilingual controls performed significantly higher semantic clusters in both English and Spanish ($P < 0.05$). The only other significant predictor of performance was once again LAR of the LUQ ($\beta = 0.222$, $t(36) = 2.06$, $P < 0.05$).

(c) Mean Semantic Switching Score. The regression analysis for mean semantic switching score for the normal subjects or participants with aphasia did not reveal any significant influence of the LAR on the categorical measures or differences between the measures. Table 4, however, showed differences between controls and patients, which was confirmed in individual t-tests; bilingual controls had a higher semantic switching score in English ($t(20) = 2.8$, $P = 0.01$) and Spanish ($t(20) = 4.96$, $P < 0.001$) than their patient counterparts.

To further understand patterns of lexical-access within each of the participant groups, data were separated and analyzed. Three ANCOVAs (with LAR as the covariate) were performed for each group for each of the dependent variable (total correct words, mean semantic cluster scores, and mean semantic switching scores).

(a) Correct Words. An ANCOVA for the bilingual control data revealed that LAR did in fact influence the effect of language and category on the correct words. Firstly, there was a significant main effect of language ($F(1, 71) = 32.8$, $P < 0.000001$) and a main effect of category ($F(2, 71) = 11.8$, $P < 0.00005$) after controlling for the LAR. Post hoc tests indicated that, for language, the total correct words were significantly greater in English than Spanish ($P < 0.0001$). For category, the total correct words for *food* items differed significantly from the *clothing* items ($P < 0.00005$) and the total correct words for *animals* differed significantly from *clothing* ($P < 0.05$). The ANCOVA was not significant for the participants with aphasia (Figure 3).

(b) Mean Semantic Cluster Score. A significant main effect of language was seen on the mean semantic cluster score on the ANCOVA ($F(1, 71) = 10.2$, $P < 0.005$) and the main effect of category was also significant ($F(2, 71) = 3.32$, $P < 0.05$). The post hoc tests for the mean semantic cluster score analysis revealed that, for language, the mean semantic cluster scores in English were significantly more than Spanish ($P < 0.01$). Additionally, for the categories, the mean semantic

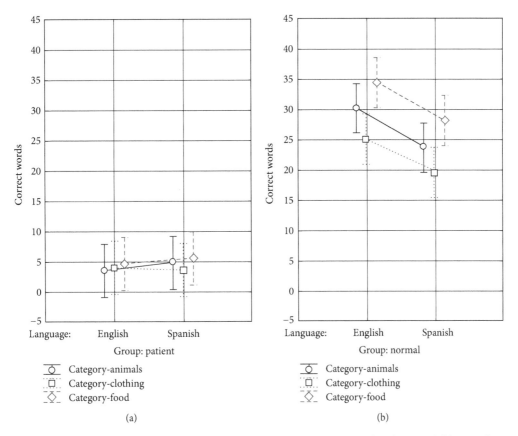

FIGURE 3: Mean number of correct words for the category generation task for (a) patients with aphasia and (b) normal controls in English and Spanish for three categories: animals, clothing, and food.

cluster scores for the *food* items were significantly higher than for the *clothing* items ($P < 0.05$). The categories of *food* items and *animals* did not show any significant difference. The ANCOVA for participants with aphasia data was not significant.

(c) Mean Semantic Switching Score. The final ANCOVA analysis on the mean semantic switching score for the normal controls or participants with aphasia did not reveal any significant influence of the LAR on the categorical measures or differences between the measures.

3.5. Individual Patient Analysis. Because the parametric statistical analysis for the patients was mostly nonsignificant, a more qualitative inspection of the data was carried out. As is evident in Figures 4 and 5 the results of the participants with aphasia showed more variation than did those of the normal controls on all three tasks (BNT, BPNT, and CG task). Individual inspection of the participant data showed that participants BA04 and BA17 produced more correct responses in English than Spanish across the three tasks. On the other hand, participants BA07, BA10, BA19, BA22, and BA23 produced more correct responses in Spanish than English in all three tasks. Two patients, BA01 and BA18, received scores that were remarkably similar in both languages, while participant BA21 produced either no correct responses or performed with very low accuracy in both languages, for

all tasks. With regards to the nature of category-specific access on the category generation task, the broad variety of responses and scores were independent of category; however, it was clear that the categories *Animals* and *Food* were easier to access than *Clothing* for most patients, a finding that was similar to the control data. Also, only two of the ten patients showed language differences in their semantic clustering ability, with BA17 producing more clusters in English and BA10 producing more clusters in Spanish. Likewise, only a few patients (BA04, BA17, and BA22) showed language-specific differences in their semantic switching scores, while other patients demonstrated similar switching patterns in English and Spanish.

3.6. Across Task Correlations. Recall that, in the introduction, we argued that the three word retrieval tasks assessed similar aspects of lexical access, but the nature of the tasks placed slightly different demands on lexical access. In the final analysis, we systematically correlated the three tasks administered with the only significant continuous predictor in the regression analysis, LAR to examine to what extent these measures actually correlated with each other. Bilingual controls and bilingual individuals with aphasia were separated for this analysis again to prevent group-driven effects in the results. The bivariate correlation analysis revealed for the bilingual controls, significant ($P < 0.05$) correlations emerged between

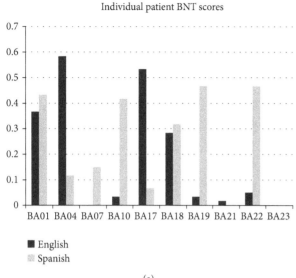

Individual patient BNT scores

(a)

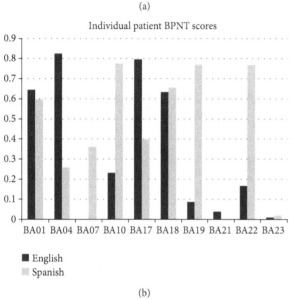

Individual patient BPNT scores

(b)

FIGURE 4: Individual patient accuracy on the two naming tasks: BNT (a) and BPNT (b) in English and Spanish.

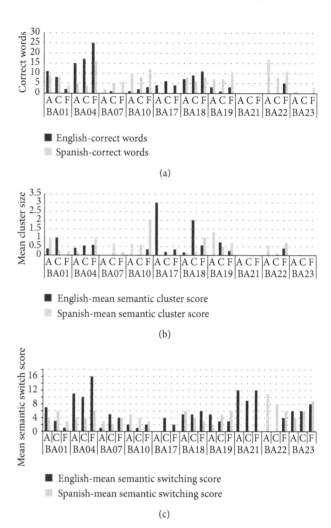

(a)

(b)

(c)

FIGURE 5: Results of category generation task for individual patients across three categories Animals (A), Food (F), and Clothing (C) in English and Spanish. (a) Correct Word Scores for the Category Generation Task in English and Spanish across each participant in the categories, (b) Mean Semantic Cluster Scores, and (c) Mean Semantic Switching Scores. Comparing each participant in their correct responses provided in English and Spanish exemplifies their dominant languages and individual differences.

LAR and correct words generated, LAR and BNT, and LAR and BPNT in English (see Table 5). Additionally, significant correlations were observed between BPNT and BNT, and correct words generated and BPNT (and BNT) responses. In Spanish, significant ($P < 0.05$) correlations emerged between correct words generated and BNT, BNT and BPNT, LAR and BNT, and LAR and BPNT. For bilingual individuals with aphasia, in English significant ($P < 0.05$) correlations emerged between correct words and BPNT, LAR, and correct words, LAR, and BNT, and LAR and BPNT. In Spanish, significant ($P < 0.05$) correlations emerged only between correct words generated and BPNT.

4. Discussion

The present study examined the nature of lexical-access in normal bilinguals and in participants with bilingual aphasia

across three different lexical-semantic access tasks (BNT picture naming, BNPT picture naming, and verbal fluency). Results are discussed in the context of the goals proposed in the study.

4.1. Comparison of the Three Lexical Retrieval Tasks. The results from the three lexical retrieval tasks revealed several similarities and some important differences. Notably, the results from the two confrontation naming tests, the BNT and BPNT, were somewhat different regarding the factors that drove performance for each test. For the BPNT, Group, LAR, Confidence, and Family Proficiency were significant determiners of performance. However, for the BNT, only Group, LAR, and Language were significant determiners of performance.

TABLE 5: Pearson correlations of BNT, BPNT, correct words on the category generation task, and LAR administered for bilingual controls and individuals with aphasia. Correlations significant at $P < 0.05$ are highlighted with an asterisk.

Group	Variable	Correct Words-E	Correct Words-S	LAR-E	LAR-S	BPNT-E	BPNT-S	BNT-E	BNT-S
Bilingual controls	Correct Words-E	1	0.277	0.892*	−0.506	0.769*	−0.385	0.818*	−0.211
	Correct Words-S		1	0.270	0.382	−0.137	0.555	−0.003	0.612*
	LAR-E			1	−0.440	0.737*	−0.207	0.787*	−0.147
	LAR-S				1	−0.337	0.846*	−0.364	0.820*
	BPNT-E					1	−0.311	0.961*	−0.118
	BPNT-S						1	−0.281	0.855*
	BNT-E							1	−0.097
	BNT-S								1
Bilingual individuals with aphasia	Correct Words-E	1	0.286	0.707*	−0.151	0.799*	0.027	0.045	−0.229
	Correct Words-S		1	0.013	0.347	0.051	0.796*	−0.386	0.254
	LAR-E			1	0.310	0.878*	0.049	0.636*	−0.183
	LAR-S				1	0.058	0.625	0.325	0.494
	BPNT-E					1	0.132	0.490	−0.428
	BPNT-S						1	−0.070	0.186
	BNT-E							1	−0.122
	BNT-S								1

As previously mentioned, the BPNT included two sets of high frequency words in English and Spanish. Many of the items on the BNT, however, are low frequency words in spontaneous speech (e.g., *abacus*) and are not translated particularly well in Spanish. Indeed previous studies that have examined BNT in Spanish and English in normal bilinguals have described lower performance accuracy [13] in Spanish. After comparing two groups of bilingual adults (Spanish/English and French/English) and monolingual English adults on the BNT, it was determined that, for both bilingual groups, mean test scores were significantly below the monolingual group while not significantly differing from each other. The study suggests variability between each bilingual group and individual participants, with less significance derived from background influences. Consequently, one would expect performance in the dominant language in bilinguals to be far greater than performance in the nondominant language for the BNT, while differences between the two languages on the BPNT would be less great due to the high frequency of the items in both languages, which was one of the findings of the study.

With respect to the category generation task, results indicated that the ability to semantically cluster, switch, and efficiently produce correct words in the task was influenced by Group, Language, and LAR. Previous studies assessing the performance of bilingual Spanish/English and monolingual English and Spanish speakers additionally demonstrated a significantly greater performance of bilingual participants in verbal fluency tasks depending on the age of acquisition and level of bilingualism without, however, an effect of language [23, 25]. Differences may have arisen between the above two studies and the data presented here based on the geographic sampling of patients and level of balanced bilingualism found within our groups (see further on individual patient analysis).

What our results indicate is that, across the three tasks, when language proficiency self-rating was controlled for, at least for the controls, performance in English was higher than performance in Spanish. These results are underscored by the fairly robust correlations between the three lexical retrieval tasks and their overall correlation with LAR.

4.2. Performance Differences between Languages. Overall, the data revealed that the normal controls were more accurate in English than in Spanish on the BNT, BPNT, and both correct words and mean semantic cluster scores on the category generation task, even when language proficiency was taken into account. In contrast, for aphasic participants, there was no significant effect across languages. This observation is interesting against the comparison of the analyses of language use and background for both groups. While both groups demonstrated greater language exposure and proficiency in Spanish than in English, the difference between the two languages was larger for the patient group than the control group. Notably, controls demonstrated an interesting split between language history (where values were generally higher in Spanish than English) and current language use (where current use was higher in English than in Spanish). Since the current lexical retrieval tasks tap into real-time lexical access, perhaps current language use may be reflective of the degree of lexical access. For patients, the overall group analysis were not significant; however, individual analyses showed that there were more patients with higher performance in Spanish than in English.

Results from the three categories, *animals*, *food*, and *clothing* on the category generation task revealed that the differences between *food* and *clothing* items for the total

TABLE 6: Description of error types and examples of errors produced in English and Spanish.

Error	Description	Example	
		English target	Spanish target
No response in nontarget language (1)	No response or response of "I don't know" in the language not being tested	Target: cabbage Response: No me recuerdo	Target: lechuga Response: I don't remember
No response in target language (1.5)	No response/response of "I don't know" in the language in session being tested	Target: glove Response: I don't know	Target: media Response: No sé
Neologism in nontarget language (2)	Unrecognized word in any dialect of the language not being tested after correcting for possible phonemic errors	Target: Counter Response: clov	Target: tiburón Response: babberi
Neologism in target language (2.5)	Unrecognized word in any dialect of the language being tested after correcting for possible phonemic errors	Target: shelf Response: crademan	Target: rastrillo Response: serame
Perseveration to a nonprobe (3)	Repetition at least three times of a neologism or word unrelated to the target and not previously presented to the subject	Target: arm Response: go go	Target: brazo Response: go go
Perseveration to a probe in session (3.5)	Repetition at least three times (in any language) of a word previously presented to the subject but unrelated to the target	Target: necklace Response: baseball (if generated at least twice before)	Target: brazo Response: ring ring (if generated at least twice before)
Unrelated word in nontarget language (4)	Word semantically and phonologically unrelated to the target word in the language not being tested	Target: counter Response: perro	Target: puerta Response: berry
Unrelated word in target language (4.5)	Word semantically and phonologically unrelated to the target word in the language being tested	Target: hook Response: coach	Target: jarra Response: ardilla
Circumlocution in nontarget language (5)	Utterance (description) providing semantic information about the target in the language not being tested	Target: hamburger Response: algo que se come	Target: oso Response: an animal
Circumlocution in target language (5.5)	Utterance (description) providing semantic information about the target in the language being tested	Target: building Response: a structure	Target: perica Response: un para hombre
Semantic error in nontarget language (6)	Semantic substitution/paraphasia in the language not being tested	Target: mop Respose: rastrillo	Target: anillo Response: diamond
Semantic error in target language (6.5)	Semantic substitution/paraphasia in the language being tested	Target: pitcher Response: coffee pot	Target: brazo Response: mano
Mixed error in nontarget language (7)	Combination of two or more errors from analysis criteria in the language not being tested	Target: sword Response: fecha	Target: mapache Response: racooco
Mixed error in target language (7.5)	Combination of two or more errors from analysis criteria in the language being tested	Target: leg Response: musolos	Target: hormiga Response: arinas
Phonemic error in nontarget language (8)	Greater than one phonemic substitution or omission in the language not being tested	Target: robe Response: bete	Target: edificio Response: build
Phonemic error in target language (8.5)	Greater than one phonemic substitution or omission in the language being tested	Target: celery Response: cerelec	Target: aspiradora Response: astirador
Correct in nontarget language (9)	Correct response (including single phoneme substitutions) in the language not being tested	Target: shelf Response: estante	Target: taburete Response: stool
Dysarthric/apractic intelligible response (9.5)	Response from a patient with known dysarthria or apraxia		
Accent influence in target language (10)	Correct response in target language but containing the phonology of the language not being tested	Target: duck Response: dok ([dog])	Target: pollo Response: polo ([powlo])
Correct in target language (10.5)	Correct response (including single phoneme substitution, addition or omission for aphasic participants only) in the language being tested	Target: giraffe Response: giraffe	Target: avestruz Response: avestruzo

correct words and mean semantic cluster score and the differences between the *animals* and *clothing* items for the total correct words also remained after controlling for LAR for the controls (and to a lesser extent for some of the patients). Therefore, the differences in performance observed for the normal controls between each category had a large cultural influence and were based on the individual's own vocabulary and lifetime experiences [23]. In contrast, Pekkala et al. [27] showed that, between two normal monolingual groups of Finnish and English-speaking subjects, differences in performance on semantic verbal fluency tasks were minimal even after normalizing for educational influences. They, therefore, suggested that cultural and language differences do not have a significant contribution to performance in monolingual normal controls. As an alternative explanation, the normal controls, in general, possessed a much greater ability of producing sequential clusters of words and the ability to switch between clusters in all categories that were tested, which was assumed to be a function of their greater level of cognition and effective semantic strategizing techniques [21].

4.3. Differences across Participant Groups. As would be expected, normal controls were significantly better at lexical retrieval on all three tasks relative to bilingual patients with aphasia. At first glance this difference between the groups may suggest that patients and normal controls perform radically differently on the picture naming tests. However, Figure 2 shows that both groups produce similar errors in both languages, with the difference being the rate of each error type between the groups. This finding suggests that despite lexical retrieval deficits associated with stroke, the basic mechanism and potential breakdown of lexical retrieval in participants with aphasia on naming tasks are no different from that of the normal controls (Figure 1). For instance, both patients and controls produced mainly semantic paraphasias and circumlocutions in the target language/nontarget language. Consistent with our findings, in a study examining the nature of semantic errors in monolingual aphasia, Dell et al. [42] found that individuals with and without aphasia performed similarly with respect to error type and that semantic paraphasias produced by aphasic individuals are a continuation of semantic substitution errors in nonaphasic speech.

With respect to the category generation task, even though bilingual controls produce many more items than bilinguals with aphasia, the differences between the two groups are smaller for the semantic cluster scores, contrary to the initial predictions of the study (Table 4). This suggests that the strategies for clustering may not be all that different for the two groups. Troyer et al. [18] found that while clustering and switching were correlated with performance on verbal fluency, there was a greater effect of switching on phonemic fluency. Although a negative correlation between semantic clustering and switching was found in the Troyer study, optimal performance requires a balance between a decrease in the number of switches and the total number of words produced. In summary, these results suggest that while bilingual individuals with aphasia may not be able to access an item

successfully, they appear to cluster their responses within appropriate semantic subcontexts. Finally, while patients with aphasia produced fewer semantic switches than their controls, the ratio of correct words to semantic switches was not all that different between patients and controls (Table 4).

4.4. Individual Patient Performance. In general, the low overall accuracy of the aphasic participant group precluded the possibility of drawing conclusions about the effect of brain damage once prestroke language proficiency was controlled. For all three tasks, it was observed that there were large individual differences creating much variation in the data to interpret. Observations of the results for BA04 and BA17 for the BNT and BPNT are especially noteworthy. Despite reporting Spanish as the L1 and near equal amounts of time speaking each language, BA04 and BA17 performed with greater accuracy in English than in Spanish on both the BNT and the BPNT. Other patients' naming accuracies were commensurate with their premorbid relative dominance in each language.

Similarly on the CG task, closer inspection of the results for individual participants revealed that participants with aphasia, like their controls, produced items within each category and each language, reflective of their relative dominance in each language. While a few participants reported they were English dominant (BA04, BA17, and BA21), only BA04 and BA17 produced more items in English. Other participants who were Spanish dominant (BA07, BA10, BA19, BA22, and BA23) produced more items in Spanish. There were also participants who showed no differences between the outputs in the two languages. These results underscore the influence of premorbid language proficiency on lexical retrieval even after brain damage and provide some validation for our reported measures of language use, exposure, and proficiency.

4.5. Influence of Language Proficiency on Lexical Retrieval. Interestingly, the initial regression analyses showed that, of all the LUQ variables, only LAR was consistently a significant predictor of performance across all five measures of lexical access (across the three tasks). This effect is due to nature of the variable: LAR is a compound, albeit subjective, judgment comprised of all the other variables of the LUQ. It therefore represents all the other variables of the LUQ combined. The results of the regression suggest that each factor of the LUQ does predict performance on the lexical retrieval tasks examined, but only when they are combined do the individual factors become significant as performance predictors. Of note is the difference between current language use and all other measures of the language exposure and proficiency for the bilingual controls. These results validate the need to obtain a multidimensional view of language use and exposure, and possibly the LAR captures some of that multidimensionality as it is a measure of the participants own judgment of their proficiency.

Importantly, LAR-English correlated with naming accuracy on BNT-English, BPNT-English, and correctly generated words in English for both the bilingual controls and bilingual patients with aphasia. Correlations between LAR-Spanish were less robust for both the controls and patients, perhaps indicating the lack of stability of this measure in obtaining a comprehensive lifespan history of Spanish language usage, of notable concern since all the patients (and several controls) were native Spanish speakers. Nonetheless, the observation that different measures of lexical retrieval correlated with a compound measure of language proficiency is an encouraging preliminary observation. The results of Kohnert et al. [12] and the present study underline the importance of independent self-reported measures of language proficiency in assessing language impairment of bilingual individuals with aphasia. While much work needs to be done in terms of delineating specific aspects of language proficiency (life time exposure, family proficiency, or education) that differentially influence various language processing tasks, the present study demonstrates that, until then, a composite albeit subjective measure of self-rated language ability is a good place to start.

5. Conclusion

The large differences in performance of the normal subjects and bilingual participants with aphasia demonstrate a fundamental lexical retrieval deficit in bilingual individuals with aphasia, but one that is further influenced by language proficiency in the two languages. The findings of our study indicate that normal controls and participants with aphasia make similar types of errors in both English and Spanish and develop similar clustering strategies despite significant performance differences between the groups.

Appendix

A. Categorization of Items on the Category Generation Task

Animals

(1) *Living Environment*

 (a) Africa

 (i) aardvark, antelope, buffalo, camel, chameleon, cheetah, chimpanzee, cobra, eland, elephant, gazelle, giraffe, gnu, gorilla, hippopotamus, hyena, impala, jackal, lemur, leopard, lion, manatee, mongoose, monkey, ostrich, panther, rhinoceros, tiger, wildebeest, warthog, zebra;

 (b) Australia

 (i) emu, kangaroo, kiwi, opossum, platypus, Tasmanian devil, wallaby, wombat

 (c) Arctic/Far North

 (i) auk, caribou, musk ox, penguin, polar bear, reindeer, seal;

 (d) Farm

 (i) chicken, cow, donkey, ferret, goat, horse, mule, pig, sheep, turkey;

 (e) North America

 (i) badger, bear, beaver, bobcat, caribou, chipmunk, cougar, deer, elk, fox, moose, mountain lion, puma, rabbit, raccoon, skunk, squirrel, wolf;

 (f) Water

 (i) Alligator, auk, beaver, crocodile, dolphin, fish, frog, lobster, manatee, muskrat, newt, octopus, otter, oyster, penguin, platypus, salamander, sea lion, seal, shark, toad, turtle, whale;

(2) *Human Use*

 (a) Beasts of Burden

 (i) Camel, donkey, horse, llama, ox

 (b) Fur

 (i) Beaver, chinchilla, fox, mink, rabbit

 (c) Pets

 (i) budgie, canary, cat, dog, gerbil, golden retriever, guinea pig, hamster, parrot, rabbit

(3) *Zoological Categories*

 (a) Bird

 (i) budgie, condor, eagle, finch, kiwi, macaw, parrot, parakeet, pelican, penguin, robin, toucan, woodpecker;

 (b) Bovine

 (i) bison, buffalo, cow, musk ox, yak;

 (c) Canine

 (i) coyote, dog, fox, hyena, jackal, wolf;

 (d) Deer

 (i) antelope, caribou, eland, elk, gazelle, gnu, impala, moose, reindeer, wildebeest;

 (e) Feline

 (i) bobcat, cat, cheetah, cougar, jaguar, leopard, lion, lynx, mountain lion, ocelot, panther, puma, tiger;

 (f) Fish

 (i) bass, guppy, salmon, trout;

 (g) Insect

 (i) ant, beetle, cockroach, flea, fly, praying mantis;

(h) Insectivores

  (i) aardvark, anteater, hedgehog, mole, shrew;

(i) Primate:

  (i) ape, baboon, chimpanzee, gibbon, gorilla, human, lemur, marmoset, monkey, orangutan, shrew;

(j) Rabbit

  (i) coney, hare, pika, rabbit;

(k) Reptile/Amphibian

  (i) alligator, chameleon, crocodile, frog, gecko, iguana, lizard, newt, salamander, snake, toad, tortoise, turtle;

(l) Rodent

  (i) beaver, chinchilla, chipmunk, gerbil, gopher, groundhog, guinea pig, hamster, hedgehog, marmot, mole, mouse, muskrat, porcupine, rat, squirrel, woodchuck;

(m) Weasel

  (i) badger, ferret, marten, mink, mongoose, otter, polecat, skunk.

The scoring system is outlined below. The only constraint utilized was for subordinate examples of a particular item. In this case, items were considered to be correct if they had distinct functions (e.g., long sleeve shirt versus short sleeve shirt) or were different species of an animal (pilgrim hawk versus red hawk).

An example of this procedure is from the pretesting task from BA01. This set of words would be grouped successively giving the following scores:

bee

dog

raccoon

ant

raccoon

raccoon

cat

rabbit

horse

bunny

raccoon.

Firstly, *bee* would be given a score of 0 because it is not semantically related to dog in any way. In the same way, *dog*, *raccoon*, and *ant* are all not semantically related, so they would each receive a score of 0. As repetitions are counted, the next two words produced, *raccoon* and *raccoon*, are semantically related (as they are the same word), so they would receive a score of 1. Of the remaining five words, *cat*, *rabbit*, *horse*, *bunny*, and *raccoon*, the first four are semantically related giving a score of 4, as *cat*, *rabbit*, *horse*,

and *bunny* are pets and *bunny* and *raccoon* are animals from North America.

$$0 + 0 + 0 + 0 + 1 + 4 = 5$$

The mean of these scores is then taken to determine an average score for each category:

$$\frac{5}{6} = 0.833. \tag{A.1}$$

This same procedure is repeated for the posttesting task, and the two values from pre- and posttesting are compared with a basic bar graph.

The semantic switching score for the example above would be 5 (5 arrows above). Again, the scores are calculated for pre- and posttesting and a bar graph is created to compare the values.

Clothing Items. The scoring system is still the same for the semantic cluster and semantic switching score as above. The subcategories for clothing are as follows:

(1) *similar weather conditions*

  (a) clothing for each season

    (i) winter (jacket, sweater, hat, etc.)
    (ii) summer (shorts, bathing suit, sunglasses, etc.);

(2) *upper body versus lower body*

  (a) upper Body

    (i) shirt, sweater, coat, vest, and so forth;

  (b) lower body

    (i) pants, shorts, capris, shoes, and so forth;

(3) *accessories*

  (a) accessories are matched to their appropriate category in the above two subcategories

    (i) sunglasses, cap, to summer clothing
    (ii) hat, scarf, gloves, mittens, to winter clothing
    (iii) necklace, earrings, rings, tie to upper body clothing;

(4) *sets of matching clothing (strong pairs)*

  (a) pairs of clothes that are usually worn together

    (i) coat and tie; sweatshirt, and sweatpants, jeans and, t-shirt, socks and shoes, and so forth;

  (b) different occasions

    (i) formal wear

      (1) suit, dress shirt, blouse, tuxedo, and so forth.

Food Items. The scoring system is the same as stated in the previous two categories. The subcategories have been grouped based on the following criteria:

(1) *beans*

(2) *beverages*

    (a) water, soda, juice, milk, and so forth

(3) *breads*

(4) *candy*

(5) *cold cereals*

(6) *condiments*

(7) *desserts*

(8) *fish*

(9) *fruits*

(10) *grains/cereals*

(11) *junk food*

(12) *meats*

    (a) cold cuts

    (b) poultry

(13) *dairy products*

(14) *nuts/seeds*

(15) *prepared foods and meals*

    (a) sandwiches, pasta, cake

(16) *seafood*

(17) *spices/herbs*

(18) *spreads*

(19) *vegetables*

(20) *ethnic foods*

    (a) spanish/mexican

        (i) beans, burrito, quesadilla, rice, and so forth

    (b) italian

        (i) pizza, pasta, spaghetti, and so forth

    (c) other ethnicities not specified

(21) *occasions*

    (a) breakfast foods (time of day)

        (i) pancakes, waffles, eggs, bacon, cereal, and so forth

    (b) birthday foods

        (i) cake, pizza, ice-cream, and so forth.

Acknowledgments

A portion of this was supported by NIDCD no. R21DC009446 and a Clinical Research grant from American Speech Language Hearing Foundation to the first author.

References

[1] H. Goodglass, "Disorders of naming following brain injury," *American Scientist*, vol. 68, no. 6, pp. 647–663, 1980.

[2] H. Goodglass, A. Wingfield, and M. R. Hyde, "The Boston corpus of aphasic naming errors," *Brain and Language*, vol. 64, no. 1, pp. 1–27, 1998.

[3] J. F. Kroll and E. Stewart, "Category interference in translation and picture naming: evidence for asymmetric connections between bilingual memory representations," *Journal of Memory and Language*, vol. 33, no. 2, pp. 149–174, 1994.

[4] J. F. Kroll, S. C. Bobb, M. Misra, and T. Guo, "Language selection in bilingual speech: evidence for inhibitory processes," *Acta Psychologica*, vol. 128, no. 3, pp. 416–430, 2008.

[5] J. F. Kroll, J. G. van Hell, N. Tokowicz, and D. W. Green, "The Revised Hierarchical Model: a critical review and assessment," *Bilingualism*, vol. 13, no. 3, pp. 373–381, 2010.

[6] A. Costa, W. La Heij, and E. Navarrete, "The dynamics of bilingual lexical access," *Bilingualism*, vol. 9, no. 2, pp. 137–151, 2006.

[7] A. Costa and M. Santesteban, "The control of speech production by bilingual speakers: Introductory remarks," *Bilingualism*, vol. 9, no. 2, pp. 115–117, 2006.

[8] J. Abutalebi and D. W. Green, "Understanding the link between bilingual aphasia and language control," *Journal of Neurolinguistics*, vol. 21, no. 6, pp. 558–576, 2008.

[9] D. W. Green, "Control, activation, and resource: a framework and a model for the control of speech in bilinguals," *Brain and Language*, vol. 27, no. 2, pp. 210–223, 1986.

[10] D. W. Green, "Mental control of the bilingual lexico-semantic system," *Bilingualism*, vol. 1, no. 2, pp. 67–81, 1998.

[11] E. Kaplan, H. Goodglass, and S. Weintraub, *Boston Naming Test*, Lippincott Williams & Wilkins, Baltimore, Md, USA, 2nd edition, 2001.

[12] K. J. Kohnert, A. E. Hernandez, and E. Bates, "Bilingual performance on the Boston Naming Test: preliminary norms in Spanish and English," *Brain and Language*, vol. 65, no. 3, pp. 422–440, 1998.

[13] P. M. Roberts, L. J. Garcia, A. Desrochers, and D. Hernandez, "English performance of proficient bilingual adults on the Boston Naming test," *Aphasiology*, vol. 16, no. 4–6, pp. 635–645, 2002.

[14] A. Ardila, F. Ostrosky-Solís, and B. Bernal, "Cognitive testing toward the future: The example of Semantic Verbal Fluency (ANIMALS)," *International Journal of Psychology*, vol. 41, no. 5, pp. 324–332, 2006.

[15] A. Acevedo, D. A. Loewenstein, W. W. Barker et al., "Category fluency test: Normative data for English- and Spanish-speaking elderly," *Journal of the International Neuropsychological Society*, vol. 6, no. 7, pp. 760–769, 2000.

[16] M. Rosselli, R. Tappen, C. Williams, J. Salvatierra, and Y. Zoller, "Level of education and category fluency task among Spanish speaking elders: number of words, clustering, and switching strategies," *Aging, Neuropsychology, and Cognition*, vol. 16, no. 6, pp. 721–744, 2009.

[17] A. K. Troyer, "Normative data for clustering and switching on verbal fluency tasks," *Journal of Clinical and Experimental Neuropsychology*, vol. 22, no. 3, pp. 370–378, 2000.

[18] A. K. Troyer, M. Moscovitch, and G. Winocur, "Clustering and switching as two components of verbal fluency: evidence from younger and older healthy adults," *Neuropsychology*, vol. 11, no. 1, pp. 138–146, 1997.

[19] J. E. Fisk and C. A. Sharp, "Age-related impairment in executive functioning: updating, inhibition, shifting, and access," *Journal of Clinical and Experimental Neuropsychology*, vol. 26, no. 7, pp. 874–890, 2004.

[20] A. K. Ho, B. J. Sahakian, T. W. Robbins, R. A. Barker, A. E. Rosser, and J. R. Hodges, "Verbal fluency in Huntington's disease: a longitudinal analysis of phonemic and semantic clustering and switching," *Neuropsychologia*, vol. 40, no. 8, pp. 1277–1284, 2002.

[21] C. Raboutet, H. Sauzéon, M.-M. Corsini, J. Rodrigues, S. Langevin, and B. N'Kaoua, "Performance on a semantic verbal fluency task across time: dissociation between clustering, switching, and categorical exploitation processes," *Journal of Clinical and Experimental Neuropsychology*, vol. 32, no. 3, pp. 268–280, 2010.

[22] A. K. Troyer, M. Moscovitch, G. Winocur, L. Leach, and M. Freedman, "Clustering and switching on verbal fluency tests in Alzheimer's and Parkinson's disease," *Journal of the International Neuropsychological Society*, vol. 4, no. 2, pp. 137–143, 1998.

[23] P. M. Roberts and G. Le Dorze, "Semantic organization, strategy use, and productivity in bilingual semantic verbal fluency," *Brain and Language*, vol. 59, no. 3, pp. 412–449, 1997.

[24] M. Rosselli, A. Ardila, K. Araujo et al., "Verbal fluency and repetition skills in healthy older Spanish-English bilinguals," *Applied Neuropsychology*, vol. 7, no. 1, pp. 17–24, 2000.

[25] M. Rosselli, A. Ardila, J. Salvatierra, M. Marquez, L. Matos, and V. A. Weekes, "A cross-linguistic comparison of verbal fluency tests," *International Journal of Neuroscience*, vol. 112, no. 6, pp. 759–776, 2002.

[26] D. Bethlehem, J. de Picciotto, and N. Watt, "Assessment of verbal fluency in bilingual Zulu-English speakers," *South African Journal of Psychology*, vol. 33, no. 4, pp. 236–240, 2003.

[27] S. Pekkala, M. Goral, J. Hyun, L. K. Obler, T. Erkinjuntti, and M. L. Albert, "Semantic verbal fluency in two contrasting languages," *Clinical Linguistics and Phonetics*, vol. 23, no. 6, pp. 431–445, 2009.

[28] D. Adrover-Roig, N. Galparsoro-Izagirre, K. Marcotte, P. Ferré, M. A. Wilson, and A. Inés Ansaldo, "Impaired L1 and executive control after left basal ganglia damage in a bilingual Basque-Spanish person with aphasia," *Clinical Linguistics and Phonetics*, vol. 25, no. 6-7, pp. 480–498, 2011.

[29] M. Kambanaros and K. K. Grohmann, "Profiling performance in L1 and L2 observed in Greek-English bilingual aphasia using the Bilingual Aphasia Test: a case study from Cyprus," *Clinical Linguistics and Phonetics*, vol. 25, no. 6-7, pp. 513–529, 2011.

[30] M. Kambanaros, L. Messinis, and E. Anyfantis, "Action and object word writing in a case of bilingual aphasia," *Behavioural Neurology*, vol. 25, no. 3, pp. 215–222, 2012.

[31] S. Kiran and R. Iakupova, "Understanding the relationship between language proficiency, language impairment and rehabilitation: evidence from a case study," *Clinical Linguistics and Phonetics*, vol. 25, no. 6-7, pp. 565–583, 2011.

[32] M. I. Koumanidi Knoph, "Language assessment of a Farsi-Norwegian bilingual speaker with aphasia," *Clinical Linguistics and Phonetics*, vol. 25, no. 6-7, pp. 530–539, 2011.

[33] M. L. Senaha and M. A. de Mattos Pimenta Parente, "Acquired dyslexia in three writing systems: study of a Portuguese-Japanese bilingual aphasic patient," *Behavioural Neurology*, vol. 25, no. 3, pp. 255–272, 2012.

[34] M. Tschirren, M. Laganaro, P. Michel et al., "Language and syntactic impairment following stroke in late bilingual aphasics," *Brain and Language*, vol. 119, no. 3, pp. 238–242, 2011.

[35] P. M. Roberts and L. Deslauriers, "Picture naming of cognate and non-cognate nouns in bilingual aphasia," *Journal of Communication Disorders*, vol. 32, no. 1, pp. 1–23, 1999.

[36] M. L. Muñoz and T. P. Marquardt, "Picture naming and identification in bilingual speakers of Spanish and English with and without aphasia," *Aphasiology*, vol. 17, no. 12, pp. 1115–1132, 2003.

[37] L. A. Edmonds and S. Kiran, "Confrontation naming and semantic relatedness judgements in Spanish/English bilinguals," *Aphasiology*, vol. 18, no. 5-7, pp. 567–579, 2004.

[38] L. A. Edmonds and S. Kiran, "Effect of semantic naming treatment on crosslinguistic generalization in bilingual aphasia," *Journal of Speech, Language, and Hearing Research*, vol. 49, no. 4, pp. 729–748, 2006.

[39] S. Kiran, E. Pena, L. Bedore, and L. Sheng, "Evaluating the relationship between category generation and language use and proficiency," in *Proceedings of the Donostia Workshop on Neurobilingualism*, San Sebastian, Spain, 2010.

[40] M. Paradis, *Bilingual Aphasia Test*, Lawrence Erlbaum Associates, New Jersey, NJ, USA, 1st edition, 1989.

[41] H. Goodglass, E. Kaplan, and S. Weintraub, *Boston Naming Test*, Lea & Febiger, Philadelphia, Pa, USA, 1983.

[42] G. Dell, D. Gagnon, M. Martin, E. Saffran, and M. Schwartz, "Lexical access in aphasic and nonaphasic speakers," *Psychological Review*, vol. 104, no. 4, pp. 801–838, 1997.

8

Variations in the Presentation of Aphasia in Patients with Closed Head Injuries

Dara Oliver Kavanagh,[1] Conor Lynam,[1] Thorsten Düerk,[1] Mary Casey,[2] and Paul W. Eustace[1]

[1] *Department of Surgery, Mayo General Hospital, Castlebar, Co Mayo, Ireland*
[2] *Department of Radiology, Mayo General Hospital, Castlebar, Co Mayo, Ireland*

Correspondence should be addressed to Dara Oliver Kavanagh, dara_kav@hotmail.com

Academic Editor: Raul Coimbra

Impairments of speech and language are important consequences of head injury as they compromise interaction between the patient and others. A large spectrum of communication deficits can occur. There are few reports in the literature of aphasia following closed head injury despite the common presentation of closed head injury. Herein we report two cases of closed head injuries with differing forms of aphasia. We discuss their management and rehabilitation and present a detailed literature review on the topic. In a busy acute surgical unit one can dismiss aphasia following head injury as behaviour related to intoxication. Early recognition with prolonged and intensive speech and language rehabilitation therapy yields a favourable outcome as highlighted in our experience. These may serve as a reference for clinicians faced with this unusual outcome.

1. Introduction

Closed head injury may result in a wide range of speech and language deficits ranging from total loss of interpersonal communication to minor flaws in word selection. They constitute a significant workload in the acute hospital setting.

Aphasia is a recognised yet under reported sequela of closed head injury. It is defined as impairment of comprehension or production of language in written or spoken forms due to an acquired lesion of the dominant cerebral hemisphere. There are many types of aphasia ranging from nonfluent (Broca's) aphasia, which is characterised by slow and incorrectly articulated speech to fluent (Wernicke's) aphasia in which the patient exhibits well-articulated speech, which lacks meaning. Broca's area as described by the French pathologist Pierre Broca lies in areas 44 and 45 of Brodman in the inferior frontal gyrus of the dominant cerebral hemisphere, usually the left cerebrum. Injury to this area will produce a Broca's aphasia [1]. Broca's (motor) aphasia is associated with a deficit in speech production or language output, often accompanied by a deficit in written communication. The patient is aware of the impairment. Wernicke's area, as described by the

German Neurologist Karl Wernicke, lies in the posterior part of area 22 in the superior temporal, gyrus of the left cerebral hemisphere. Wernicke's (sensory) aphasia is characterised by impaired comprehension of spoken and written words, associated with effortless, articulated but paraphasic, speech and writing. Circumlocution can be a feature. More aggressive forms are characterised by incomprehensible speech. The patient is frequently unaware of the deficit. The speech centres are linked by the arcuate fasciculus. This curves around the posterior end of the lateral fissure within the white matter deep to the supramarginal gyrus [2].

The current series represents the experience of a district general hospital. Over 2000 annual referrals are evaluated in the emergency department. Of these, two hundred and seventy-one (range 251–317) met the criteria for acute admission to the Surgical Unit based on Advanced Trauma Life Support (ATLS) guidelines. Nine (range 9–12) patients were transferred to the National Neurosurgical Centre at Beaumont Hospital for more detailed neurosurgical management. Herein, we report two differing forms of aphasia following significant closed head injuries with favourable outcomes.

2. Case 1

A 27-year-old english-speaking right-handed Irish male was involved in a road traffic accident in which he was projected thirty meters from his motorbike following a head-on collision with an approaching vehicle at 1700 hours. He was wearing a helmet and full protective clothing. On arrival in the accident and emergency department at 1830 hours his Glasgow coma scale (GCS) was 4/15. He was intubated and ventilated. His pupils were equal and reactive to light. His vital signs were within normal limits. He had bilateral periorbital haematomas (Racoon eyes) and a right-sided hemiparesis.

Computed Axial Tomography (CT) scan as shown in Figure 1 revealed an intracerebral haemorrhage in the left temporal lobe corresponding to Wernicke's area. Other radiological findings included fractures of the base of the right thumb, the right radial styloid, the right ulnar styloid, the radial and ulnar diaphyses, and comminuted fractures of the right humerus and femur. Following discussion with the National Neurosurgical Centre he underwent operative fixation of his orthopaedic injuries. He was managed initially in the intensive care unit and was gradually weaned off sedation. His GCS returned to 15/15 on the 16th day. He had significant expressive difficulties (Wernicke's aphasia). His speech was fluent but contained paraphasias and jargon. He was unaware of these abnormalities. He was unable to read text aloud and understand written language. A speech and language assessment reported severe comprehensive difficulties. The patient gave inaccurate yes/no answers to either personal or general orientation questions. He required extra-verbal cues to facilitate auditory comprehension. His lack of awareness of his reduced communicative abilities resulted in frustration. It was difficult to ascertain whether semantic memory compromise was evident. At the time of discharge his receptive aphasia had improved slightly and he was referred for further speech and language rehabilitation. A formal psychological evaluation was unavailable. He was seen at two-week intervals by the speech therapist. His speech and language improved but he demonstrated decreased attention and tangential speech with compromised reading ability (40% reading comprehension of single words). He also had a significant reduction in fluency with pronunciation difficulties and circumlocution. His receptive function was unaffected. His short-term memory was also impaired. Categorisation and odd-one-out activities were used to stimulate semantic processing and representations. At six-month follow-up his fluency of speech had improved significantly. He was able to construct complete sentences with occasional circumlocution. His comprehension of single words improved to 90%. He produced errors only during higher level semantic tasks. He continues to improve.

3. Case 2

A 32-year-old english-speaking right-handed intoxicated Irish male presented following a fall onto a concrete path with a GCS score of 9/15. Both pupils were equal and reactive

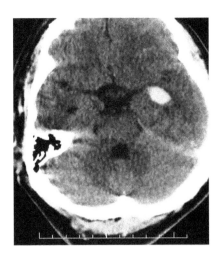

FIGURE 1: There is an area of high attenuation involving the left temporal lobe anterosuperiorly corresponding with Wernicke's area.

to light. His blood alcohol levels were 383 mcg per litre, which clouded the clinical picture (a serum alcohol level >80 mcg per litre is equivalent to 2 units of alcohol). His vital signs were within normal limits. He had multiple facial abrasions and a soft tissue swelling on the left occipital region and blood was seen emanating from his left ear. Auroscopy revealed haemotympanum. He was commenced on prophylactic intravenous antibiotics. CT brain (Figure 2) demonstrated a haematoma of the left frontal, temporal and parietal lobes superimposed upon a previous haematoma along with subarachnoid extension with slight midline shift to the right and evidence of air in the posterior cranial fossa. The National Neurosurgical Centre recommended supportive therapy and serial clinical assessments. The following morning his GCS deteriorated to 7/15 and he was intubated and ventilated. A right-sided hemiparesis was noted. His pupils and haemodynamic parameters were unchanged. A follow-up CT brain was unchanged. He was transferred to National Neurosurgical Unit in view of this clinical deterioration. A craniotomy was performed with evacuation of the temporal lobe haematoma and insertion of an intracranial pressure monitor. He was extubated on the 14th postoperative day and initially obeyed commands. He returned to our institution for further rehabilitation. Initially he had features of a motor aphasia (Broca's). He was able to respond nonverbally by blinking his eyelids. Assessment of auditory comprehension was difficult but appeared intact. As his clinical condition improved his expressive capabilities improved but did not fully recover. After 12 weeks he successfully made his first verbal response. He was transferred to the National Rehabilitation Centre. At 3-month follow-up he had ongoing circumlocution and reported difficulty with reading and writing. He reported persistence of posttraumatic amnesia. His mobility problems related to hemiparesis had resolved and he was independent in all activities of daily living.

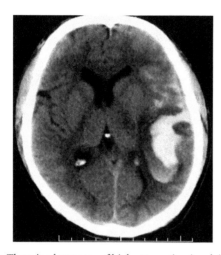

FIGURE 2: There is a large area of high attenuation involving the left frontal, temporal and parietal lobes incorporating Broca's area with subarachnoid extension and fresh haemorrhage in the suprasellar cistern.

4. Discussion

Aphasia is the primary language abnormality in adults and has multiple causes including trauma, infection, brain tumours, hypoxia, and obstructive hydrocephalus. Although the association between language disorders and head trauma has been known for millenniums, descriptions of such cases were scarce until World Wars I and II, when head injuries were, for the most part, penetrating wounds [1]. In contrast with these aphasias secondary to penetrating wounds, there are still few detailed descriptions of aphasia after closed head injuries. They can be challenging clinically. The absence of significant other neurological signs can result in cases being misdiagnosed as a transient ischemic attack or cerebrovascular accident [3]. They can be dismissed as intoxication, confusion, and psychosis or even malingering. In particular it has been noted that fluent aphasia can be elusive to nonneurologically orientated physicians [4]. The availability of a neurologist allows detection of more subtle deficits. The incidence of language disturbance is 1 per 1000 emergency referrals. They highlight the clinical challenge one is sometimes faced with when initially evaluating the intoxicated head injured patient. They reinforce the need to determine the mechanism of injury and thereby an appropriately high index of suspicion. The cases presented in this paper illustrate clear examples of both motor and sensory aphasias associated with a closed head injury and provide a guide to clinicians as to the presentation, management, and prognosis of such cases.

The severity of head injury can be scored on numerous parameters such as GCS on arrival, neurological deficit, and/or CT findings. One of the most consistent prognostic markers used in the medical literature is the presence of posttraumatic amnesia (PTA), where PTA for longer than one week predicts a severe head injury. There has been a growing debate in the neuropsychiatric literature on the question of whether patients who sustain a blunt head injury can develop symptoms of acute stress disorder (ASD) and posttraumatic stress disorder (PTSD). These are typically characterised by fear and intrusive recollections of the event. Speech deficits do not tend to be a major component of these sequelae. Over the last few years there have been many publications in the field of military medicine reporting cases of mild traumatic head injury due to blasts experiencing [5–7]. PTSD is less evident in the setting of severe head injury as described in the current series. Data disputing an association between traumatic brain injury and PTSD comes from Warden et al. among others [8]. He examined 47 patients with moderately severe TBI and found that although a minority of subjects endorsed the avoidance and autonomic arousal symptoms of PTSD, none reported any reexperiencing. A study of victims of road traffic accidents reached similar conclusions after finding a dearth of PTSD symptoms in a subgroup of patients who had briefly lost consciousness [9]. Feinstein et al. report symptoms of PTSD in a sample of head-injured patients assessed within a couple of months of injury and stratified for severity of head injury on the basis of duration of PTA. However, when PTA extended beyond one hour, symptoms of reexperiencing the traumatic event (intrusive phenomena) and avoidant behaviour occurred significantly less often. We need to recognize that irrespective of the mechanism involved, symptoms of PTSD may occur across the full range of head injury severity and demand our prompt attention [10].

Subtle changes in speech can also be evident. The spontaneous speech of head injured patients can be inappropriate in length, confused, lacking informational content, and slow. Language deficits may not be the sole cause for impairments in discourse. Normal discourse also requires adequate social and cognitive abilities, and these abilities are frequently impaired in closed head injured patients. The prognosis for recovery of language functioning is good but residual deficits, especially in naming, may persist over many years. Subjective reports of language problems in head injured patients are not as frequent as the reports of memory problems.

Aphasia associated with head injury can develop hours or even weeks after the initial precipitating event. It is most commonly associated with right blunt orbito-frontal trauma with a contre-coup left temporo-parietal injury [3, 11, 12]. This type of impact imparts a shearing force to the head which causes motion of the cerebral hemispheres within the closed cranium. Peripheral areas are more susceptible to direct impact with the cranium.

Menon et al. describe their experience with 31 consecutive patients with closed head injuries over a two-year period. The mean age was 36 years old. They demonstrated that poor outcome in relation to speech occurred more frequently in the presence of severe head injury (GCS < 8) on arrival or a prolonged comatosed state (>132 hours). Both patients in the current series had similar ages and had GCS scores of 4 and 9, respectively. Paradoxically case 1 (GCS = 4) had a better functional outcome. However, case 1 was comatosed for 72 hours while case 2 was comatosed for 168 hours perhaps explaining the differing functional outcomes [13]. Overall, communication disability tends to recover well especially during the first 6 months and to a lesser extent over the next three years regardless of severity of the injury [14–16]. Dahlberg et al. identified a volunteer sample of 52 people with closed head injury who were at least 1 year post injury [17]. They had received rehabilitation and had persistent social communication deficits one year post injury. Patients were randomised to receive treatment or not. Subjects who received social communication skills training had improved communication skills that were maintained on follow-up. Overall life satisfaction for participants was improved. In fact, it has been suggested that recovery can continue up to 10 years [18]. Few cases recover their premorbid status. Alajouanine et al. report a more favourable outcome with posttraumatic aphasias than with aphasias related to cerebrovascular disease.

Even mild brain injury (GCS > 12) can result in subtle long-term impairment of speech. Whelan et al. compared a detailed language profile of a 19-year-old woman, 2 years following a mild brain injury with a matched normative cohort of 10 participants with no neurological impairment. Deficits in attention, lexical access, complex lexical-semantic manipulation, response monitoring, and organization were revealed. Thus lending support for the hypotheses pertaining to neuronal fallout mechanisms within the frontal lobes as a consequence of mild neurological insult [19]. Others have proposed that long-term speech deficits and other functional deficits have therapeutic potential other than speech therapy. It has been hypothesised that "idle" or "recoverable" injured neurons may be evaluated with SPECT imaging prior to administration of hyperbaric oxygen. These were subsequently evaluated with SPECT imaging post therapy, demonstrating perfusion. This hypothesis has not gained popularity despite initial enthusiasm. Early goal directed therapy in the treatment of the trauma patients with adequate cerebral oxygenation and prevention of hypotension is paramount to ensure a patient reaches a stage, where rehabilitation is possible [20]. Future work is essential to optimise outcome from this socially debilitating deficit as the incidence of blunt trauma due to motor vehicle injuries continues to rise.

5. Conclusion

Patients who sustain closed head injuries are susceptible to a variety of functional and psychological impairments. Speech is one of the cardinal factors that determine the outcome of a prolonged illness and intensive rehabilitation. It determines whether one can integrate into daily life at home and at work. These cases highlight that despite significant initial deficits in speech and language following closed head injuries favourable long-term outcomes can be achieved with prolonged and intensive rehabilitation.

References

[1] S. Nishio, N. Takemura, Y. Ikai, and T. Baba, "Sensory aphasia after closed head injury," Journal of Clinical Neuroscience, vol. 11, no. 4, pp. 442–444, 2004.

[2] M. J. T. Fitzgerald, Neuroanatomy, Basic and Clinical, WB Saunders, 3rd edition, 1996.

[3] S. O. Dell, R. Batson, D. L. Kasdon, and T. Peterson, "Aphasia in subdural hematoma," Archives of Neurology, vol. 40, no. 3, pp. 177–179, 1983.

[4] J. L. Stone, J. R. Lopes, and R. A. Moody, "Fluent aphasia after closed head injury," Surgical Neurology, vol. 9, no. 1, pp. 27–29, 1978.

[5] M. Vukovic, J. Vuksanovic, and I. Vukovic, "Comparison of the recovery patterns of language and cognitive functions in patients with post-traumatic language processing deficits and in patients with aphasia following a stroke," Journal of Communication Disorders, vol. 41, no. 6, pp. 531–552, 2008.

[6] S. W. Hoffman and C. Harrison, "The interaction between psychological health and traumatic brain injury: a neuroscience perspective," Clinical Neuropsychologist, vol. 23, no. 8, pp. 1400–1415, 2009.

[7] R. D. Vanderploeg, H. G. Belanger, and G. Curtiss, "Mild traumatic brain injury and posttraumatic stress disorder and their associations with health symptoms," Archives of Physical Medicine and Rehabilitation, vol. 90, no. 7, pp. 1084–1093, 2009.

[8] D. L. Warden, L. A. Labbate, A. M. Salazar, et al., "Posttraumatic stress disorder in patients with traumatic brain injury and amnesia for the event?" The Journal of Neuropsychiatry & Clinical Neurosciences, vol. 9, no. 1, pp. 18–22, 1997.

[9] R. Mayou, B. Bryant, and R. Duthie, "Psychiatric consequences of road traffic accidents," British Medical Journal, vol. 307, no. 6905, pp. 647–651, 1993.

[10] A. Feinstein, S. Hershkop, D. Ouchterlony, A. Jardine, and S. McCullagh, "Posttraumatic amnesia and recall of a traumatic event following traumatic brain injury," The Journal of Neuropsychiatry & Clinical Neurosciences, vol. 14, no. 1, pp. 25–30, 2002.

[11] W. A. Lishman, "Psychiatric disability after head injury: the significance of brain damage," Proceedings of the Royal Society of Medicine, vol. 59, no. 3, pp. 261–266, 1966.

[12] M. Groher, "Language and memory disorders following closed head trauma," Journal of Speech and Hearing Research, vol. 20, no. 2, pp. 212–223, 1977.

[13] E. B. Menon, S. Ravichandran, and E. S. Tan, "Speech disorders in closed head injury patients," Singapore Medical Journal, vol. 34, no. 1, pp. 45–48, 1993.

[14] K. M. Heilman, A. Safran, and N. Geschwind, "Closed head trauma and aphasia," Journal of Neurology Neurosurgery and Psychiatry, vol. 34, no. 3, pp. 265–269, 1971.

[15] M. R. Bond and D. N. Brooks, "Understanding the process of recovery as a basis for the investigation of rehabilitation for the brain injured," Scandinavian Journal of Rehabilitation Medicine, vol. 8, no. 3-4, pp. 127–133, 1976.

[16] T. Najenson, L. Mendelson, I. Schechter, C. David, N. Mintz, and Z. Groswasser, "Rehabilitation after severe head injury," Scandinavian Journal of Rehabilitation Medicine, vol. 6, no. 1, pp. 5–14, 1974.

[17] C. A. Dahlberg, C. P. Cusick, L. A. Hawley, et al., "Treatment efficacy of social communication skills training after traumatic brain injury: a randomized treatment and deferred treatment controlled trial," Archives of Physical Medicine and Rehabilitation, vol. 88, no. 12, pp. 1561–1573, 2007.

[18] T. Alajouanine, P. Castaigne, F. Lhermitte, R. Escourolle, and B. De Ribaucourt, "43 cases of post traumatic aphasia: anatomical and clinical data and evolutionary aspects," L'Encéphale, vol. 46, no. 1, pp. 1–45, 1957.

[19] B.-M. Whelan, B. E. Murdoch, and N. Bellamy, "Delineating communication impairments associated with mild traumatic brain injury: a case report," *Journal of Head Trauma Rehabilitation*, vol. 22, no. 3, pp. 192–197, 2007.

[20] R. A. Neubauer, S. F. Gottlieb, and N. H. Pevsner, "Hyperbaric oxygen for treatment of closed head injury," *Southern Medical Journal*, vol. 87, no. 9, pp. 933–936, 1994.

9

Production of Verb Tense in Agrammatic Aphasia

Yasmeen Faroqi-Shah[1] and Laura Friedman[2]

[1]*University of Maryland, College Park, MD, USA*
[2]*University of Wisconsin-Madison, Madison, WI, USA*

Correspondence should be addressed to Yasmeen Faroqi-Shah; yfshah@umd.edu

Academic Editor: Annalena Venneri

In a majority of languages, the time of an event is expressed by marking tense on the verb. There is substantial evidence that the production of verb tense in sentences is more severely impaired than other functional categories in persons with agrammatic aphasia. The underlying source of this verb tense impairment is less clear, particularly in terms of the relative contribution of conceptual-semantic and processing demands. This study aimed to provide a more precise characterization of verb tense impairment by examining if there is dissociation *within* tenses (due to conceptual-semantic differences) and an effect of experimental task (mediated by processing limitations). Two sources of data were used: a meta-analysis of published research (which yielded 143 datasets) and new data from 16 persons with agrammatic aphasia. Tensed verbs were significantly more impaired than neutral (nonfinite) verbs, but there were no consistent differences between past, present, and future tenses. Overall, tense accuracy was mediated by task, such that picture description task was the most challenging, relative to sentence completion, sentence production priming, and grammaticality judgment. An interaction between task and tense revealed a past tense disadvantage for a sentence production priming task. These findings indicate that verb tense impairment is exacerbated by processing demands of the elicitation task and the conceptual-semantic differences between tenses are too subtle to show differential performance in agrammatism.

1. Introduction

Agrammatic aphasia is a cluster of language symptoms following damage to left hemisphere peri-Sylvian regions. The core feature of agrammatic aphasia is severely impoverished sentence production: utterances consist of words strung together in an ungrammatical sequence, or, at best, simple canonical sentences (e.g., subject-verb-object, in English) [1–3]. Associated features of agrammatic aphasia include difficulty with verbs (both in sentences and single word recall) and with grammatical morphemes (both free standing and inflectional morphemes) [4–6]. Further, many (but not all) individuals with agrammatic speech production present with asyntactic comprehension [7]. This refers to difficulty interpreting syntactically complex sentences (such as the passive and object relatives), particularly in semantically reversible contexts. Whereas sentence production impairment is the

hallmark of agrammatism, there is considerable individual variability in the extent of other deficits [8, 9].

Crosslinguistically, sentence production difficulty in agrammatism is often characterized by exceptional difficulty producing certain types of morphosyntactic structures, such as tense marking, relative to other structures, such as agreement and mood marking (e.g., in English [10–13]; in Hebrew [14]; in German [15]; but see conflicting results in [16]; in Spanish [17, 18]; in Dutch [19, 20]; and in Greek [21–23]). The crosslinguistic data also demonstrate that the tense disadvantage occurs even when morphological complexity of the verb, such as affixation and additional free grammatical morphemes, is held constant [12, 24].

Accounts of Tense Production Deficits in Agrammatism. Given the prominence of tense deficits in agrammatism, there are numerous tense-centric theoretical accounts of agrammatic aphasia [12, 14, 15, 19]. Some accounts are based on the syntactic theory of generative grammar [25, 26], according to which certain syntactic nodes hosting complementizers, along with other functional categories, such as tense, are located higher in the syntactic tree than others (e.g., agreement, mood, and aspect). Syntactic accounts, such as the Tree Pruning Hypothesis [14], propose that this hierarchical relation between different morphosyntactic categories is observed in agrammatism such that impairment of any node implies impairment of higher nodes as well (also [27]). However, most crosslinguistic evidence has found that breakdown of functional categories does not consistently follow the pattern of morphosyntactic hierarchy (e.g., [11, 15, 16, 21, 22, 28]).

Another family of tense-centric accounts of agrammatism draws attention to the fact that, in addition to its morphosyntactic role, verb tense interfaces with semantics of the event. That is, tense is an "interpretable" syntactic feature [15]. The tense underspecification account suggests that the tense features (+/− PAST) are inadequately specified in functional category representations of persons with agrammatic aphasia [15]. The diacritical encoding hypothesis uses the framework of language production models and claims difficulties in encoding semantic components of the message onto inflectional morphology [12]. Some of these accounts include difficulties with verb aspect, which also represents the temporal state of an event [21, 22, 29–31]. Support for differentiating between the syntactic and semantic components of tense morphology in agrammatic individuals comes from better performance on knowledge of syntactic well-formedness constraints (e.g., *is walking* versus *will walking*) than on knowledge of the correspondence between verb forms and their time reference [12, 32]. The argument is that, unlike subject-verb agreement which serves a purely morphosyntactic function, verb tense serves a deictic function because it refers to the temporal relationship between the event being described and the time of speaking [12, 19, 21, 23, 31, 33, 34]. These deictic implications of verb tense confer additional conceptual-semantic complexity in its formulation and comprehension.

Further, it has been proposed that reference to past events is "selectively impaired in agrammatic aphasia" such that past tense and perfect aspect are particularly challenging to produce compared to present tense and imperfect aspect [19, 35]. In the past discourse linking hypothesis (PADILIH), Bastiaanse and colleagues have used the greater temporal mismatch between speaking and event time to explain why their studies found worse performance on sentences eliciting the past compared to the present [19, 29, 36, 37]. Other authors have noted that discourse linking is not restricted to past events and that reference to the future is also discourse linked because it is a projection to a subsequent time point [38–40]. It is currently unclear whether production of past events is actually selectively impaired or worse than present and future events because numerous other studies have reported no accuracy differences between past and present/future [11, 12, 15, 16, 20, 21, 31, 41, 42].

There are other theoretical accounts of agrammatic production that identify more general sources of difficulty. Resource limitation accounts propose an interaction between computational demands and performance success, especially for syntactic computations. Empirical support for the impact of limited processing resources on agrammatic production comes from the influence of task complexity [20] and syntactic complexity ([33]; see [43] for agrammatic comprehension). Kok and colleagues [20] demonstrated the effect of task complexity on successful production of verb morphology by comparing success on two tasks: sentence completion, in which participants had to inflect a nonfinite verb, and anagram ordering, in which individual words had to be sequenced to form a sentence *and* the verb had to be inflected. Agrammatic participants performed significantly worse on the more demanding anagram ordering task, suggesting an effect of computational load in computation of verb morphology.

To summarize, a variety of accounts have been proposed to characterize the difficulty with production of tense morphology in agrammatism. A majority of the more recent accounts incorporate some reference to the semantics of time, one account proposes further dissociation within temporal morphology, and some accounts allow for performance variation based on task processing demands. Although there is substantial empirical data on agrammatic tense production, it is unclear whether tense morphology is modulated by semantic (or any other) variables. Actually, a precise characterization of the verb tense deficit in agrammatism is lacking, which is a precursor to developing a reasonable explanation for this symptom. This study aims to further our understanding of verb tense performance by investigating the influence of two variables: temporal category (past, present, or future) and the elicitation task. A brief background on these two variables is provided before describing the current study.

Linguistic and Cognitive Representation of Time. Most of the world's languages have some mechanism of conveying the unfolding of events over time. *Tense* refers to grammatically expressing the linear temporal relationship between the moment of speaking (S), the moment of the event (E) being described, and, sometimes, another reference point (R) [44–47]. For example, a sentence such as "*He signed the papers*" refers to an event that occurred before the time of speaking as shown in Table 1 (adapted from [45]). This contrasts with simple present, where the speaking and event time are simultaneous, and simple future, where the speaking time occurs prior to the event (see Table 1). Time is also depicted by *aspect*, which refers to the temporal distribution of an event, irrespective of event time [48]. Hence, an event may be completed or perfective as in "*He had signed the papers/He has signed the papers*," or ongoing and imperfective as in "*He was signing the papers/He will be signing the papers*" (Table 1). There is considerable variability across and within languages in how tense and aspect are denoted [49]. For example, tense and aspect may be conflated, occurring on the same grammatical morpheme, which is frequently a verb affix; for example, the preterite −*Ó* in Spanish refers to past and perfect. Within a language, some tense/aspectual morphemes may be conjugated on the verb, while others may be free morphemes (often preverbal auxiliaries), such as the contrast between

TABLE 1: Temporal distance (—) between speaking time (S), reference time (R), and event time (E).

Tense/aspect	Example	Linear ordering
Simple past	He signs the papers	E, R—S
Simple present	He signed the papers	S, E, R
Simple future	He will sign the papers	S—R, E
Present progressive	He will be signing the papers	S, E~, R
Past progressive	He was signing the papers	E~, R—S
Present perfect	He has signed the papers	E—S, R
Past perfect	He had signed the papers	E—R—S

present/past (*verb + s/verb + d*) and future in English (*will + verb*) as shown in Table 1. Temporal relationships may also be represented by adverbs, such as "*earlier*" or "*yesterday.*" And in some languages such as Mandarin, adverbs are the only mechanism of denoting temporal relations.

Empirical investigations of tense and aspect processing in neurologically healthy adults have mostly examined the extent to which different sentences evoke a mental representation of the event. For example, Magliano and Schleich [50] presented participants with short stories in which a critical sentence in the middle of the story described an action in past progressive or simple past (*Stephanie was changing/changed the flat tire*). This was followed by a yes/no probe question about the event (*Is Stephanie back on her way to the airport yet?*). Participants' response times to the probe questions were faster for imperfective sentences. Similar findings of faster response times for imperfectives compared to perfectives have been found in sentence-picture matching [51], self-paced reading [52], and action execution [53]. As for tense processing, monitoring for a word following a short paragraph was faster when the target word occurred in sentences with present tense compared to past tense in Spanish [54]. The interaction between tense and aspect was examined using six sentence types (past and present tense in simple, progressive, and perfect aspects) in a sensibility judgment task [55]. Response times were influenced by verb aspect, with the fastest responses to simple aspect (. . .*closed/closes the drawer*) and slowest responses to perfectives (. . .*had closed/has closed the drawer*), but there was no effect of verb tense on response times.

To summarize, data from neurologically healthy adults shows that sentences in the imperfective aspect are consistently faster than perfectives, while present tense is faster than past only when aspect is held constant as in Carreiras et al. [54]. This implies that mental representation of events is constructed more rapidly if the event is construed as ongoing (imperfective) and occasionally if there is temporal overlap between speaking time and event time (present tense). This finding is often explained using the embodied cognition framework, according to which sentence processing evokes sensorimotor simulations, which are probably more vivid for ongoing events [50, 51]. It is also possible that evoking mental representations of completed events (i.e., past/perfective sentences) places additional demands on memory for perceptual

details [40]. Using a similar logic of perceptual detail, evoking mental representations of the future (tense) is argued to be more challenging (greater abstraction) because the event has not yet occurred [40, 56, 57]. For example, Pinker's [57] analysis of the semantics of tense differentiates between events that have actually taken place or are ongoing (*realis*) and events that are hypothetical and future (*irrealis*). Empirical findings have been consistent with less robust (or more abstract) mental simulation of future events compared to past and present events: Zwaan et al. [58] found faster self-paced reading times for present and past events compared to future events. A functional neuroimaging study that compared past, present, and future tense sentences in Hebrew found activation of sensorimotor regions for past and present but not for future [40]. Sentences in the future activated ventromedial prefrontal regions, and this contrast between activation instances for present/past versus future sentences mirrored that for concrete versus abstract sentences.

On the basis of these processing differences observed in healthy adults, one could predict that verb tense/aspect with a greater mismatch between speaking, event, and reference times will be more vulnerable to the effects of aphasia (Table 1). In other words, past and future tenses and perfect aspect would be more impaired than present tense and imperfective aspect. Few studies of agrammatism have compared perfect and imperfect aspect to glean the influence of grammatical aspect on sentence production (but see [29]). In some studies, tense and aspect are conflated, where simple past was compared with present progressive, rather than with simple present ([36] in English). In some languages, controlling the aspect made for unnatural sentences for one tense more than other tenses: in Dutch, past tense is typically used with perfect aspect, and requiring participants to use imperfect aspect with past tense was unnatural [20]. In order to examine if conceptual differences (i.e., in the mental representation of temporal reference) can account for tense impairment, it is important to first determine if there is a consistent performance difference between tenses.

Influence of Elicitation Task on Performance. A variety of experimental paradigms have been used to examine performance on tense and other functional categories. The primary motivation behind the various paradigms is to manipulate which specific tense needs to be produced and to indicate this unambiguously to the participant. The various paradigms are also used to circumvent cooccurring limitations in lexical retrieval, word ordering, and working memory. For instance, participants may be required to complete a sentence fragment, the word to be inflected is provided, or multiple words are given in a forced-choice structure [10–12, 15, 59]. This sentence completion paradigm places minimal lexical retrieval demands, hence tapping the morphosyntactic abilities of the person (e.g., *Yesterday the man. . .the apple* [eats, will eat, ate]). However, this task is unnatural and does not approximate *sentence production* in its true sense [20]. In the sentence production priming paradigm used in the Test for Assessing Reference of Time (TART, [60]), the tester models the target sentence for a photograph and the participant is required to produce the same sentence structure for a slightly different photograph (*For this picture you can say the man ate the apple. For this picture you can say the man...* [peeled the apple]). In this paradigm, lexical retrieval demands are minimal, while there may be additional demands on working memory compared to the sentence completion task. Notably, the photographs used to elicit past tense in TART often do not portray the target action because the action has already been completed. For example, the photograph of a man looking at an empty plate is used to elicit "*The man ate an apple.*" In contrast, the photographs used to elicit present tense portray the action, which could potentially create confoundedness of greater difficulty for past tense sentences.

A third experimental task provides the content words in random order and requires the participant to produce the sentence; a picture may or may not be used to aid the sentence [20, 42]. This task places additional demands on syntactic formulation of the entire sentence but more closely approaches sentence production. Finally, grammaticality or goodness judgment tasks are used, which tap linguistic competence rather than sentence production [15, 32, 61]. A crucial calculation in the interpretation of grammaticality judgment performance is an estimate of response bias, which refers to the possibility that a participant may push the *yes* or *no* button for most of the trials showing little sensitivity to the construct being tested [62]. Unfortunately, most studies on tense deficits using grammaticality judgment task fail to report measures of response bias (A-prime or D-prime). Further, some studies have only reported findings on the ungrammatical sentences (e.g., [63], for Arabic) while others compute accuracy over both grammatical and ungrammatical sentences. The role of task differences on performance was demonstrated by Kok et al. [20] for a group of Dutch speaking aphasic participants: performance on the same set of sentences was worse when the entire sentence had to be produced compared to sentence completion, in which only the inflected verb had to be produced. Therefore, in order to determine whether true differences exist across tenses, it is important to evaluate whether tense differences exist irrespective of the experimental manipulation.

To summarize, a theoretical account of tense impairment in agrammatism has been elusive. An impairment in the cognitive representation of time or in conveying temporal reference on verb morphology is currently a promising explanation. In order to evaluate this explanation and further our understanding of tense deficits, we need to unambiguously determine whether there are differences in performance across tenses that supersede crosslinguistic and methodological differences.

The Present Study. This study aims to provide a more precise characterization of verb tense impairment in agrammatism by examining whether there is dissociation within tenses such that any one tense is more impaired than other tenses. The basis for this question comes from (1) sentence comprehension findings in healthy adults, showing that a mismatch between the time of speaking and the occurrence of an event (as in past tense and perfect aspect) incurs a processing cost compared to when the speaker refers to an ongoing event (as in present tense and imperfect aspect), (2) recent mixed

findings across studies about the relative impairment of past tense compared to other tenses, and (3) the potential for methodological differences to produce different patterns of results across studies. In the present study, we compared whether past, present, and future tenses show differential levels of impairment using two approaches: (1) a meta-analysis of prior studies and (2) reporting new data from a group of 16 persons with agrammatic aphasia using an experimental task that has been relatively less frequently used in prior research. Given that there have been numerous studies of verb tense in agrammatism, it is worth reexamining the substantial corpus of existing data to synthesize the existing findings on tense deficits. It should be noted that although different tenses have been elicited in prior studies, a comparison of tenses was not the primary focus of most prior studies (with the exception of Bastiaanse et al. series using TART). Rather, the focus was on comparing tense with other functional categories (e.g., [10, 14, 16, 28]). Hence, the meta-analysis of prior studies presents these data in a different perspective.

This study posed two research questions. First, we asked whether there is a difference in performance across different tenses (past versus present versus future) and relative to tense-neutral stimuli. Although we initially intended to compare perfect versus imperfect aspect, this question could be not addressed because of the small number of studies reporting aspectual comparisons. Second, we asked whether there is an interaction between elicitation task and tense performance. Based on sentence comprehension data from healthy adults and the differences in speaking and event time for past tense, we hypothesized that past tense performance would be worse than present tense. Additionally, we hypothesized that this difference would be evident in select experimental tasks, such as sentence production, but not in grammaticality judgment, due to the more complex computation demands of production tasks.

2. Meta-Analysis of Published Studies

2.1. Methods. Published articles in English peer-reviewed journals reporting investigations of functional categories in persons with aphasia were identified using the key words aphasia, morphology, functional categories, tense, aspect, and agrammatism. The electronic databases used for the search were Science Citation Index, Medline (PubMed), PsycInfo, and Academic Search Premier. In addition, citation lists of identified articles were combed for further sources. The search was restricted to research studies available electronically between 1980 and December 2013. This identified approximately 60 potential articles for the review. We read the abstracts of these articles for relevance and excluded several studies based on content, narrowing the number of potential articles down to 38. After reading the text of the remaining articles, we used the following predetermined inclusionary criteria to identify the studies that qualified for the meta-analysis: (1) the study reported original data from participants with a diagnosis of sudden onset aphasia (not progressive); (2) language profile was described in adequate detail to determine the specific symptomatology of the patient (e.g., agrammatic, nonfluent, and fluent); (3) native language performance was reported, although the participants could have been multilingual; (4) the study provided data for individual participants, with breakdown of scores for the various tense types; (5) task/stimuli were presented as sentences (i.e., not single word repetition); (6) syntactically simple sentences were used to minimize the confoundedness of syntactic complexity with tense encoding; (7) the study presented data for some combination of past, present, and future tense stimuli to enable within-subjects comparison (i.e., not just a single tense). Other functional categories such as agreement, mood, and aspect were noted. Reports that duplicated data, such as conference proceedings and full articles, were included only once. Multiple datasets from individual patients were included in the meta-analysis only if each dataset was original to the study. This resulted in a final set of twelve articles, with 106 individual participants totaling to 143 datasets.

2.1.1. Coding and Data Analyses. All studies were coded for language of testing, description of aphasia profile, description of lesion information, the experimental task, response type (e.g., verbal), the number of stimuli used, raw scores, proportion accuracy, and the conclusions of the authors. Four different experimental tasks were used in the studies reviewed: (1) sentence production priming (SPP), in which participants were provided with a pair of pictures (the examiner modeled the target sentence for the first picture and asked the participant to describe the second picture using a sentence similar to the model); (2) sentence completion (SC), in which participants were required to complete a sentence fragment using the correct form of a given word from among a forced choice (e.g., *Speaks, Speak,* and *Spoke*); (3) sentence production using picture description (SPPic), in which participants had to describe a single picture using temporal adverbs as prompts (e.g., *Yesterday, Nowadays*); (4) grammaticality judgment (GJ), in which the participant decided whether a sentence was grammatical or not. The stimuli used in studies were coded for tense into the following four categories: present, past, future, and neutral. Tense-neutral stimuli were verbs that did not require tense marking, because these occurred in embedded clauses or other syntactic structures where tense was marked on a different main verb (e.g., Sheila wanted to *move* to the city). When different aspects were used, such as simple present and present progressive, these were combined into the corresponding tense. For studies where raw scores were not reported, these were computed from the relevant figures or percentage scores. Raw scores were converted to standard (z) scores and statistically compared using analysis of variance with tense and task as the independent factors.

2.2. Results. The meta-analysis included 143 total datasets elicited from seven different languages. Sixty-eight of these datasets included three tenses (past, present, and future) while 75 datasets included two of the three tenses. Sentence completion task was used for 60 of the datasets, sentence production priming was used for 49 datasets, sentence production with pictures was used for eight datasets, and 26 datasets used grammaticality judgment. The average age of participants was 55.53 years and the average time following onset was 74.85 months. Of the 106 participants, 77 were male, 26 were female, and three participants' gender was not reported. The majority of the patients had a left cerebrovascular accident. Individual participant data from each study are presented in Table 2. Across all tasks, accuracy was 47.7% (SD = 13.2).

Analysis of variance revealed statistically significant main effects of sentence type ($F(3, 392) = 16.78$, $p < 0.001$) and task ($F(3, 382) = 9.35$, $p < 0.001$). There was no significant task by tense interaction ($p > 0.05$). Tamhane's post hoc statistics indicate that the past, present, and future tenses are all significantly lower in accuracy than neutral tense ($p < 0.001$). Additionally, past tense and present tense were significantly different from each other ($p = 0.01$; mean difference = −0.9; SE = 0.028). The difference between past versus future and present versus future was not statistically significant ($p > 0.05$). Tamhane's post hoc analyses of the effect of experimental tasks showed that the sentence production picture task was significantly less accurate than the three other tasks: sentence production priming, sentence completion, and grammaticality judgment ($p < 0.001$).

In order to more precisely examine tense differences for each task, four separate ANOVAs were computed for each task. An a priori decision was made to use a more conservative p value to account for the multiple ANOVAs (one-fourth of 0.05 yielded a significant p of <0.0125). No significant differences were found between the tenses for sentence production with pictures ($F(2, 21) = 0.121$, $p = 0.88$, $p > 0.05$), grammaticality judgment ($F(2, 59) = 2.8$, $p > 0.05$), or sentence completion ($F(2, 134) = 2.7$, $p > 0.05$). There was a significant difference across tenses for sentence production priming ($F(3, 159) = 9.3$, $p < 0.001$). Post hoc comparisons with Bonferroni correction revealed significantly lower accuracy of past and future sentences compared to neutral sentences (mean difference > 0.25, $p < 0.0125$). Comparisons of present versus neutral (mean difference = 0.2, $p = 0.04$) and past versus present tense (mean difference = 0.17, $p = 0.02$) approached the significance threshold of $p < 0.0125$.

To summarize, the analysis of 143 published datasets revealed an effect of task on overall accuracy: sentence production with pictures yields significantly lower accuracy than the other three experimental tasks. While there was consistent superiority for neutral sentences over tensed sentences, the differences between past, present, and future sentences were inconsistent across tasks and primarily driven by the sentence production priming task.

3. Tense Production Using Elicited Picture Description

In order to further inform our understanding of how persons with agrammatic aphasia are affected by verb tense, we examined previously acquired data from participants reported in our prior studies [32, 66–71]. The data reported here are from the intake protocol regularly used to determine the presence of agrammatic aphasia. Although these data were

TABLE 2: Individual participant data from the studies included in the meta-analysis.

Reference	Language	Task and response	Patient	Age/gender	MPO	Lesion/aphasia	Number correct/total			
							Neutral	Past	Present	Future
Bastiaanse et al. (2004), page 129 (Table 1) [64]	Dutch	SC, verbal	B1	NR	NR	NR/Broca's		14/30	18/30	
			B2	NR	NR	NR/Broca's		15/30	21/30	
			B3	NR	NR	NR/Broca's		18/30	10/30	
Bastiaanse et al. (2011), pages 671-672 (Appendices 3 and 4) [36]	Chinese	SPP, verbal	C1	42/M	127	LCVA/Broca's	20/20	11/20	1/20	1/20
			C2	22/M	96	TBI/Broca's	20/20	12/20	6/20	6/20
			C3	50/M	97	LCVA/Broca's	19/20	13/20	13/20	18/20
			C4	41/M	180	LCVA/Broca's	18/20	0/20	1/20	0/20
			C5	55/M	92	LCVA/Broca's	20/20	10/20	7/20	16/20
			C6	65/M	204	LCVA/Broca's	20/20	2/20	0/20	0/20
			C7	33/M	125	LCVA/Broca's	16/20	16/20	20/20	20/20
			C8	55/M	156	LCVA/Broca's	17/20	5/20	8/20	8/20
			C10	50/M	177	LCVA/Broca's	20/20	0/20	0/20	0/20
			C11	51/M	212	LCVA/Broca's	11/20	5/20	6/20	4/20
	English	SPP, verbal	E1	52/M	59	LCVA/Broca's	16/20	13/20	19/20	19/20
			E2	47/M	55	LCVA/Broca's	17/20	18/20	16/20	20/20
			E3	64/M	220	LCVA/Broca's	19/20	3/20	13/20	12/20
			E4	48/F	23	LCVA/Broca's	3/20	12/20	19/20	12/20
			E5	53/M	108	LCVA/Broca's	20/20	12/20	18/20	19/20
			E6	60/F	61	LCVA/Broca's	19/20	6/20	4/20	7/20
			E7	53/M	43	RCVA/Broca's	20/20	14/20	19/20	19/20
			E8	68/M	180	TBI/Broca's	3/20	4/20	12/20	4/20
			E9	74/F	36	LCVA/Broca's	16/20	6/20	20/20	19/20
			E10	54/M	39	LCVA/Broca's	18/20	17/20	16/20	13/20
			E11	58/M	226	LCVA/Broca's	16/20	12/20	20/20	20/20
			E12	37/M	34	LCVA/Broca's	4/20	2/20	12/20	3/20
	Turkish	SPP, verbal	T1	68/M	2	LCVA/Broca's		6/20	17/20	17/20
			T2	54/M	5	LCVA/Broca's		4/20	9/20	7/20
			T3	49/F	84	LCVA/Broca's		11/20	15/20	18/20
			T4	43/F	4	LCVA/Broca's		10/20	20/20	15/20
			T5	68/M	1	LCVA/Broca's		11/20	16/20	18/20
			T6	39/F	7	LCVA/Broca's		10/20	16/20	18/20
			T7	65/M	12	LCVA/Broca's		6/20	4/20	17/20
			T8	59/M	2	LCVA/Broca's		13/20	18/20	18/20
Clahsen and Ali (2009), page 446 (Table 6) [11]	English	SC, pointing	BG	36/M	60*	NR/Broca's		8/10	10/10	
			JS	65/M	96*	NR/Broca's		2/10	8/10	
			KC	78/M	96*	NR/Broca's		3/10	6/10	
			RC	77/M	24*	NR/Broca's		8/10	6/10	
			JP	68/M	60*	NR/Broca's		10/10	7/10	
			KS	66/M	18*	NR/Broca's		9/10	6/10	
			PB	82/M	36*	NR/Broca's		6/10	5/10	
			BM	52/M	36*	NR/Broca's		9/10	5/10	
			BR	82/M	36*	NR/Broca's		6/10	3/10	
		GJ, verbal	BG			NR/Broca's		15/20	15/20	
			JS			NR/Broca's		11/20	12/20	
			KC			NR/Broca's		13/20	12/20	
			RC			NR/Broca's		12/20	11/20	
			JP			NR/Broca's		18/20	16/20	
			KS			NR/Broca's		13/20	14/20	
			PB			NR/Broca's		17/20	11/20	
			BM			NR/Broca's		11/20	11/20	
			BR			NR/Broca's		15/20	14/20	

TABLE 2: Continued.

Reference	Language	Task and response	Patient	Age/gender	MPO	Lesion/aphasia	Number correct/total			
							Neutral	Past	Present	Future
Dickey et al. (2008) [61]	English	GJ, keyboard	A01	60/F	180*	NR/Broca's	27/30	26/60	16/30	11/30
			A02	63/F	132*	NR/Broca's	28/30	44/60	29/30	29/30
			A03	56/F	168*	NR/Broca's	26/30	36/60	14/30	15/30
			A04	57/F	48*	NR/Broca's	21/30	27/60	14/30	15/30
			A05	50/M	108*	NR/Broca's	18/30	24/60	14/30	14/30
			A06	36/F	36*	NR/Broca's	19/30	30/60	14/30	14/30
			A07	68/F	144*	NR/Broca's	23/30	32/60	14/30	16/30
			A08	66/F	84*	NR/Broca's	23/30	39/60	16/30	18/30
			A09	57/M	48*	NR/Broca's	7/30	4/60	4/30	4/30
			A10	36/F	24*	NR/Broca's	24/30	37/60	14/30	14/30
Dragoy and Bastiaanse (2013), page 127 (Appendix 3) [29]	Russian	SPP, verbal	1	31/F	35	NR/nonfluent		27/40	15/20	8/20
			2	32/F	29	NR/nonfluent		31/40	11/20	10/20
			3	33/F	20	NR/nonfluent		20/40	12/20	5/20
			4	35/M	70	NR/nonfluent		23/40	17/20	5/20
			5	36/F	29	NR/nonfluent		19/40	17/20	10/20
			6	46/M	16	NR/nonfluent		20/40	14/20	15/20
			7	68/M	29	NR/nonfluent		20/40	15/20	18/20
Duman and Bastiaanse (2008), page 9 (Appendix A)[37]	Turkish	SC, verbal	B1	66/F	2.5	LCVA/agrammatic	16/30			15/30
			B2	70/M	6	LCVA/agrammatic	4/30			18/30
			B3	44/F	16	LCVA/agrammatic	14/30			13/30
			B4	47/F	26	LCVA/agrammatic	11/30			12/30
			B5	40/M	28	LCVA/agrammatic	13/30			15/30
			B6	26/F	120	TBI/agrammatic	16/30			16/30
			B7	75/M	20	LCVA/agrammatic	3/30			19/30
Faroqi-Shah and Thompson (2004), page 492 (Figure 3) [42]	English	SPPi, verbal	CH	56/M	90	LCVA/Broca's		2/17	14/17	1/17
			MK	54/M	12	LCVA/Broca's		3/17	0/17	7/17
			MR	44/F	45	LCVA/Broca's		3/17	13/17	2/17
			JP	65/M	30	LCVA/Broca's		1/17	2/17	10/17
			MD	62/M	120	LCVA/Broca's		3/17	9/17	3/17
			JO	69/M	88	LCVA/Broca's		7/17	3/17	7/17
			RH	64/M	100	LCVA/Broca's		9/17	2/17	0/17
			LD	52/F	14	LCVA/Broca's		6/17	0/17	10/17
Faroqi-Shah and Thompson (2007), pages 139-140 (Figures 2 and 3) [12]	English	SC, verbal	B1	55/M	156*	LCVA/Broca's	11/15	19/30	14/15	
			B2	58/M	48*	LCVA/Broca's	15/15	18/30	14/15	
			B3	59/M	168*	LCVA/Broca's	13/15	17/30	5/15	
			B4	64/M	60*	LCVA/Broca's	10/15	17/30	8/15	
			B5	55/F	108*	LCVA/Broca's	11/15	14/30	5/15	
			B6	68/M	120*	LCVA/Broca's	9/15	11/30	5/15	
			B7	59/F	96*	LCVA/Broca's	12/15	12/30	10/15	
			B8	63/M	108*	LCVA/Broca's	12/15	20/30	5/15	
			B9	66/M	60*	LCVA/Broca's	14/15	14/30	8/15	
			B10	55/F	72*	LCVA/Broca's	15/15	11/30	5/15	
		SC, verbal	B1			LCVA/Broca's		3/15	10/15	7/15
			B2			LCVA/Broca's		5/15	8/15	8/15
			B3			LCVA/Broca's		10/15	8/15	9/15
			B4			LCVA/Broca's		5/15	9/15	10/15
			B5			LCVA/Broca's		7/15	10/15	7/15
			B6			LCVA/Broca's		8/15	7/15	7/15
			B7			LCVA/Broca's		8/15	5/15	8/15
			B8			LCVA/Broca's		8/15	8/15	9/15
			B9			LCVA/Broca's		3/15	9/15	8/15
Fyndanis et al. (2012), page 1140 (Table 4) [31]	Greek	SC, verbal	GT	44/M	4.5	LCVA/agrammatic	8/21	12/16	12/19	
			GL	59/M	38	LCVA/agrammatic	2/21	8/16	9/19	

TABLE 2: Continued.

Reference	Language	Task and response	Patient	Age/gender	MPO	Lesion/aphasia	Number correct/total			
							Neutral	Past	Present	Future
Jonkers and de Bruin (2009), page 1265 (Appendix 2) [65]	Dutch	SC, verbal	B1	80/M	26	NR/Broca's		16/20	14/20	
			B2	70/M	12	NR/Broca's		2/20	16/20	
			B3	41/F	4	NR/Broca's		10/20	19/20	
			B4	55/M	3	NR/Broca's		19/20	19/20	
			B5	41/M	49	NR/Broca's		5/20	2/20	
			B6	78/M	42	NR/Broca's		11/20	20/20	
			B7	41/F	4	NR/Broca's		16/20	13/20	
Nanousi et al. (2006), pages 220, 223, and 226 (Tables 6, 8, and 10) [21]	Greek	SPP, verbal	DS	66/M	48*	LCVA/Broca's		31/60	25/60	15/30
			PA	61/M	48*	LCVA/Broca's		29/60	32/60	13/30
			ZA	41/M	36*	LCVA/Broca's		25/60	19/60	9/30
			AS	38/M	96*	LCVA/Broca's		28/60	28/60	15/30
			AJ	55/M	72*	LCVA/Broca's		23/60	19/60	10/30
			RS	46/M	108*	LCVA/Broca's		25/60	25/60	12/30
		SPP, verbal	DS			LCVA/Broca's	19/60			21/60
			PA			LCVA/Broca's	23/60			32/60
			ZA			LCVA/Broca's	11/60			20/60
			AS			LCVA/Broca's	23/60			33/60
			AJ			LCVA/Broca's	2/60			18/60
			RS			LCVA/Broca's	15/60			25/60
		SC, verbal	DS			LCVA/Broca's	26/48	34/48	13/24	
			PA			LCVA/Broca's	34/48	35/48	11/24	
			ZA			LCVA/Broca's	25/48	27/48	12/24	
			AS			LCVA/Broca's	30/48	32/48	16/24	
			AJ			LCVA/Broca's	26/48	30/48	10/24	
			RS			LCVA/Broca's	29/48	27/48	14/24	
Wenzlaff and Clahsen (2004), page 64 (Table 4) [15]	German	SC, verbal	DB	58/F	276*	LCVA/Broca's		14/20	14/20	
			EL	49/F	264*	LCVA/Broca's		19/20	14/20	
			KM	84/F	24*	LCVA/Broca's		12/20	17/20	
			MH	59/M	180*	LCVA/Broca's		12/20	15/20	
			HM	66/M	144*	LCVA/Broca's		17/20	13/20	
			WH	70/M	192*	LCVA/Broca's		8/20	17/20	
			OP	69/M	24*	LCVA/Broca's		12/20	7/20	
		GJ, verbal	DB			LCVA/Broca's		10/20	10/20	
			EL			LCVA/Broca's		10/20	10/20	
			KM			LCVA/Broca's		12/20	11/20	
			MH			LCVA/Broca's		12/20	11/20	
			HM			LCVA/Broca's		18/20	17/20	
			WH			LCVA/Broca's		10/20	10/20	
			OP			LCVA/Broca's		10/20	10/20	

GJ: grammaticality judgment; LCVA: left cerebrovascular accident; MPO: months post onset; NR: not reported; RCVA: right cerebrovascular accident; SC: sentence completion; SPP: sentence production priming; SPPi: sentence production with picture description; TBI: traumatic brain injury; *months post onset calculated from years in the original study.

collected previously, these data have not been reported in any prior study or included in the meta-analysis reported in the previous section.

3.1. Methods

3.1.1. Participants. Sixteen participants (10 men, 6 women) with a medical history of left cerebrovascular accident were included in the study. The participants ranged in age from 39 to 70 years (mean = 54.06) and, at the time of testing,

and ranged from 14 to 163 months from onset of their left hemisphere damage (mean = 52.56). All participants were native speakers of English and premorbidly right-handed (except AP10 who was left-handed). None of the participants reported a history of any significant speech-language, psychiatric, or neurological diagnoses prior to the onset of left hemisphere damage. Demographic and language profiles of all sixteen participants are reported in Table 3. All participants provided informed consent prior to participation in the study.

TABLE 3: Demographic and language data of participants in the sentence production task.

Patient	Age, gender, hand	Educ. years	MPO	Aphasia	Western Aphasia Battery-Revised				Narrative speech analysis					
					AQ	Spont. Speech	Compr.	Naming	WPM	MLU	Prop. Sent.	Prop. Gram. Sent.	Open : Closed	Noun : Verb
AP1	59/M/R	24	29	Broca's	66.8	13	7.6	6.4	39.04	4.08	0.43	0.11	1.09	0.96
AP3	65/M/R	17	73	Broca's	65.9	11	8.8	6.1	24.67	5.76	0.52	0.31	1.15	1.7
AP5	64/F/R	19	75	Broca's	57.2	11	7.6	5.3	48.24	2.78	0.52	0.35	2.29	2.75
AP6	70/F/R	17	163	Broca's	65.9	14	6.35	7.8	53.44	3.68	0.22	0.1	1.26	5.25
AP8	55/F/R	17	114	Mixed	90.4	18	10	8.6	34.41	5.88	0.84	0.57	1.07	2.06
AP9	56/M/R	14	23	Broca's	83.6	15	9.5	7	60.3	5.89	0.8	0.63	0.9	1.87
AP10	40/M/L	18	115	Broca's	77.4	14	8.5	8.4	29.19	3.83	0.48	0.5	1.35	1.93
AP12	61/M/R	16	15	Broca's	57.2	11	6.6	6.5	68	5.4	0.76	0.36	0.67	0.61
AP14	44/M/R	19	14	Broca's	71.6	13	9.3	7.6	32.56	1.95	0.2	0	5	1.41
AP15	55/M/R	13	16	Mixed	80.5	13	9.45	8.6	75.82	3.41	0.36	0.39	1.8	4.23
AP17	44/F/R	17	15	Mixed	45.4	7	6.3	6	11.11	1.67	0.1	0	58	6.57
AP18	39/M/R	18	26	Broca's	71.8	13	6.8	8.5	36	3.16	0.36	0.5	1.1	5
AP19	55/M/R	19	14	Broca's	61.8	11	9.2	6.5	23.12	1.64	0.1	0	4.07	3.67
AP23	47/M/R	12	33	Broca's	68.8	11	7.9	7.1	13.76	2.68	0.18	0.44	1.18	1.79
AP24	62/F/R	15	61	Broca's	61.2	12	6.25	5.6	28.09	2.93	0.5	0.16	2.3	2.47
AP26	49/F/R	14	55	Mixed	80.3	15	9.05	8.5	31.63	31.24	0.1	0	6.1	5.5

AQ: aphasia quotient (max = 100); Compr.: comprehension score (max = 10); Noun : Verb: ratio of nouns to verbs; MLU: mean length of utterance in words; MPO: months post onset; Open : Closed: ratio of open to closed class words; Prop. Gram. Sent.: proportion of grammatically accurate sentences; Prop. Sent.: proportion of sentences; Spont. Speech: spontaneous speech; WPM: words per minute.

3.1.2. Background Speech, Language, and Cognitive Information. All participants were given a battery of speech and language tests and screening for hearing, visual, and cognitive status. This included elicitation of narratives of the cookie theft picture and selected narrative story cards [72], Western Aphasia Battery-Revised (WAB-R, [73]), inventory of articulatory characteristics of the Apraxia Battery of Adults [74], verbal and nonverbal agility subtests of the Boston Diagnostic Aphasia Examination-3rd Edition (BDAE-3rd Edition, [75]). All participants had a clinical profile of Broca's aphasia (nonfluent speech, relatively preserved comprehension, and impaired repetition). Four participants (AP8, AP15, AP17, and AP26) were unclassifiable as per the subtest scores of the WAB-R although they had nonfluent speech because they were relatively mildly impaired in terms of overall severity. Narrative speech data revealed a morphosyntactic production profile consistent with agrammatism for all sixteen participants with low proportion of complete sentences, low proportion of grammatically accurate sentences, and high noun : verb ratio (see Table 3). None of the participants had significant verbal apraxia, defined as fewer than four features in the apraxia inventory of Apraxia Battery for Adults-2nd Edition and score higher than 8 on the verbal agility subtest of BDAE-3rd Edition. All participants could successfully read single words and passed a hearing screening at 40 dBHL in both ears (except AP1 who used hearing aids) and a vision screen (at least 20/40 corrected or uncorrected vision in both eyes).

3.1.3. Materials and Procedure. The stimuli consisted of twenty black and white line drawings of transitive ($N = 15$) and intransitive ($N = 5$) action sequences. There were an equal number of regular and irregular verbs (ten each). A sequence of three action pictures, depicting future, present, and past tense, was used (see Figure 2). In order to elicit sentences with different tenses, a variety of temporal adverbs were printed on one of the three pictures in the sequence (*Yesterday, In a moment, Tomorrow, Right now,* and *Nowadays*). The nouns and verb pertaining to the action were also printed on each picture to alleviate the impact of lexical retrieval failure on sentence production. Participants were instructed to describe each picture using a single sentence beginning with the temporal adverb and using the words printed on the picture. Two practice items were provided during which the experimenter clarified the use of present progressive and simple present for "*Right now*" and "*Nowadays,*" respectively. Five sentences each were elicited in the simple present (verbs), present progressive (is verb-*ing*), simple past (verb-*ed*), and future tense (will verb) (total $N = 20$). There was no response time limit and participants were allowed to self-correct spontaneously.

Responses were transcribed by the experimenter during the session and later scored for accuracy. The final self-corrected response was scored as correct if it unambiguously matched the target tense elicited by the appropriate adverb. Hence, a response such as "*Yesterday the girl will peel the potatoes*" is scored as incorrect. Word order errors (e.g., noun-noun-verb as in "*Yesterday...the girl...potatoes...peeling*") were ignored and only verb morphology was scored for

TABLE 4: Individual tense accuracy data for sentence production task.

Participant	Past	Present		Future
		Simple	Progressive	
AP1	0.4	0.8	0.0	0.0
AP3	0.0	0.0	0.2	1.0
AP5	0.0	0.0	0.0	0.0
AP6	0.0	0.0	0.0	1.0
AP8	0.6	0.0	0.6	0.2
AP9	1.0	0.0	0.2	0.0
AP10	0.0	0.3	0.0	1.0
AP12	0.2	0.0	0.4	0.0
AP14	0.0	0.0	0.8	0.4
AP15	0.0	0.0	1.0	0.0
AP17	0.0	0.0	0.6	0.2
AP18	0.2	0.0	0.0	0.0
AP19	0.0	0.0	0.2	1.0
AP23	0.4	0.4	0.2	0.0
AP24	0.2	0.0	0.0	0.0
AP26	0.0	0.6	0.6	0.0
Mean (SD)	0.19 (0.28)	0.22 (0.3)		0.30 (0.4)

accuracy of tense. In order to be consistent with studies that were included in the meta-analysis of the previous section of this paper, scores of simple present and present progressive were combined to get the present tense score (the pattern of performance across tenses was unchanged irrespective of whether present tense was considered separately (simple present versus present progressive) or when these two scores were combined). Accuracy scores for each participant for each tense were converted to standard (z) scores for statistical analysis. Errors were categorized into *incorrect tense* (e.g., *peels* for *peeled*), *unmarked* in which the verb lacks any clear tense or agreement marking (e.g., *peeling* or *peel produced without an auxiliary or modal*), *others*, which included omissions of the verb, and *no responses*.

3.2. Results. One-way analysis of variance found no main effect of tense (mean (SD) present = 0.22 (0.19), past = 0.19 (0.29), and future = 0.30 (0.43), $F(2, 45) = 0.535$, $p = 0.59$). Planned pairwise comparisons yielded no significant differences between any two tense categories ($p > 0.05$). Individual participant data, which are provided in Table 4, show that overall most participants had zero accuracy for at least one tense. Four participants scored 100% on future tense (AP3, AP6, AP10, and AP19), and two participants each scored 100% on present and past tense (AP15 and AP9). The distribution of errors for individual participants is given in Table 5. There was preponderance of *unmarked verb* substitutions (75.4% of all errors) across all participants, with the exception of AP9. *Incorrect tense* errors were produced 15.8% of the time and *other* errors were produced in 8.7% of the instances.

TABLE 5: Distribution of errors for each participant in the sentence production task.

Participant	Incorrect tense	Unmarked	Others	Total errors
AP1	7	7	0	14
AP3	0	13	1	14
AP5	0	19	1	20
AP6	0	14	1	15
AP8	4	8	1	13
AP9	12	1	1	14
AP10	4	3	0	7
AP12	5	9	3	17
AP14	0	10	4	14
AP15	0	15	0	15
AP17	0	15	1	16
AP18	2	16	1	19
AP19	0	11	3	14
AP23	3	9	3	15
AP24	1	17	1	19
AP26	0	14	0	14

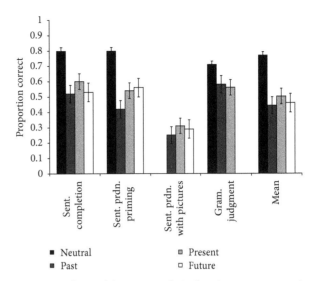

FIGURE 1: Findings of the meta-analysis showing mean proportion accuracy sorted by tense and experimental task. The number of datasets for each tense is $N = 42$ (neutral), $N = 143$ (past), $N = 130$ (present) and $N = 81$ (future).

4. Discussion

The aim of this study was to further characterize the tense deficit in persons with agrammatic aphasia in terms of differential impairment across temporal reference and experimental task. This was achieved in two ways: by synthesizing the existing published evidence on tense deficits in 143 datasets of persons with agrammatic aphasia and by contributing new data from sixteen participants using a picture description task. The obvious advantage of analyzing a large dataset, as was done in this study, is to minimize the influence of different sources of variability arising in small group studies: individual variability which can skew group averages, language-specific morphosyntactic patterns, and the experimental manipulations (task instructions, stimuli) which could inadvertently impact one experimental condition. There were three main findings of the meta-analysis. First, the aphasic participants were significantly impaired in the experimental tasks, with an overall accuracy of just 47%. Second, we found a significant effect of experimental task on performance accuracy. Third, there was no striking accuracy difference with respect to temporal reference, but with one exception: only in the sentence production priming task was the past tense worse than present and future tenses (by 12 and 14 percent, resp.). The new data from picture description found no difference among tense types, replicating the findings of the meta-analysis. In the following sections, we will consider the question of between-tense differences, followed by a discussion of the current understanding of verb tense impairment in agrammatism.

4.1. Is There a Differential Tense Impairment? As outlined in the Introduction, there were two compelling reasons to predict worse performance on past and future tense compared to present tense for agrammatic aphasic speakers. The first is a divergence between speaking time and reference time for past and future, but not present tense (Table 1, [44, 45, 47, 57]). Additionally, neurologically healthy speakers process sentences referring to ongoing events faster than completed or hypothetical events [50–55]. And developmentally, children acquire past tense later than present tense [76, 77] and show a past tense disadvantage in specific language impairment [78]. If these differences in temporal reference influenced sentence processing in agrammatism, we should have found a consistent disadvantage for past and future across all experimental tasks. This prediction was not confirmed. Moreover, if one were to argue that differences in processing temporal reference are subtle and observable only when agrammatic persons' syntactic mechanism is sufficiently taxed, then we should have observed the predicted pattern in the most challenging experimental task, sentence production with pictures. Unlike for sentence completion, priming, and grammaticality judgment, producing sentences with pictures task employs syntactic structure building in addition to computation of verb tense [20]. Not surprisingly, performance was 22 to 27 percent worse on sentence production with pictures compared to the other experimental tasks (Figure 1). However, the prediction of *differential* tense performance in this challenging task was not confirmed, both in the meta-analysis and new empirical data. Thus, this study found that although computation of verb tense was generally impaired in agrammatism, there was little variability among tense types for three out of four experimental tasks, including the task that had the lowest overall accuracy.

The reason for the past tense disadvantage specifically in the sentence production priming task is unclear [29, 36, 37, 64]. There are three noteworthy considerations in interpreting this result. First, the magnitude of the past tense disadvantage (12–14%) is relatively modest in comparison to the significant difficulty with computing tense (47% accuracy) in agrammatism. Hence, any theoretical

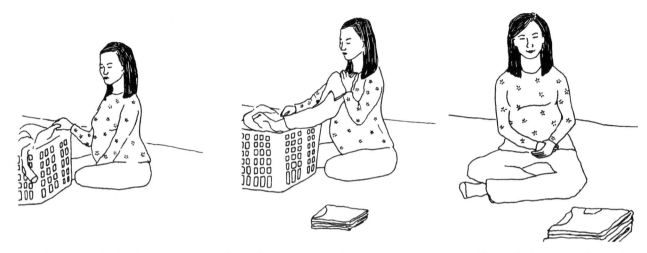

FIGURE 2: An example of a picture sequence used to elicit different tenses. The picture shows the action "folding." The action is about to begin in the first (future), ongoing in the second (present), and completed in the third (past) picture of the sequence.

account of agrammatism must account for the overarching tense difficulty foremost before accounting for the relative differences in a specific task. Second, given the broader pattern of a lack of differential tense performance in other experimental tasks, the most parsimonious explanation for the past tense disadvantage is the specific demands of the sentence production priming (SPP) task. The elicitation sentences used in SPP and sentence completion are analogous (e.g., Now the man is... [eating an apple]), but SPP also includes a precedent sentence (e.g., Now the man is peeling an apple) [29]. It is plausible that the need to mentally switch actions (*peeling* to *eating* in this example) increases processing demands, which are then specifically detrimental to completed actions because the stimulus pictures do not actually show the action. For instance, a sentence such as "*The man has poured the milk*" is elicited using a picture of a man sitting in front of a full glass of milk [60, 79]. Two other findings that are consistent with the SPP task-specific interpretation are a disadvantage for perfect aspect using the SPP task in which stimuli did not depict the action [29, 37] and a similar performance disadvantage in fluent (nonagrammatic) aphasia [29]. Further research is necessary to verify whether verb tense production in such pictured elicitation tasks is affected by the consistency with which the action is (not) depicted in the elicitation stimuli.

4.2. How Can We Characterize the Verb Tense Impairment in Agrammatism? Collective data from 122 persons with agrammatic aphasia (PWAA) analyzed in this study show (1) an overwhelming difficulty in production and processing of verb tense, (2) individual differences in accuracy of different tenses (see the appendix and Table 3), and (3) a hierarchy of task difficulty. The first finding reiterates the view that verb tense impairment is a *core* symptom of agrammatism. In fact, not a single PWAA showed unimpaired performance, although a handful scored well above chance (e.g., patients EL and HM in Wenzlaff [15], C7 in Bastiaanse et al. [36]; see the appendix). Other studies have reported that PWAA perform poorly on judgment of verb tense violations (e.g., *John

slept tomorrow), while they are sensitive to judgment of structural syntactic violations (e.g., *Father sleeping brother) [10, 12, 32, 80]. Further, accuracy of elicited tense production is found to correlate significantly with tense judgment in PWAA [32]. This greater difficulty of tense compared to structural syntactic judgments and correlation with sentence production further supports the centrality of verb tense difficulties to agrammatism.

Numerous theoretical accounts over the past two decades suggest a difficulty in the semantics to morphosyntax interface as the most parsimonious account of verb tense deficits of agrammatism. These include a distinction between interpretable and uninterpretable syntactic features [21, 23, 31], referential and nonreferential syntax [33], encoding message features onto morphosyntax [12], and mapping between functional and grammatical elements [3, 81].

The second noteworthy point of verb tense performance is the intraindividual variability across tense types; that is, many PWAA's accuracy was widely different across tenses (e.g., JS scored 0.3 and 0.8 for past and present tense, [11]; see the Appendix). Without comparisons with a control group, it is unclear whether any of these differences is an actual dissociation [82, 83]. In some instances, the small numbers of stimuli for each tense condition preclude meaningful statistical comparisons to examine neuropsychological dissociations. However, prior investigations have analyzed patterns of intraindividual variability for verb tense. It was found that PWAA's verb tense errors typically favor verb forms that are more accessible. That is, the target verb form is substituted by another verb form that is more frequent (hence more accessible) than the target [42, 84–86]. Further, individual participants tend to overuse a single verb form, giving a near-perfect accuracy for the verb tense corresponding to that verb form ([42]; see also Table 3). For example, AP9 in this study overused the past form (verb + ed) and AP15 overused progressive verbs, resulting in 100% accuracy for these tenses, but close-to-zero accuracy for other tenses (accuracy in Table 3 and substitution errors in Table 4). To summarize, the most likely source of individual variability in tense production is different strategies of verb form accessibility adopted by individual participants. That is, when faced with the challenge of transitioning from semantic representations to morphosyntactic representations, the agrammatic system resorts to using the most accessible elements. While the current data cannot directly address tense dissociations, future research comparing performance with a normal control group could help elucidate whether there are any dissociations among tense types.

Finally, we found a robust effect of task difficulty on accuracy, with significantly worse performance on overt production (sentence production priming and sentence production with pictures) compared to selection (grammaticality judgment and sentence completion). This task differential is consistent with the computational accounts of agrammatism proposed by Avrutin [38] and Kok et al. [20]. These accounts propose that mapping of conceptual-semantic representations onto morphosyntax involved in tense marking is challenging for PWAA, primarily because it involves more computations and strictly structural operations such as verb agreement. Further, the number of linguistic computations has an additive effect on performance [20]. It is noteworthy that Kok et al. [20] observed that a hierarchy of task difficulty is seen for most, but not all, PWAA (e.g., patients NU and WO in their study). Hence, computational load is one factor (but not the entire source) of the symptom complex of agrammatism.

4.3. Conclusions. The data accrued from this study and the past three decades of agrammatism research emphasize that difficulties in processing and producing verb tense are best considered as one of the crucial components of the symptom profile of agrammatism. While mapping of conceptual-semantic representations onto morphosyntax for tense marking is particularly challenging, this is likely to be mediated by processing limitations and accessibility of specific verb forms. At present, there is little evidence of a differential tense impairment; however, future research specifically aimed at examining double dissociations in individual participants and the effect of stimulus manipulations may shed more light on tense differentials. It is also crucial to establish whether a disadvantage for temporally complete events is a general pattern found across several populations or is a core characteristic of agrammatic aphasia, because a parsimonious theory of agrammatism really needs to account for symptoms that are unique to the condition. Data from other populations indicate that the disadvantage for past events is not unique to agrammatism and is found in healthy adults and children, fluent aphasia, and specific language impairment [29, 50–55, 76–78].

Disclosure

Findings from this study were presented at the 2013 Academy of Aphasia Conference in Lucerne, Switzerland.

Acknowledgments

The authors thank Melissa Stockbridge for assistance with data scoring and coding.

References

[1] L. Menn and L. Obler, Eds., *Agrammatic Aphasia: A Cross-language Narrative Sourcebook*, Benjamins, Amsterdam, The Netherlands, 1990.

[2] L. Menn and L. Obler, Eds., *Agrammatic Aphasia: A Cross-Language Narrative Sourcebook*, Benjamins, Amsterdam, The Netherlands, 1990.

[3] E. M. Saffran, M. F. Schwartz, and O. S. M. Marin, "The word order problem in agrammatism. II. Production," *Brain and Language*, vol. 10, no. 2, pp. 263–280, 1980.

[4] G. Miceli, M. C. Silver, G. Villa, and A. Caramazza, "On the basis for the agrammatic's difficulty in producing main verbs," *Cortex*, vol. 20, no. 2, pp. 207–220, 1984.

[5] E. M. Saffran, R. S. Berndt, and M. F. Schwartz, "The quantitative analysis of agrammatic production: procedure and data," *Brain and Language*, vol. 37, no. 3, pp. 440–479, 1989.

[6] L. B. Zingeser and R. S. Berndt, "Retrieval of nouns and verbs in agrammatism and anomia," *Brain and Language*, vol. 39, no. 1, pp. 14–32, 1990.

[7] D. Caplan and N. Hildebrandt, *Disorders of Syntactic Comprehension*, MIT Press, Cambridge, Mass, USA, 1988.

[8] R. Sloan Berndt, C. C. Mitchum, A. N. Haendiges, and J. Sandson, "Verb retrieval in aphasia: 1. Characterizing single word impairments," *Brain and Language*, vol. 56, no. 1, pp. 68–106, 1997.

[9] A. Caramazza, E. Capitani, A. Rey, and R. S. Berndt, "Agrammatic Broca's aphasia is not associated with a single pattern of comprehension performance," *Brain and Language*, vol. 76, no. 2, pp. 158–184, 2001.

[10] M. Arabatzi and S. Edwards, "Tense and syntactic processes in agrammatic speech," *Brain and Language*, vol. 80, no. 3, pp. 314–327, 2002.

[11] H. Clahsen and M. Ali, "Formal features in aphasia: tense, agreement, and mood in English agrammatism," *Journal of Neurolinguistics*, vol. 22, no. 5, pp. 436–450, 2009.

[12] Y. Faroqi-Shah and C. K. Thompson, "Verb inflections in agrammatic aphasia: encoding of tense features," *Journal of Memory and Language*, vol. 56, no. 1, pp. 129–151, 2007.

[13] M. W. Dickey, L. H. Milman, and C. K. Thompson, "Perception of functional morphology in agrammatic Broca's aphasia," *Brain and Language*, vol. 95, no. 1, pp. 82–83, 2005.

[14] N. Friedmann and Y. Grodzinsky, "Tense and agreement in agrammatic production: pruning the syntactic tree," *Brain and Language*, vol. 56, no. 3, pp. 397–425, 1997.

[15] M. Wenzlaff and H. Clahsen, "Tense and agreement in German agrammatism," *Brain and Language*, vol. 89, no. 1, pp. 57–68, 2004.

[16] F. Burchert, M. Swoboda-Moll, and R. De Bleser, "The left periphery in agrammatic clausal representations: evidence from German," *Journal of Neurolinguistics*, vol. 18, no. 1, pp. 67–88, 2005.

[17] M. J. Benedet, J. A. Christiansen, and H. Goodglass, "A cross-linguistic study of grammatical morphology in Spanish- and English-speaking agrammatic patients," *Cortex*, vol. 34, no. 3, pp. 309–336, 1998.

88

Aphasia: A Cognitive Neuropsychological Approach

[18] A. Gavarró and S. Martínez-Ferreiro, "Tense and agreement impairment in Ibero-romance," *Journal of Psycholinguistic Research*, vol. 36, no. 1, pp. 25–46, 2007.

[19] R. Bastiaanse, "Production of verbs in base position by Dutch agrammatic speakers: inflection versus finiteness," *Journal of Neurolinguistics*, vol. 21, no. 2, pp. 104–119, 2008.

[20] P. Kok, A. van Doorn, and H. Kolk, "Inflection and computational load in agrammatic speech," *Brain and Language*, vol. 102, no. 3, pp. 273–283, 2007.

[21] V. Nanousi, J. Masterson, J. Druks, and M. Atkinson, "Interpretable vs. uninterpretable features: evidence from six Greek-speaking agrammatic patients," *Journal of Neurolinguistics*, vol. 19, no. 3, pp. 209–238, 2006.

[22] S. Stavrakaki and S. Kouvava, "Functional categories in agrammatism: evidence from Greek," *Brain and Language*, vol. 86, no. 1, pp. 129–141, 2003.

[23] S. Varlokosta, N. Valeonti, M. Kakavoulia, M. Lazaridou, A. Economou, and A. Protopapas, "The breakdown of functional categories in Greek aphasia: evidence from agreement, tense, and aspect," *Aphasiology*, vol. 20, no. 8, pp. 723–743, 2006.

[24] S. Fix and C. K. Thompson, "Morphophonological structure and agrammatic regular/irregular past-tense production," *Brain and Language*, vol. 99, no. 1-2, pp. 166–167, 2006.

[25] N. Chomsky, *Lectures on Government and Binding*, Foris, Dordrecht, The Netherlands, 1981.

[26] J. Y. Pollock, "Verb movement, universal grammar and the structure of IP," *Linguistic Inquiry*, vol. 20, no. 3, pp. 365–424, 1989.

[27] H. Hagiwara, "The breakdown of functional categories and the economy of derivation," *Brain and Language*, vol. 50, no. 1, pp. 92–116, 1995.

[28] M. Lee, "Dissociations among functional categories in Korean agrammatism," *Brain and Language*, vol. 84, no. 2, pp. 170–188, 2003.

[29] O. Dragoy and R. Bastiaanse, "Aspects of time: time reference and aspect production in Russian aphasic speakers," *Journal of Neurolinguistics*, vol. 26, no. 1, pp. 113–128, 2013.

[30] A. Economou, S. Varlokosta, A. Protopapas, and M. Kakavoulia, "Factors affecting the production of verb inflections in Greek aphasia," *Brain and Language*, vol. 103, pp. 53–54, 2007.

[31] V. Fyndanis, S. Varlokosta, and K. Tsapkini, "Agrammatic production: interpretable features and selective impairment in verb inflection," *Lingua*, vol. 122, no. 10, pp. 1134–1147, 2012.

[32] Y. Faroqi-Shah and M. W. Dickey, "On-line processing of tense and temporality in agrammatic aphasia," *Brain and Language*, vol. 108, no. 2, pp. 97–111, 2009.

[33] S. Avrutin, "Weak syntax," in *Broca's Region*, Y. Grodzinsky and K. Amunts, Eds., pp. 49–62, Oxford University Press, New York, NY, USA, 2006.

[34] M. Wenzlaff and H. Clahsen, "Finiteness and verb-second in German agrammatism," *Brain and Language*, vol. 92, no. 1, pp. 33–44, 2005.

[35] R. Bastiaanse, "Why reference to the past is difficult for agrammatic speakers," *Clinical Linguistics & Phonetics*, vol. 27, no. 4, pp. 244–263, 2013.

[36] R. Bastiaanse, E. Bamyaci, C.-J. Hsu, J. Lee, T. Y. Duman, and C. K. Thompson, "Time reference in agrammatic aphasia: a cross-linguistic study," *Journal of Neurolinguistics*, vol. 24, no. 6, pp. 652–673, 2011.

[37] T. Y. Duman and R. Bastiaanse, "Time reference through verb inflection in Turkish agrammatic aphasia," *Brain and Language*, vol. 108, no. 1, pp. 30–39, 2009.

[38] S. Avrutin, "Comprehension of discourse-linked and non-discourse-linked questions by children and Broca's aphasics," in *Language and the Brain*, Y. Grodzinsky, L. Shapiro, and D. Swinney, Eds., pp. 295–315, Academic Press, San Diego, Calif, USA, 2000.

[39] V. Fyndanis, C. Manouilidou, E. Koufou, S. Karampekios, and E. M. Tsapakis, "Agrammatic patterns in Alzheimer's disease: evidence from tense, agreement, and aspect," *Aphasiology*, vol. 27, no. 2, pp. 178–200, 2013.

[40] M. Gilead, N. Liberman, and A. Maril, "The language of future-thought: an fMRI study of embodiment and tense processing," *NeuroImage*, vol. 65, pp. 267–279, 2013.

[41] K. Patterson and R. Holland, "Patients with impaired verb-tense processing: do they know that yesterday is past?" *Philosophical Transactions of the Royal Society B: Biological Sciences*, vol. 369, no. 1634, Article ID 20120402, 2014.

[42] Y. Faroqi-Shah and C. K. Thompson, "Semantic, lexical, and phonological influences on the production of verb inflections in agrammatic aphasia," *Brain and Language*, vol. 89, no. 3, pp. 484–498, 2004.

[43] M. Garraffa and N. Grillo, "Canonicity effects as grammatical phenomena," *Journal of Neurolinguistics*, vol. 21, no. 2, pp. 177–197, 2008.

[44] B. Comrie, *Tense*, Cambridge University Press, Cambridge, UK, 1985.

[45] N. Hornstein, "Towards a theory of tense," *Linguistic Inquiry*, vol. 8, pp. 521–557, 1977.

[46] H. C. van Riemsdijk and E. Williams, *Introduction to the Theory of Grammar*, MIT Press, Cambridge, Mass, USA, 1986.

[47] K. Zagona, "Some effects of aspect on tense construal," *Lingua*, vol. 117, no. 2, pp. 464–502, 2007.

[48] B. Comrie, *Aspect*, Cambridge University Press, Cambridge, UK, 1976.

[49] R. I. Binnick, Ed., *The Oxford Handbook of Tense and Aspect*, Oxford University Press, New York, NY, USA, 2012.

[50] J. P. Magliano and M. C. Schleich, "Verb aspect and situation models," *Discourse Processes*, vol. 29, no. 2, pp. 83–112, 2000.

[51] C. J. Madden and R. A. Zwaan, "How does verb aspect constrain event representations?" *Memory and Cognition*, vol. 31, no. 5, pp. 663–672, 2003.

[52] C. J. Madden and D. J. Therriault, "Verb aspect and perceptual simulations," *The Quarterly Journal of Experimental Psychology*, vol. 62, no. 7, pp. 1294–1303, 2009.

[53] B. Bergen and K. Wheeler, "Grammatical aspect and mental simulation," *Brain and Language*, vol. 112, no. 3, pp. 150–158, 2010.

[54] M. Carreiras, N. Carriedo, M. A. Alonso, and A. Fernández, "The role of verb tense and verb aspect in the foregrounding of information during reading," *Memory & Cognition*, vol. 25, no. 4, pp. 438–446, 1997.

[55] M. Payne and Y. Faroqi-Shah, "Mental representation of events: an investigation of agrammatic aphasia," *Procedia—Social and Behavioral Sciences*, vol. 94, pp. 155–156, 2013.

[56] R. J. Anderson and S. A. Dewhurst, "Remembering the past and imagining the future: differences in event specificity of spontaneously generated thought," *Memory*, vol. 17, no. 4, pp. 367–373, 2009.

[57] S. Pinker, *The Stuff of Thought: Language as a Window into Human Nature*, Viking, New York, NY, USA, 2007.

[58] R. A. Zwaan, L. J. Taylor, and M. Boer, "Motor resonance as a function of narrative time: further tests of the linguistic focus hypothesis," *Brain and Language*, vol. 112, no. 3, pp. 143–149, 2010.

[59] M. Penke and G. Westermann, "Broca's area and inflectional morphology: evidence from Broca's aphasia and computer modeling," *Cortex*, vol. 42, no. 4, pp. 563–576, 2006.

[60] R. Bastiaanse, R. Jonkers, and C. K. Thompson, *Test for Assessing Reference of Time (TART)*, University of Groningen, Groningen, The Netherlands, 2008.

[61] M. W. Dickey, L. H. Milman, and C. K. Thompson, "Judgment of functional morphology in agrammatic aphasia," *Journal of Neurolinguistics*, vol. 21, no. 1, pp. 35–65, 2008.

[62] D. M. Green and J. A. Swets, *Signal Detection Theory and Psychophysics*, John Wiley & Sons, New York, NY, USA, 1966.

[63] S. Diouny, "Tense/agreement in Moroccan Arabic: the tree-pruning hypothesis," *SKY Journal of Linguistics*, vol. 20, pp. 141–169, 2007.

[64] R. Bastiaanse, A. Sikkema, and R. van Zonneveld, "Verb inflection in Broca's aphasia: influence of movement, finiteness, tense, and regularity," *Brain and Language*, vol. 91, no. 1, pp. 128–129, 2004.

[65] R. Jonkers and A. de Bruin, "Tense processing in Broca's and Wernicke's aphasia," *Aphasiology*, vol. 23, no. 10, pp. 1252–1265, 2009.

[66] Y. Faroqi-Shah, "A comparison of two theoretically-driven treatments for verb inflection deficits in aphasia," *Neuropsychologia*, vol. 46, no. 13, pp. 3088–3100, 2008.

[67] Y. Faroqi-Shah, "Can verb morphology be primed in agrammatic aphasia?" in *Proceedings of the Clinical Aphasiology Conference*, Jackson Hole, Wyo, USA, 2008.

[68] Y. Faroqi-Shah, "Selective treatment of regular versus irregular verbs in agrammatic aphasia: efficacy data," *Aphasiology*, vol. 27, no. 6, pp. 678–705, 2013.

[69] Y. Faroqi-Shah and L. E. Graham, "Treatment of semantic verb classes in aphasia: acquisition and generalization effects," *Clinical Linguistics and Phonetics*, vol. 25, no. 5, pp. 399–418, 2011.

[70] Y. Faroqi-Shah and C. R. Virion, "Constraint-induced language therapy for agrammatism: role of grammaticality constraints," *Aphasiology*, vol. 23, no. 7-8, pp. 977–988, 2009.

[71] Y. Faroqi-Shah, E. Wood, and J. Gassert, "Verb impairment in aphasia: a priming study of body part overlap," *Aphasiology*, vol. 24, no. 11, pp. 1377–1388, 2010.

[72] N. Helm-Estabrooks and M. Nicholas, *Narrative Story Cards*, PRO-ED, Austin, Tex, USA, 6th edition, 2003.

[73] A. Kertesz, *Western Aphasia Battery—Revised*, Pearson Education, San Antonio, Tex, USA, 2006.

[74] B. Dabul, *Apraxia Battery for Adults—Second Edition (ABA-2)*, PRO-ED, Austin, Tex, USA, 2000.

[75] H. Goodglass, E. Kaplan, and B. Barresi, *Boston Diagnostic Aphasia Examination*, Lippincott Williams & Wilkins, Philadelphia, Pa, USA, 3rd edition, 2001.

[76] P. A. Broen and S. A. Santema, "Children's comprehension of six verb-tense forms," *Journal of Communication Disorders*, vol. 16, no. 2, pp. 85–97, 1983.

[77] J. McShane and S. Whittaker, "The encoding of tense and aspect by three- to five-year-old children," *Journal of Experimental Child Psychology*, vol. 45, no. 1, pp. 52–70, 1988.

[78] L. B. Leonard and P. Deevy, "Tense and aspect in sentence interpretation by children with specific language impairment," *Journal of Child Language*, vol. 37, no. 2, pp. 395–418, 2010.

[79] R. Bastiaanse, L. Bos, L. Stowe, and O. Dragoy, "Time-reference and tense teased apart," *Procedia—Social and Behavioral Sciences*, vol. 61, pp. 39–40, 2012.

[80] M. C. Linebarger, M. F. Schwartz, and E. M. Saffran, "Sensitivity to grammatical structure in so-called agrammatic aphasics," *Cognition*, vol. 13, no. 3, pp. 361–392, 1983.

[81] M. F. Schwartz, E. M. Saffran, R. B. Fink, J. L. Myers, and N. Martin, "Mapping therapy: a treatment programme for agrammatism," *Aphasiology*, vol. 8, no. 1, pp. 19–54, 1994.

[82] J. R. Crawford, P. H. Garthwaite, and C. D. Gray, "Wanted: fully operational definitions of dissociations in single-case studies," *Cortex*, vol. 39, no. 2, pp. 357–370, 2003.

[83] K. R. Laws, T. M. Gale, V. C. Leeson, and J. R. Crawford, "When is category specific in Alzheimer's disease?" *Cortex*, vol. 41, no. 4, pp. 452–463, 2005.

[84] L. K. Obler, K. Harris, M. Meth, J. Centeno, and P. Mathews, "The phonology-morphosyntax interface: affixed words in agrammatism," *Brain and Language*, vol. 68, no. 1-2, pp. 233–240, 1999.

[85] M. Penke, U. Janssen, and M. Krause, "The representation of inflectional morphology: evidence from Broca's aphasia," *Brain and Language*, vol. 68, no. 1-2, pp. 225–232, 1999.

[86] B. A. O'Connor Wells, "Tense-mood-aspect frequency, verb-form regularity and context-governed choice in agrammatism: evidence from Spanish ser and estar," *Dissertation Abstracts International: Section B: The Sciences and Engineering*, vol. 72, no. 5, p. 2745-B, 2011.

10

Psychosocial Well-Being in Persons with Aphasia Participating in a Nursing Intervention after Stroke

Berit Arnesveen Bronken,[1,2] **Marit Kirkevold,**[1,3] **Randi Martinsen,**[1,2]
Torgeir Bruun Wyller,[4,5] **and Kari Kvigne**[2]

[1] Department of Nursing Science, Faculty of Medicine, Institute of Health and Society, University of Oslo,
P.O. Box 1130 Blindern, 0318 Oslo, Norway
[2] Department of Nursing and Mental Health, Faculty of Public Health, Hedmark University College, P.O. Box 400,
2418 Elverum, Norway
[3] Institute of Public Health, University of Århus, Nordre Ringgade 1, 8000 Århus C, Denmark
[4] Faculty of Medicine, Institute of Clinical Medicine, University of Oslo, P.O. Box 1171 Blindern, 0318 Oslo, Norway
[5] Department of Geriatric Medicine, Oslo University Hospital, P.O. Box 4956 Nydalen, 0424 Oslo, Norway

Correspondence should be addressed to Berit Arnesveen Bronken, b.a.bronken@medisin.uio.no

Academic Editor: Kim Usher

The psychosocial adjustment process after stroke is complicated and protracted. The language is the most important tool for making sense of experiences and for human interplay, making persons with aphasia especially prone to psychosocial problems. Persons with aphasia are systematically excluded from research projects due to methodological challenges. This study explored how seven persons with aphasia experienced participating in a complex nursing intervention aimed at supporting the psychosocial adjustment process and promoting psychosocial well-being. The intervention was organized as an individual, dialogue-based collaboration process based upon ideas from "Guided self-determination." The content addressed psychosocial issues as mood, social relationships, meaningful activities, identity, and body changes. Principles from "Supported conversation for adults with aphasia" were used to facilitate the conversations. The data were obtained by participant observation during the intervention, qualitative interviews 2 weeks, 6 months, and 12 months after the intervention and by standardized clinical instruments prior to the intervention and at 2 weeks and 12 months after the intervention. Assistance in narrating about themselves and their experiences with illness, psychological support and motivation to move on during the difficult adjustment process, and exchange of knowledge and information were experienced as beneficial and important by the participants in this study.

1. Introduction

Aphasia, an acquired language disorder caused by brain damage, affects about one-third of the stroke population [1, 2]. About 40% continues to have significant language impairment at 18 months after stroke [3]. Aphasia ranges from mild, involving difficulties in finding words, to severe, involving severe impairment of all language modalities and leading to problems with expressions and comprehension of speech, reading, and writing and the use of language as a flexible tool in everyday life [4]. Language is the most important tool for human interplay, social participation, and community, and we make sense of life events and experiences through language [5].

The sudden and dramatic onset of aphasia following stroke is associated with major disruptions of everyday life and affects all dimensions of quality of life [4, 6]. The psychosocial adjustment process is complicated and protracted [7], and persons with aphasia (PWA) are especially prone to psychosocial problems, such as anxiety and depression [4, 8, 9], threatened identity [10], changes in their relationships with their significant others [11, 12], reduced social networks and social isolation/exclusion [13], unemployment, and abandonment of leisure activities [14]. The emotional and psychosocial factors have a marked impact on recovery, the psychosocial adjustment process, and the response to rehabilitation [4, 15, 16].

Several studies have sought to prevent and treat psychosocial problems in stroke survivors in general [17–20], but the outcomes differ substantially and the theoretical foundations of the effective components are unclear [21, 22]. However emotional support, information, and practical assistance are documented as important [21]. Two randomized controlled studies [23, 24] demonstrated that a systematic followup of stroke survivors with counseling [23] and "motivational interviewing" [24] significantly improved mood during the first year after a stroke. PWA were not focused on explicitly in these studies, and in the Watkins study, persons with severe communication problems were excluded.

Interventions that include PWA pose methodological challenges due to the communicative barriers. This has resulted in a systematic exclusion of this target group outside the field of speech-and-language therapy [25, 26]. In a meta-synthesis of 293 qualitative research reports concerning chronic illness, Paterson, Thorne, Canam, and Jillings found that only two studies involved informants with impaired verbal communication [27]. In a systematic review of nursing rehabilitation of stroke patients with aphasia [28], the authors reviewed 24 papers relevant to nursing-specific interventions. Their key finding was that the integration of speech-and-language interventions and functional communication training into daily care could improve the effectiveness of speech-and-language therapy. The major focus was on functional communication training and screening tools to detect aphasia. In contrast, Hjelmblink and colleagues [29] found that the defined language impairment misled both the health care professionals and the PWA to focus only on language therapy, hence leaving the participant unsupported in other important aspects of rehabilitation.

Nurses have a key role in stroke rehabilitation [24, 30, 31], and they have a unique possibility to follow patients over time and thereby secure continuity. We believe that nursing interventions tailored to assist PWA and their relatives in coping with psychosocial consequences of the stroke need to be targeted explicitly. In response to this, we developed a complex clinical intervention [32] aimed at supporting the psychosocial adjustment process and promoting psychosocial well-being the first year after stroke [33]. In this paper we focus on the experiences of the participants with aphasia which were included in the study. The aims of this study were to explore how the participants with aphasia experienced participating in the intervention and its impact on their recovery process and psychosocial well-being during and after the intervention.

2. Materials and Methods

2.1. Design. The current study was part of a larger study comprising 25 cases of stroke survivors followed during the first year after stroke. The larger study had a development and evaluation design guided by the UK Medical Research Council Framework [32], which is a recommended framework for developing and evaluating complex clinical interventions in health care. The development of the current theoretically and empirically informed intervention is reported in depth elsewhere [33]. In seven of the cases the participants had moderate-to-severe aphasia. These cases are explored further in depth in this paper. A qualitative multiple case approach was seen to be appropriate to explore the context-sensitive and multidimensional aspects of the individual recovery process such as coping resources, social network, age, gender, culture, and meaning attached to individual values and life concerns and how the intervention interacted with the individual challenges and needs [34].

2.2. Description of the Intervention. The recovery process following a stroke has been referred to as a demanding journey in which the stroke survivor moves through different phases as various challenges unfold [35, 36]. We used a metaphor translated to "The great trial of strength," which refers to a prestigious and demanding bicycle race in Norway (lasting 15–20 hours), known by most Norwegians. Healthy and well-trained bicycle riders are followed by an escort car, which provides the support and equipment that the riders need. We assumed that a stroke survivor also needed an "escort car" to address different needs as they arose during the "recovery journey" after the stroke. Each session was conceptualized as a "pit stop" in this unpredictable "race" toward recovery.

The intervention was organized as an individual, dialogue-based, collaboration and problem-solving process between the stroke survivor and a trained nurse. Ideas from the approach "Guided self-determination" [37] were applied to assist the participants in developing new life skills to cope with psychosocial consequences of the stroke. The intervention addressed four dimensions of psychosocial well-being: Basic emotional state, meaningful activities, social relationships and self-concept [38], all of which are threatened by stroke [7, 14, 39, 40]. For each encounter we constructed worksheets addressing topics described as challenging in the stroke literature (related to the aforementioned dimensions of psychosocial well-being). The worksheets were adjusted linguistically for PWA. We used principles from the method "Supported conversations for adults with aphasia" [41] to facilitate the conversations. The intervention was planned to consist of eight encounters, each lasting about 1 hour, to be conducted during the first 6 months after a stroke. Table 1 shows an overview of the guiding topical outline of the encounters and the topics of the associated worksheets which were planned for each encounter. Further information is available upon request.

2.3. Inclusion Criteria and Presentation of the Participants. The study was conducted in Norway in the period 2007–2009.

Inclusion criteria were adult persons (18 years or above) having suffered a stroke during the previous twelve weeks, medically stable, with sufficient cognitive functioning to participate (assessed by their physician/stroke team), interested in participating, and Norwegian speaking. Persons diagnosed

TABLE 1: Topical outline of the intervention (guiding structure).

Encounter	Aim	Worksheet
One	To establish a relationship for collaboration in an early phase after the stroke.	1a: Invitation to collaboration 1b: The stroke—what happened?
Two	To gather knowledge about personal values, interests, and goals as a common platform for further collaboration. (Who are you (identity), which life is interrupted by the stroke?). To prepare for further collaboration after home coming.	2a: Life line—Personal background, values and interests 2b: Metaphor—"The great trial of strength"
Three	To support the participant in their process of adjusting to a changed situation "from healthy to stroke survivor in everyday life." To support the participant in clarifying setting goals (short terms) and opportunities.	3a: Personal metaphor of your life as a stroke survivor 3b: Mood in everyday life (unfulfilled sentences)
Four	Invitation to narrate about bodily experiences and changes. Support in making sense of the new experiences and mobilize available recourses. Renegotiate new roles and identity adjustment.	4a: Me and my life (unfulfilled sentences) 4b: My body (graphical illustration of a woman/man)
Five	Identify goals to focus and sort out what has to be done by whom to reach the goals. Support to identify personal resources and significant resources in their network.	5a: Problem-solving process 5b: Daily activities in everyday life (unfulfilled sentences) 5c: Relationship with others (unfulfilled sentences)
Six	Help to integrate illness and life in a way that appear manageable for the participant. Support to promote health and build up resistance resources (i.e., sleep, social relationships, meaningful activities, food, physical activity). Support to develop new life skills that are necessary to live well with changes caused by the stroke.	6a: Illness and life 6b: Choice of aims to focus 6c: Balance in everyday life 2b: Metaphor (How is the terrain you are moving in now? What kind of support do you need from the "escort car")
Seven	Talk about experiences and support the coping process. Assistance to be conscious about personal recourses and recourses in their network/environment.	7a: Coping in everyday life 7b: Habits I need to change/should change 7c: Network
Eight	Negotiating perspectives and goals for the further recovery process. Summarizing the collaboration process.	2b: Metaphor (past-present-future)

with aphasia were broadly included due to the exploratory design.

Seven persons, one woman and six men, with moderate-to-severe aphasia were included. Their ages ranged from 33 to 72 years. A speech-and-language therapist assessed their language impairment and described their ability to produce speech, comprehend language, read, and write prior to the intervention. The participants entered the intervention program 4 to 12 weeks after stroke onset. Table 2 gives a brief presentation of the participants in terms of medical and demographic data (prior to the intervention).

2.4. Duration and Context of the Intervention. The frequency of the encounters and the duration of the intervention period were initially planned to be eight encounters over 6 months. Among the participants with aphasia we had to prolong the intervention to complete the program because the participants needed more time, the trajectories differed, and medical complications necessitated adjustments. During a period lasting from 9.5 to 14.5 months, 10 to 16 encounters were carried out in each case, lasting from 40 minutes to 2 hours. The encounters took place in various locations depending on where the participants were in their trajectories, including the hospital, the rehabilitation unit, and the home.

2.5. Methodological Consideration and Data Collection. Traditional methods for gaining self-reported data, such as interviews and questionnaires, are less suitable for PWA because of the presence of language impairment. Linguistic data from interviews are affected by changes in the syntactic, semantic, and pragmatic use of the language [13, 42, 43]. Questionnaires can also pose problems that result from the presence of nonlinguistic cognitive symptoms, such as apraxia, neglect, visuospatial problems [44], paresis, and vision disturbances [45]. In an attempt to meet these challenges, we assumed that triangulating various approaches would provide us with a more nuanced and complete picture of the experiences, given the limited ability of the participants to produce rich interview text [46]. Triangulation is recommended by several authors to improve trustworthiness of case studies [34, 47, 48]. The data were obtained by the following methods and data sources.

2.5.1. Participant Observation. We used participant observation during the intervention to achieve an insider's view of the process. In total, 89 individual encounters between each of the participants and the same intervention nurse were completed. The nurse wrote down systematic notes (referred to as log notes) after each session. The log notes described content of the dialogues, activity and interplay, the

TABLE 2: Medical and demographic information describing the participants.

Participants	Physical extent of the stroke	Language ability	Civil status	Work
Man, 53 years	Hemorrhagia of the left hemisphere. Paresis in right side. Can walk. Visuospatial neglect.	Word production and understanding seriously affected, no functional reading or writing ability.	Lived together with wife and three children (teenagers).	Full time
Man, 72 years	Thrombosis of the left hemisphere. Hemiplegic right side. Paralysis in right arm. Not able to walk alone.	Speech production and speech understanding seriously affected. No functional reading or writing ability. Good situational understanding.	Lived together with wife. One grown child and one grandchild.	Retired
Man, 63 years	Thrombosis of the left hemisphere. No visible motor symptoms. Independent of help.	Speech production seriously affected. Speech apraxia. Disability in reading and writing. Good understanding.	Lived alone. Two grown children and one grandchild.	Full time
Man, 43 years	Thrombosis of the left hemisphere. Slight numbness and reduced strength in right side. Diplopia.	Expressive and impressive difficulties. Understanding better than production of speech. Reading and writing disability. Good situational understanding.	Lived partly alone. Two children (teenagers).	Full time
Man, 60 years	Thrombosis of the left hemisphere. Hemiplegic right side, some neglect. Can walk short distances with a stick.	Understanding is better than production of speech. Requires time to find words. Reading and writing disability.	Lived alone. Two grown up children and two grandchildren	Full time
Woman, 33 years	Thrombosis of the left hemisphere. Paresis in right side.	Serious expressive and impressive difficulties. Sound and word paraphasia. Strongly reduced reading and writing disability. Situational understanding is good.	Lived alone.	Full time
Man, 64 years	Hemorrhagia in the left hemisphere. Reduced strength in right side. Can walk with a roller. Reduced ADL function. Reduced vision. Concentration and memory affected.	Good speech production and understanding, reading and writing disability, dysarthria.	Lived in a nursing home after stroke onset. No children.	Disability benefit

use of worksheets and communication resources, context, duration, and reflections.

2.5.2. Qualitative Thematic Interviews. The participants took part in three individual qualitative followup interviews at 2 weeks, 6 months, and 12 months after the intervention had ended (21 in total). The interviews were recorded on video to extend the limited verbal expressions with nonverbal data. The first interview focused on the experiences of participating in the intervention program and the perceived impact of the program on psychosocial well-being (i.e., mood, relationships, activity, and self-esteem). The second and the third interview were followup interviews based on the same themes and relevant topics that had been discussed during the intervention and in the previous interview(s). The interviews took place mainly in the participants' home (15), but some of them were conducted in a conference room at the hospital (5) and a rehabilitation unit (1). The interviews lasted from 50 minutes to 2 hours.

2.5.3. Standardized Clinical Instruments. We applied four standardized clinical instruments addressing different aspects of subjective psychosocial well-being. The Stroke and Aphasia Quality of Life (SAQOL-39) is a disease-specific quality-of-life scale that measures a stroke's impact on the "physical", "psychosocial," "communication," and "energy" domains [49]. Cantril's Ladder Scale more globally addresses

satisfaction with life [50]. The Faces Scale measures the affective experience of happiness/sadness [51], whereas the Hopkins Symptom Check List (short version, HSCL-8) addresses symptoms of depression and anxiety [52]. All instruments were deemed to be appropriate for PWA because of the use of visuals [50, 51] and adjusted and simple text [52, 53]. The instruments were used three times: prior to the intervention (T1), two weeks after the intervention (T2), and one year after the intervention (T3). The instruments are further described in Table 3.

2.6. Data Analysis. The qualitative data was analyzed from a hermeneutic-phenomenological approach inspired by Ricoeur and Kvale [55–61]. This approach aims to understand the meaning of lived experiences through the interpretation of text. The text included verbatim transcripts of interviews, written expressions on the worksheets, drawings, images, pictograms, and log notes. According to Ricoeur [56], the metaphorical process plays a semantic role and contributes value to the meaning of a text through its ability to stimulate imagination and emotion. In this study the use of metaphorical thinking supported our interpretation and understanding throughout the analytical process, especially when the participants used single syllables, few words, drawings, artwork, nonverbal communication, or exchanged words.

TABLE 3: Standardized clinical instruments.

Type	Instrument	Concepts	Scores
Health-related quality of life	Stroke and Aphasia Quality of life SAQOL-39 [49]	Disease specific quality of life	39 items. Four dimensions rating the extent to which the informants struggle with different functions. Scoring: total score and four subscores (physical function, communication ability, psychosocial life, and energy). Range: 5–1, "no trouble at all" (5) to "could not do it at all" (1).
Global evaluation	Faces Scale [51]	Emotional well-being	Seven visual faces whose expressions vary from very happy to very sad. The scale does not have verbal labels, but each face was given numerical values for the purpose of graphical illustration. The most happy face was given the numerical value 7 and the most sad face was given the numerical value 1.
Global evaluation	Cantril's Ladder Scale [50]	Life satisfaction	Visual ladder with ten steps and 11 numbers ranging from 10 to 0: step ten at the top of the ladder depicts the highest level of satisfaction, and step one depicts the lowest. The scale does not have verbal labels, but was given numerical values for the purpose of graphical illustrations. Step ten was given the numerical value 10, step 1 the numerical value 0.
Symptom specific	Hopkins Symptom Check List—8 items [52, 54]	Psychological distress/mental health	Eight statements related to common symptoms of anxiety and depression with scores ranging from 4 to 1: "not bothered" (4) to "very bothered" (1).

The analytical process encompassed three main phases: naive reading, structural analysis, and comprehensive understanding [62]. In the first phase, the entire text from all cases was read to provide an overall impression. In the structural phase, each case was explored in depth, and each data source was analyzed separately as described below.

The interviews that had been recorded on video were viewed and transcribed verbatim. The transcripts were read separately and together with the video records several times to confirm the meaning of the text. The video supplemented the text with nonverbal expressions which were important to provide a richer interview text. Meaning units related to the aims of the study were identified and structured into themes. The log notes from all the encounters were further explored to extend the meaning of the themes that emerged from the interviews. For example, when the participants referred to events and experiences from the intervention, the log notes provided more detailed information about the content, the circumstances, and the actions associated with these sessions as well as where and when they took place.

Data obtained from the standardized clinical instruments were organized with a computer software program (PASW Statistics 18) to create graphical plot diagrams from all instruments to explore changes in the participants' statements over time. The Faces Scale and the Cantril's Ladder Scale are visual scales without verbal labels. We gave each face in the Faces Scale and each step in the Cantril's Ladder Scale numerical values to create graphical illustrations by the use of the computer software program. Secondly, the statements were interpreted in relation to the analyses of the qualitative data, ending in a summary (case record) for each case [47]. The data from the interviews, log notes, and instruments complemented each other.

In the last phase, we compared the similarities and differences as well as the patterns across the cases in relation to the purpose of the study. Four of the authors

(Berit Bronken, Marit Kirkevold, Randi Martinsen, and Kari Kvigne) conducted the analysis. Disagreements were discussed and led to further analysis, which was completed when the findings were redefined or confirmed.

2.7. Ethical Considerations. A language therapist or a specially trained nurse outside the research group had obtained written informed consent from the participants before the study began. Oral and written information was communicated through the use of adjusted language and illustrated communication resources. A separate written informed consent was obtained before the postintervention followup interviews, that were recorded on video. The project was approved by The Regional Committee for Medical and Health Research Ethics and The Norwegian Social Science Data Services.

PWA are vulnerable to harm because of their reduced ability to express their meanings and reservations [63]. Autonomy, self-determination, respect, and ethical sensitivity were emphasized at all stages of the research process, considering the asymmetric relationship between the participants and the intervention nurse with regard to role, knowledge, language, and health condition. During the intervention, clinical care and security had priority over research goals. There was no conflict between the therapeutic goals and research goals. Small samples could compromise confidentiality [64]. To counteract this possibility, we have modified descriptions that might identify the participants.

3. The Participants' Experiences of Participating in the Intervention and Its Perceived Impact on Their Recovery Process

Our findings are presented in two main sections; 3 and 4. First we present the participants' experiences of participating in the intervention and its perceived impact on their recovery process (3). In Section 4 we describe how the participants expressed their psychosocial well-being before, during, and after the intervention.

3.1. Assistance to Narrate about Themselves and Their Experiences.

The participants expressed a great need to talk about events and experiences in their new life situation and about unfamiliar reactions and symptoms caused by the stroke. The long-lasting partnership made it possible to gradually coconstruct and frame their stories, which could be shared and further developed and discussed over time. The topics introduced by the worksheets were experienced as useful starting points for the subsequent conversations and stories. The stories were gradually constructed through an interactive process of talking, writing, using nonverbal expressions, drawings, and communication resources during the intervention ("toolbox" with illustrated materials). The stories were written down after each encounter (by the intervention nurse) and followed up in later encounters depending on the participant's individual wishes and needs. The interactive process of coconstructing stories is described elsewhere [65]. The content of the stories varied considerably and mirrored the individual life situation, needs, and goals of each participant. Individualization and flexibility were mentioned as important elements of the intervention, which was expressed like: "I felt free to decide myself what to talk about, no pressure or anything like that."

All of them appreciated to tell who they used to be before they were hit by the stroke and how they struggled to adjust to their compromised roles as a partner, father, grandfather, friend, and worker after the stroke. They were all concerned about being perceived as competent adult persons, but difficulties in expressing themselves led to frustration and misunderstanding both in themselves and others in their close network. Facilitation to construct stories about events and experiences, receiving response, and discussing coping strategies were expressed as beneficial. The following quotes represent the sentiment among the participants: (The encounters) "lifted me up" and "raised me up." The topics of the worksheets were experienced as relevant and important to talk about and described as beneficial in terms of "something concrete to focus on," "interesting," "systematic," "awareness-raising," and "helped to structure thoughts and feelings."

For several of the participants, "the great trial of strength" metaphor, which was applied throughout the intervention, was experienced as a meaningful figurative representation of the recovery process and a beneficial "tool" to use when communicating about the ups and downs of recovery, energy, endurance, the physical challenge of negotiating difficult environments, meeting needs, and performing movements. One participant expressed it in this way:

> The metaphor has been meaningful because it [the trajectory] has been a great trial of strength. Now I am not in Oslo, and I am quite tired. If I had to cycle back, I would be very down [depressed. Pointing down to the ground]. One time [one stroke] is enough [smiling ironic]. I am

at Lillehammer [half way of the race], and I still need one more year before I am back home again [healthy].

3.1.1. Reserved Time for Talking (Provided Opportunities to Talk).

Time to talk and give attention to psychosocial consequences of the stroke and aphasia was underscored as important to the participants. Most of them lacked conversation partners in their natural environment who were able to understand their situation and condition. The language impairment, as well as the emotional and cognitive symptoms, the tiredness, and the bodily experiences were difficult to explain to others and difficult for others to understand, which can be exemplified by this quote:

> We talk very little, very little... I think they [family and others] believe that there is something wrong with me, and that hurts me a lot... It is difficult for me to initiate a conversation and know what to talk about, which is difficult for others to understand.

Several participants mentioned difficulties with initiating a conversation, not knowing what to talk about or how to express themselves. By specifically designating a time to discuss their psychosocial challenges, the participants were encouraged to tell about their daily experiences and life concerns, as expressed in this quote: "With the physiotherapist, I exercise; with the speech- and language therapist, I learn to talk, read and write. Here, I talk about me and my life." The participant drew a picture of a sun and pointed to the rays, each representing a significant person or source of support. Another explained it in his way: "On one hand, it is difficult to walk. On the other hand, it is difficult to talk. I can walk or talk not both things at the same time. Time to talk is important!" He struggled immensely and took time to explain and underscore these important points.

3.1.2. Confidence to Talk.

Several of the participants expressed embarrassment about their language disability outside of "treatment sessions." They were afraid of being regarded as incompetent, drunk, or childish. One participant expressed it in the following way: "To talk like a child, when you are an adult; it does something to you!" Some of the participants had, in addition to their aphasia, problems with their voices, articulation, and speech apraxia. The following situation from one of the interviews illustrates this:

> During one of the interviews, a friend came by to invite the participant for a walk. The participant stopped talking and changed to nonverbal communication. He smiled, pulled his lips together and pointed, first at the intervention nurse and then at the watch, to indicate that he had to come back later. After the friend had left, the nurse asked why he had stopped talking and just pointed to his friend. [The intervention nurse was quite surprised, as this participant talked quite well if he had time to express himself].

This participant said that he often avoided talking because he was afraid of making a fool of himself. He had been judged as drunk several times, which he was upset and offended about. The first time, a taxi driver assumed that he was drunk when the stroke first occurred. Later, during a call from a business connection, the associate quickly ended the conversation by saying, "I will call you back when you are sober." Loss of the language as a tool to maintain positions and roles as professionals, competent family members, or friends often resulted in avoiding "exposing" situations. The encounters during the intervention were experienced as a "safe" place to communicate experiences related to the illness and daily life. Confidence, acknowledgement, respect, and knowledge were described as important elements in the collaboration process.

3.2. Psychological Support

3.2.1. Expressions of Thoughts and Feelings.
All participants included in this study were enrolled after experiencing their first stroke. The sudden change from being healthy to being seriously ill and unable to talk about their condition was experienced as very difficult. The disruption of a well-functioning life caused by the stroke resulted in a condition characterized by fear, uncertainty, despair, and frustration. The importance of having a person available to support them in expressing their thoughts and feelings and communicate about them was emphasized by all of the participants, expressed like: "It helped me to put words on some of my thoughts and feelings, which were the most difficult for me." At times, the seriousness of their strained situation was precarious to some of them, as illustrated by this quote: "Without x [the intervention nurse] and y [the speech and language therapist], I would have ended up at z [a mental hospital]!" During the encounters the participants' fear of suffering another stroke was recurrent, expressed in phrases like: "I was afraid of exercising and walking outdoors alone," "I had to check that I could move and talk several times during the night," "I'm still alive," and "[....], if I don't have another stroke."

The discrepancy between the participants' increased needs to talk and their reduced abilities is illustrated by the following quotes:

> I didn't understand what it was. I never had reactions like this before, but I couldn't say it! My language! It's not my, my... [pointing at his head], my language!

> I was in coma for two days. When I woke up I didn't understand anything, anything. But the worst of all,...I couldn't talk.... It was terrible, terrible!

The participants expressed experiences of being locked in like: "I was completely alone" or "I was in a bubble, and in that bubble it was just me." Assistance to verbalize experiences helped breaking through the wall of experienced loneliness.

The participants appreciated having their reactions confirmed as "normal" by communicating about these topics during the encounters, which provided some confidence and order in an otherwise confusing situation. Taking part in the intervention helped them to handle affective and cognitive strain by communicating with a knowledgeable professional from the field of stroke and aphasia. The participants said that they felt understood in terms of their compromised language and their situation as a "stroke survivor with aphasia," as expressed in the two following quotes: "x [the intervention nurse] understood my language. I think we understood each other... mutually. Very good!" and "x [the intervention nurse] knows what it can be like to have aphasia and stroke."

3.2.2. Motivation to Endure and Continue.
The long-lasting difficulties and the uncertainty about the duration and outcome of rehabilitation threatened the participants' confidence and future prospects. They had concerns about how they should sustain themselves personally, perform their future roles, and manage economically. The encounters were something that the participants looked forward to as a place where they could share their experiences and receive encouragement and response to continue. Their experiences of the encounters were expressed through statements like: "Raised me up," "lifted me up," "helped us to endure," and "inspired me to not give up." A middle-aged man explained it in the following way: "It's easy to just stay on the sofa and go down [expressed by a downward spiral hand gesture toward the floor]." Another participant, a man with comprehensive physical disability, severe aphasia, and a complicated clinical trajectory, described the importance of his participation in the intervention with two words: "Alpha and omega." His wife, who took part in nearly every session, included the following comment:

> Without these sessions, my husband would never have returned home. I didn't think it was possible! I didn't know anything about stroke and have learned a lot. X [the intervention nurse] provided a contrast to all of the negative information that we got from the health care system. She believed in improvement and helped us to endure. We looked forward to the visits.

The participants experienced the feeling of talking, despite their aphasia. Even the participant with the most severe expressive disability responded that "talking" was what he appreciated the most during the intervention. The following quote represent a sentiment: "To talk is very important. You need that in a situation like this."

3.3. Exchange of Knowledge and Information Based on Individual Experiences.
The opportunity to gain knowledge was underscored by all of the participants as an important aspect of the sessions. The exchange of knowledge and information based on the participants' own experiences was viewed as a help for the participants' self-understanding of the situation and to learn about stroke, aphasia, common

reactions and trajectories, their rights, where to get help, and how to utilize the available coping resources. Limitations in speaking, reading, and writing made it difficult for the participants to gain information and navigate the health care system on their own. The importance of receiving feedback from professionals was mentioned by a number of the participants, as illuminated by the following quote: "Talking with someone with knowledge about my experiences, discussing them and getting some suggestions were helpful for me."

Two of the youngest participants explicitly valued their roles as "co-researchers"; they felt useful and hoped that their experiences would help others with aphasia and stroke. Generally, the participants experienced the intervention as an important supplement to the other services they received, and they recommended that this form of intervention be made available to others with aphasia in the future.

4. The Participants' Expressed Perception of Their Psychosocial Well-Being and Life Situation before, during, and after the Intervention

In this section, we present how the participants expressed their life situation both in terms of qualitative data collected from the interviews and log notes and from their self-reported statements expressed by the standardized clinical instruments.

4.1. The Road Has Been Hard. The "road" (recovery process) had been hard, long, and demanding for all of the participants. The consequences of the stroke changed their lives, and several described a "totally new world," which they aspired to adjust to. Language difficulties and their consequences, such as tiredness, social barriers, and uncertainty, remained challenging. The relationships within families had been changed, and, in several cases, friendships had been lost [66]. Some of the participants also related the changes in their social activities to personal reasons, such as feelings of isolation, difficulties engaging with others and participating in arguments and discussions, and difficulties associated with concentration, understanding, self-expression, and maintaining their earlier roles. The following quote illustrates a perceived experience of being met as different: "They [family, friends and employer] think I am sick, but I'm not. I'm 80% healthy. I have problems with my language."

4.2. I Am Doing Quite Well, but It Is a New World. At the end of the intervention, all but one of the participants described their life situation as quite well, even though the days fluctuated with ups and downs and there were still challenges in everyday life, as illuminated in the two following quotes.

> Now I'm doing relatively well, but it is the damn language. It bothers me all the time. It is another world than the one that I came from.

> I have been sick for about one week now [flu], but otherwise I mostly think it is going quite well.

> The fact that I can walk [with a stick and a lot of struggle] and sit here and... [pointing at the video camera] is fantastic! To talk is very important!... The road has been long and hard, and I still need one more year to get healthy.

One of the participants experienced a setback in his recovery caused by a frightening attack of epilepsy. Psychological distress and anxiety were reactivated, and he struggled with unwanted side effects of medication, which affected his entire life situation.

4.3. The Participants' Self-Reported Statements on the Standardized Clinical Instruments. In Table 4, we present the participants' statements on three of the standardized instruments: Cantril's Ladder Scale, the Faces Scale, and the Hopkins Symptom Check List across the three times of data collection. The statements are presented in numericals.

Figure 1 demonstrates changes over time on the SAQOL-39; total score (a), physical function (b), communication (c), psychosocial function (d), and energy (e).

First Assessment (T1). At baseline, the participants self-rated their perceived global life satisfaction from middle to very good (Table 4, Cantril). Emotionally, all of the participants but one expressed themselves to be quite happy (Table 4, Faces), and they were slightly bothered by psychological distress (HSCL-8). There was great variation in the physical affection of the stroke. Two of the participants struggled significantly or were unable to perform the functions that the questions asked for. In one case, statements for the physical dimension of the SAQOL-39 are missing because there were several activities that this participant had not yet tried. All of the participants struggled a lot with communication, with scores between 1.25 and 2.25 (Figure 1(c)). The participants rated their psychosocial situations quite well (Figure 1(d)). In one case, the statements were lower than in the other cases. This man expressed himself as extremely sad and dissatisfied with his life situation (Table 4, Faces and Cantril).

Second Assessment (T2). Two weeks after the intervention, about one year after the stroke, the participants' statements of their life satisfaction generally changed in a positive direction in four of the cases, were unchanged in two cases, and declined in one case compared with statements at T1 (Table 4, Cantril). Two participants stated themselves as happier at T2 than at T1, but in five of the cases the emotional statements tended to drop slightly. However none of them tended to be sad (Table 4, Faces). Five participants were slightly bothered with psychological distress, while two had bothersome symptoms; one participant was anxious and tired, and one was tired all the time (Table 4, HSCL-8). Changes expressed by the SAQOL-39 showed slight improvements in six of the cases and decline in one (Figure 1(a)). The degree of the relative changes in scores for the different subdimensions in each case varied substantially. Physical function improved slightly in most of the cases and markedly in one. Communication improved

TABLE 4: The participants' statements on the Cantril, Faces, and HSCL instruments.

Case	Cantril			Faces			HSCL-8		
	T1	T2	T3	T1	T2	T3	T1	T2	T3
1	7	9	9	5	7	5	3.25	4.00	3.75
2	7	8	9	7	4	7	4.00	3.75	3.88
3	7	7	6	7	4	7	4.00	3.86	3.75
4	8	9	6	7	6	5	3.75	2.00	3.13
5	8	6	6	6	5	6	3.88	3.75	3.63
6	6	6	5	5	4	4	3.50	3.25	2.75
7	3	5	4	1	4	5	3.63	3.75	3.86

Cantril: Cantril's Ladder Scale, life satisfaction (global).
Presents a picture of a ladder with 10 steps and 11 numbers (0–10).
Step ten at the top of the ladder depicts the highest level of satisfaction (10), and step one at the bottom depicts the lowest (0).
Faces: Faces Scale, affective experience of happiness/sadness.
Presents seven visual faces whose expressions vary from very happy (7) to very sad (1).
HSCL-8: Hopkins Symptom Check List with 8 items, symptoms of psychological distress (depression and anxiety). Range score: 4–1. Score 4 is not bothered, 3 is to a less degree bothered, 2 is quite bothered, and 1 is very bothered.
Time
T1: before the intervention (5–12 weeks after stroke).
T2: 2 weeks after the intervention (about 1 year after stroke).
T3: 12 months after the intervention (about 2 years after stroke).

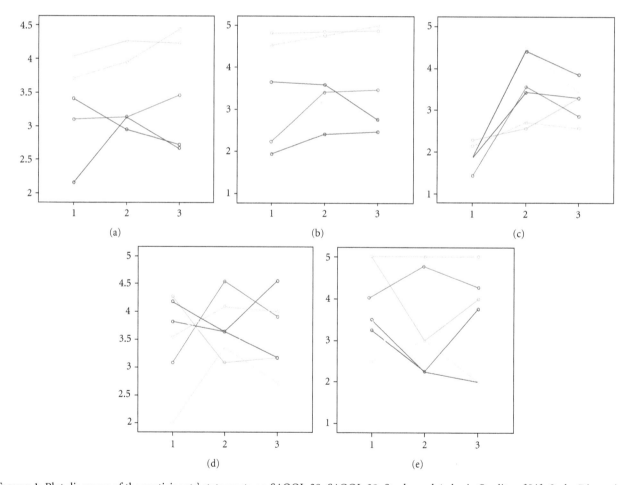

FIGURE 1: Plot diagrams of the participants' statements on SAQOL-39. SAQOL-39: Stroke and Aphasia Quality of Life Scale. Dimensions: (a) total score; (b) physical function; (c) communication; (d) psychosocial functioning, and (e) energy. *Value scores (y-axis)*. Range score: 5-1. Score 5 is no trouble at all; score 4 is a little trouble; score 3 is some trouble; score 2 is a lot of trouble; score 1 is could not do it at all. *Time (x-axis)* Time 1: T1, before the intervention (5–12 weeks after stroke). Time 2: T2, two weeks after the intervention (about 1 year after stroke). Time 3: T3, 12 months after the intervention (about 2 years after stroke).

markedly in most of the cases, slightly in one and was almost unchanged in one (Figure 1(c)). Three participants showed psychosocial improvement, one remained relatively unchanged, and three declined (Figure 1(d)). Low energy and tiredness were marked in four of the cases, while the scores improved or remained unchanged in the three remaining cases (Figure 1(e)). In the case where the total score on the SAQOL-39 declined, the energy level dropped critically from 3.50 to 1.50, which probably explained the other scores (Figure 1(e)).

Third Assessment (T3). At the long-term followup, one year after the intervention and about two years following the stroke, the participants' general satisfaction with life varied; two were very satisfied, but most of them reported that they were moderately satisfied. One had a score that was below the middle of the scale (Table 4, Cantril). Emotional well-being was generally stated as quite well; two were very happy, one was happy, three were somewhat happy, and one was neither happy nor unhappy (Table 4, Faces). In five of the cases, the total scores on the SAQOL-39 declined between T2 and T3, which may be explained by the surprising decline in ratings for communication in five of the cases and decline in psychosocial function in four cases (Figures 1(c) and 1(d)). Two participants reported that they continued to have some bothersome symptoms with tiredness and some psychological distress (Table 4, HSCL-8).

In summary, from baseline (T1) through the follow up, the participants' self-rated statements on the instruments varied. The total score measured by SAQOL-39 improved in six of the cases and declined in one. Tiredness and low energy explained most of the changes in this subject, which probably impacted the other scores. During the intervention, this participant was admitted to the hospital with suspicion of a new stroke, which delayed his recovery.

4.4. Integration of Data from the Interviews, the Log Notes, and the Instruments. The complicated recoveries of the participants were to some extent mirrored by the changes in their statements on the standardized clinical instruments, and the range of the statements (scores) was described and explained based on the qualitative data provided by the participants during the intervention. Within the first weeks following the stroke (T1), all but one of the participants were still inpatients at the hospital or in a rehabilitation unit, that is, in safe environments with access to professionals. They were happy about surviving and had an attitude that the extent of the stroke could have been worse (referring to others). They believed that their language difficulties would resolve after a period of active training. At this time, the participants were mainly optimistic, with the exception of one who experienced deep grief, not because of the stroke, but because a close friend had recently died from a serious illness.

The evolving consequences of the language disorder and the stroke became gradually clearer to them as the challenges of everyday life, family, work, and society arose after returning home. The long-lasting problems and the

uncertainty about the outcomes of the rehabilitation were difficult to understand and handle.

In four of the cases, one or several medical complications negatively impacted the recovery processes; two participants experienced frightening attacks of epilepsy, three were readmitted to the hospital because of symptoms of a new stroke (confirmed in one case), and one fell and incurred a complicated hip fracture resulting in a prolonged trajectory.

Profound life events within the family and/or at work, such as illness of a close family member, partner crises, and unfair dismissal from work, occurred in three of the cases. For example, one participant was surprisingly fired from work before even being offered a chance to try (two weeks before measurement T2). In another case, the participant's colleagues noted and documented mistakes (behind his back) to legitimate a dismissal of him. All of these events were difficult to handle for people who lacked a "normal" ability to defend themselves on top of other challenges. Loss of energy was explained by the participants' continuous efforts to concentrate, understand, and express themselves and by externally induced energy loss caused by waiting, difficulties obtaining information from health and social services, and, in some cases, unclear messages from employers.

In summary, the information obtained from the various data sources complemented each other and provided a nuanced picture of the participants' experiences of their recovery process and their subjective psychosocial well-being during and after the intervention. The qualitative data provided detailed information about the meaning of the challenges and changes that the participants experienced over time, which also were expressed by the statements on the standardized clinical instruments.

5. Discussion

To the best of our knowledge, there has been no similar psychosocial nursing intervention tailored to stroke survivors with aphasia. Participation in the intervention was experienced by the participants as an important source of support during the adjustment process. The intervention promoted their sense of psychosocial well-being through facilitating their expressions as they talked about themselves and their experiences in a new and changed life situation. The intervention also provided psychological help in terms of affective, cognitive, and motivational support during a demanding and hard "journey" of recovery. Exchange of knowledge and information was also emphasized as an important aspect of taking part in the intervention program. All these elements are documented as key elements for a successful recovery process in other studies as well [67, 68]. Our findings also correspond with findings from studies focusing on a life-coaching approach to aphasia, which highlight that learning to live well with aphasia takes time, aphasia concerns the whole family, and the goal is to help PWA to fit the consequences of stroke and aphasia into their changed lives [69].

The way the intervention was tailored and organized enhanced the participants' experiences of "talking" and sharing their stories. Storytelling is in general considered to be essential to self-understanding and sensemaking [5, 70, 71], and the act of narrating and sharing stories about experiences with illness is generally acknowledged [72] and considered as a valuable part of the recovery process after stroke [73–76]. For people with aphasia, the normally taken-for-granted ability of language is seriously disrupted [6] by their reduced ability to transform experiences, thoughts, and feelings into language and stories. The participants in the present study experienced fewer options for expressing themselves, being listened to, and being met with understanding than they were used to before stroke onset. According to Frank [77], stories are intentional, meaning that they are told with the intent that they will be listened to, and acted upon. PWA need support to tell their stories, be listened to, and interact socially.

The method "Supported conversation for adults with aphasia" points to the responsibility and the skills of the nonaphasic conversation partner to facilitate conversations with people with aphasia [41]. Clinical interventions that can support and promote the narrative processes of people with aphasia are repeatedly called for in other studies [78, 79]. Simmons-Mackie and her colleagues [80] found that partner training was effective in improving communication activities and/or participation when individuals with aphasia interact with trained communication partners. They highlighted the need for nurses to be particularly capable in communicating information about aphasia and its course to PWA and their families. The role of skilled nurses working with PWA is also highlighted in other studies [81–83]. Professional acknowledgement of unfamiliar symptoms and reactions, as well as further discussions about ways to handle them, was experienced as beneficial. The value of professional legitimization of common reactions to changes caused by chronic illness in general was outlined by Bury in 1982 [6].

The exchange of personal and professional knowledge based on the contextualized real life experiences of the participants formed the basis for the active collaborative partnership between the intervention nurse and the participants in our intervention. According to the theoretical foundation of this intervention [33], professional competence (nurse) and personal competence (participants) were regarded as different but equally important, and they were considered complementary sources of knowledge exchanged through dialogues and mutual active participation [37]. Ellis and colleagues [21] found that knowledge provision and teaching, combined with self-study, and individualized counseling, and support were more effective than passive approaches for important outcomes such as depression and anxiety. PWA were not mentioned explicitly in that review, but the findings appear to be transferable to this group and are in line with our approach.

The statements on the standardized instruments mirrored the real-life experiences of challenges and coping expressed in the qualitative data during and after the intervention. Support during the difficult process of adjusting to change was perceived as helpful and beneficial. Several of them expressed that they needed support to endure. Depression and psychological distress in PWA after stroke are common and vary over time [9, 84]. In Kauhanen's study

[9], severe depression increased from 11% at three months to 33% at twelve months after stroke. We measured symptoms of psychological distress using the Hopkins Symptom Check List (HSCL-8). According to this instrument, only one participant reached the suggested cut-off score (at T3) used in other studies [54]. In our study findings both from the qualitative data and from statements on the instruments suggest that the participants are quite happy and relatively satisfied with life. We have reflected on whether participating in the intervention program contributed to the prevention of depression, but we cannot answer this question based on data from this small group. However, it would be of interest to evaluate this hypothesis in a larger, controlled study.

The changes in the scores on the SAQOL-39 (Figures 1(b) and 1(c)) tended to remain the same between T2 and T3, and for some items, there was a slight decrease. This might be associated with the absence of the "intervention sessions" during this period, as several of the participants lacked conversation partners with whom they could communicate well. Reduced levels of energy to maintain social connections also led to social isolation. Social support and interaction with others are acknowledged as essential for sensemaking, self-image, and identity adjustment [71], all of which are threatened in PWA [10, 85], and social support has been identified as a critical factor in living successfully with aphasia [67, 69, 86, 87]. Associations between lack of social support and psychological distress in PWA are also reported by others [84].

Adequate measurement and assessment of the outcomes of intervention studies is generally difficult [32] and probably even more challenging in studies including PWA [68, 88]. The triangulation of data from several sources in the present study helped us to understand the meaning behind the participants' expressions gathered by participant observation, interviews and clinical instruments. The reality of living with aphasia was still challenging, and the life situations of the participants were not ideal, but nonetheless, they were quite happy and satisfied. Participation in the intervention program was expressed as an important contribution to their psychosocial well-being during the first year after stroke.

5.1. Strengths and Limitations. The longitudinal design, with data collection both during the intervention and during three followup sessions, using triangulation of data as well as the designated methods, is thought to extend our understanding and improve the validity of the findings [46, 47]. Findings from the log notes, the interviews, and the standardized clinical instruments provided us with a significant amount of data from a group with reduced production of speech.

The same nurse performed the encounters and the followup interviews, and we believe that this was the best way to maximize the information from the participants considering their individual ways of communicating and their vulnerable situation. Trust and confidence in each case was developed over time, and the longitudinal design contributed to a continuity which allowed for a better understanding of the participants' recovery process, and the development of increasing richness and depth of the data over time. Both active participant observation and interviews with PWA present particular risks related to the subjective selection of quotes because this group often needs support to initiate conversations and assistance in keeping conversations going. This might be a potential source of bias [61]. The participants confirmed that they had expressed what was important to them during the interviews, but some of them also commented that they not were able to express themselves in the way they wanted to. Videotapes of the postintervention followup interviews were valuable for the transcription of the interviews (total communication) and the analytical process. They also enhanced the transparency between the authors who took part in the reflexive and analytical process and analyzed the text for competing interpretations. During the intervention, however, we opted not to tape the encounters due to ethical and pragmatic reasons, as the participants were included in an early phase after stroke when they were still inpatient in acute care hospitals or rehabilitation units. Doing so would probably have enhanced the analysis of the field notes but would also have distracted the attention during the dialogues and increased the costs.

The participants in this study were younger than the average stroke survivor, which is about 76 years old (75.3 for men and 77.7 for women) in Norway [67], and only one woman participated. Generalization from this small group is not possible, and nor was it intended, but our findings correspond with comparable findings from other studies, and we believe that knowledge from our study can be transferable to others engaged in psychosocial rehabilitation to PWA following stroke. The participants also received therapy from other health care professionals, which they also underscored as important. More investigation is needed to explore the interplay between different services.

6. Conclusion

Facilitating PWA with narration about themselves and their experiences, the provision of psychological support during a demanding recovery process, and the exchange of knowledge and information were experienced as beneficial to the recovery process in seven participants of a clinical intervention program. We believe it would be worthwhile to test this intervention in a larger context in future research.

Acknowledgments

The authors thank the participants with aphasia, health care professions, and experts for invaluable contribution to the study. They also thank Helge Ness, AR Smith Grafisk, for helping them with the layout of the worksheets. The authors received grants from the Norwegian Extra Foundation for Health and Rehabilitation (the Norwegian Aphasia Association) and Norwegian Women's Public Health Association. In addition, the study was supported by the University of Oslo and Hedmark University College.

References

[1] S. T. Engelter, M. Gostynski, S. Papa et al., "Epidemiology of aphasia attributable to first ischemic stroke: incidence, severity, fluency, etiology, and thrombolysis," *Stroke*, vol. 37, no. 6, pp. 1379–1384, 2006.

[2] C. Code and B. Petheram, "Delivering for aphasia," *International Journal of Speech-Language Pathology*, vol. 13, no. 1, pp. 3–10, 2011.

[3] A. C. Laska, A. Hellblom, V. Murray, T. Kahan, and M. Von Arbin, "Aphasia in acute stroke and relation to outcome," *Journal of Internal Medicine*, vol. 249, no. 5, pp. 413–422, 2001.

[4] C. Code and M. Herrmann, "The relevance of emotional and psychosocial factors in aphasia to rehabilitation," *Neuropsychological Rehabilitation*, vol. 13, no. 1-2, pp. 109–132, 2003.

[5] D. E. Polkinghorne, *Narrative Knowing and the Human Sciences*, State University of New York Press, Albany, NY, USA, 1988.

[6] M. Bury, "Chronic illness as biographical disruption," *Sociology of Health and Illness*, vol. 4, no. 2, pp. 167–182, 1982.

[7] S. Parr, *Living with Severe Aphasia—The Experience of Communication Impairment After Stroke*, Joseph Rowntree Foundation, Pavillion, Wyo, USA, 2004.

[8] F. J. Carod-Artal and J. A. Egido, "Quality of life after stroke: the importance of a good recovery," *Cerebrovascular Diseases*, vol. 27, no. 1, supplement, pp. 204–214, 2009.

[9] M. L. Kauhanen, J. T. Korpelainen, P. Hiltunen et al., "Aphasia, depression, and non-verbal cognitive impairment in ischaemic stroke," *Cerebrovascular Diseases*, vol. 10, no. 6, pp. 455–461, 2000.

[10] B. B. Shadden, "Aphasia as identity theft: theory and practice," *Aphasiology*, vol. 19, no. 3–5, pp. 211–223, 2005.

[11] M. C. Hallé, F. Duhamel, and G. Le Dorze, "The daughter-mother relationship in the presence of aphasia: how daughters view changes over the first year poststroke," *Qualitative Health Research*, vol. 21, no. 4, pp. 549–562, 2011.

[12] G. Le Dorze and F. H. Signori, "Needs, barriers and facilitators experienced by spouses of people with aphasia," *Disability and Rehabilitation*, vol. 32, no. 13, pp. 1073–1087, 2010.

[13] S. Parr, "Living with severe aphasia: tracking social exclusion," *Aphasiology*, vol. 21, no. 1, pp. 98–123, 2007.

[14] C. Code, "The quantity of life for people with chronic aphasia," *Neuropsychological Rehabilitation*, vol. 13, no. 3, pp. 379–390, 2003.

[15] M. Cruice, L. Worrall, L. Hickson, and R. Murison, "Finding a focus for quality of life with aphasia: social and emotional health, and psychological well-being," *Aphasiology*, vol. 17, no. 4, pp. 333–353, 2003.

[16] K. Brown, L. Worrall, B. Davidson, and T. Howe, "Snapshots of success: an insider perspective on living successfully with aphasia," *Aphasiology*, vol. 24, no. 10, pp. 1267–1295, 2010.

[17] J. Smith, A. Forster, A. House, P. Knapp, J. Wright, and J. Young, "Information provision for stroke patients and their caregivers," *Cochrane Database of Systematic Reviews*, no. 2, Article ID CD001919, 2008.

[18] P. Knapp, J. Young, A. House, and A. Forster, "Non-drug strategies to resolve psycho-social difficulties after stroke," *Age and Ageing*, vol. 29, no. 1, pp. 23–30, 2000.

[19] M. L. Hackett, C. S. Anderson, A. House, and C. Halteh, "Interventions for preventing depression after stroke,"

Cochrane Database of Systematic Reviews, no. 3, Article ID CD003689, 2008.

[20] M. L. Hackett, C. S. Anderson, A. House, and J. Xia, "Interventions for treating depression after stroke," *Cochrane Database of Systematic Reviews*, no. 4, Article ID CD003437, 2008.

[21] G. Ellis, J. Mant, P. Langhorne, M. Dennis, and S. Winner, "Stroke liaison workers for stroke patients and carers: an individual patient data meta-analysis," *Cochrane Database of Systematic Reviews*, vol. 5, Article ID CD005066, 2010.

[22] J. Redfern, C. McKevitt, and C. D. A. Wolfe, "Development of complex interventions in stroke care: a systematic review," *Stroke*, vol. 37, no. 9, pp. 2410–2419, 2006.

[23] C. Burton and B. Gibbon, "Expanding the role of the stroke nurse: a pragmatic clinical trial," *Journal of Advanced Nursing*, vol. 52, no. 6, pp. 640–650, 2005.

[24] C. L. Watkins, M. F. Auton, C. F. Deans et al., "Motivational interviewing early after acute stroke: a randomized, controlled trial," *Stroke*, vol. 38, no. 3, pp. 1004–1009, 2007.

[25] C. Pound, "Reciprocity, resources, and relationships: new discourses in healthcare, personal, and social relationships," *International Journal of Speech-Language Pathology*, vol. 13, no. 3, pp. 197–206, 2011.

[26] K. Hilari and S. Byng, "Health-related quality of life in people with severe aphasia," *International Journal of Language and Communication Disorders*, vol. 44, no. 2, pp. 193–205, 2009.

[27] E. Carlsson, B. L. Paterson, S. Scott-Findlay, M. Ehnfors, and A. Ehrenberg, "Methodological issues in interviews involving people with communication impairments after acquired brain damage," *Qualitative Health Research*, vol. 17, no. 10, pp. 1361–1371, 2007.

[28] I. E. Poslawsky, M. J. Schuurmans, E. Lindeman, and T. B. Hafsteinsdóttir, "A systematic review of nursing rehabilitation of stroke patients with aphasia," *Journal of Clinical Nursing*, vol. 19, no. 1-2, pp. 17–32, 2010.

[29] F. Hjelmblink, C. B. Bernsten, H. Uvhagen, S. Kunkel, and I. Holmström, "Understanding the meaning of rehabilitation to an aphasic patient through phenomenological analysis— a case study," *International Journal of Qualitative Studies on Health and Well-Being*, vol. 2, no. 2, pp. 93–100, 2007.

[30] M. Kirkevold, "The role of nursing in the rehabilitation of stroke survivors: an extended theoretical account," *Advances in Nursing Science*, vol. 33, no. 1, pp. E27–E40, 2010.

[31] C. Burton, *Developing Stroke Services: A Key Role for Nursing and Nurses*, Wiley-Blackwell, Oxford, UK, 2010.

[32] P. Craig, P. Dieppe, S. Macintyre, S. Mitchie, I. Nazareth, and M. Petticrew, "Developing and evaluating complex interventions: the new medical research council guidance," *British Medical Journal*, vol. 337, no. 7676, pp. 979–983, 2008.

[33] M. Kirkevold, B. A. Bronken, R. Martinsen, and K. Kvigne, "Promoting psychosocial well-being following a stroke: developing a theoretically and empirically sound complex intervention," *International Journal of Nursing Studies*, vol. 49, no. 4, pp. 386–397, 2012.

[34] M. Q. Patton, *Qualitative Research & Evaluation Methods*, SAGE, Thousand Oaks, Calif, USA, 2002.

[35] K. L. Easton, "The poststroke journey: from agonizing to owning," *Geriatric Nursing*, vol. 20, no. 2, pp. 70–76, 1999.

[36] M. Kirkevold, "The unfolding illness trajectory of stroke," *Disability and Rehabilitation*, vol. 24, no. 17, pp. 887–898, 2002.

[37] V. Z. Knudsen, *Guided Self-determination: A Life Skills Approach Developed in Difficult Type 1 Diabetes*, Department of Nursing Science, University of Aarhus, Aarhus, Denmark, 2004.

[38] S. Næss, "Quality of life as psychological well-being," *Tidsskr Nor Lægeforen*, vol. 16, no. 121, pp. 1940–1944, 2001.

[39] C. Code, G. Hemsley, and M. Herrmann, "The emotional impact of aphasia," *Seminars in Speech and Language*, vol. 20, no. 1, pp. 19–31, 1999.

[40] B. Fure, T. B. Wyller, K. Engedal, and B. Thommessen, "Emotional symptoms in acute ischemic stroke," *International Journal of Geriatric Psychiatry*, vol. 21, no. 4, pp. 382–387, 2006.

[41] A. L. Holland, "Why can't clinicians talk to aphasic adults? Comments on supported conversation for adults with aphasia: methods and resources for training conversational partners," *Aphasiology*, vol. 12, no. 9, pp. 844–847, 1998.

[42] J. S. Damico, N. Simmons-Mackie, M. Oelschlaeger, R. Elman, and E. Armstrong, "Qualitative methods in aphasia research: basic issues," *Aphasiology*, vol. 13, no. 9-11, pp. 651–665, 1999.

[43] J. S. Damico and N. N. Simmons-Mackie, "Qualitative research and speech-language pathology: a tutorial for the clinical realm," *American Journal of Speech-Language Pathology*, vol. 12, no. 2, pp. 131–143, 2003.

[44] T. B. Wyller and U. Sveen, "Non-verbal cognitive symptoms after stroke," *Tidsskr Nor Lægeforen*, vol. 122, no. 6, pp. 627–630, 2002.

[45] R. Riise, B. Gundersen, S. Brodal, and P. Bjerke, "Visual problems in cerebral stroke," *Tidsskrift for den Norske Laegeforening*, vol. 125, no. 2, pp. 176–177, 2005.

[46] T. Farmer, K. Robinson, S. J. Elliott, and J. Eyles, "Developing and implementing a triangulation protocol for qualitative health research," *Qualitative Health Research*, vol. 16, no. 3, pp. 377–394, 2006.

[47] R. E. Stake, *Multiple Case Study Analysis*, The Guilford Press, New York, NY, USA, 2006.

[48] R. K. Yin, *Case Study Research: Design and Methods*, Sage, Los Angeles, Calif, USA, 2009.

[49] K. Hilari, S. Byng, D. L. Lamping, and S. C. Smith, "Stroke and aphasia quality of life scale-39 (SAQOL-39): evaluation of acceptability, reliability, and validity," *Stroke*, vol. 34, no. 8, pp. 1944–1950, 2003.

[50] H. Cantril, *The Patterns of Human Concerns*, Rutgers University Press, New Brunswick, NJ, USA, 1965.

[51] J. P. Robinson, P. R. Shaver, and L. S. Wrightsman, *Measures of Personality and Social Psychological Attitudes*, Academic Press, San Diego, Calif, USA, 1991.

[52] K. Tambs, Ed., *Choice of Questions in Short Form Questionnairs of Established Psychometric Instruments. Proposed Procedure and Some Examples*, Universtitetet i Oslo, Oslo, Norway, 2004.

[53] K. Hilari and S. Byng, "Measuring quality of life in people with aphasia: the stroke specific quality of life scale," *International Journal of Language and Communication Disorders*, vol. 36, no. 1, pp. 86–91, 2001.

[54] B. H. Strand, O. S. Dalgard, K. Tambs, and M. Rognerud, "Measuring the mental health status of the Norwegian population: a comparison of the instruments SCL-25, SCL-10, SCL-5 and MHI-5 (SF-36)," *Nordic Journal of Psychiatry*, vol. 57, no. 2, pp. 113–118, 2003.

[55] P. Ricoeur, *Interpretation Theory: Discourse and the Surplus of Meaning*, Texas Christian University Press, Fort Worth, Tex, USA, 1976.

[56] P. Ricoeur, "The metaphorical process as cognition, imagination, and feeling," *Critical Inquiry*, vol. 5, no. 1, pp. 143–159, 1978.

[57] P. Ricoeur, "Narrative time," *Critical Inquiry*, vol. 7, no. 1, pp. 169–190, 1980.

[58] S. Kvale, *Det Kvalitative Forskningsintervju*, Ad notam Gyldendal, Oslo, Norway, 1997.

[59] S. Kvale, *Doing Interviews*, vol. 2, Sage, London, UK, 2007.

[60] K. Malterud, "The art and science of clinical knowledge: evidence beyond measures and numbers," *Lancet*, vol. 358, no. 9279, pp. 397–400, 2001.

[61] K. Malterud, "Qualitative research: standards, challenges, and guidelines," *Lancet*, vol. 358, no. 9280, pp. 483–488, 2001.

[62] A. Lindseth and A. Norberg, "A phenomenological hermeneutical method for researching lived experience," *Scandinavian Journal of Caring Sciences*, vol. 18, no. 2, pp. 145–153, 2004.

[63] V. Lloyd, A. Gatherer, and S. Kalsy, "Conducting qualitative interview research with people with expressive language difficulties," *Qualitative Health Research*, vol. 16, no. 10, pp. 1386–1404, 2006.

[64] J. M. Morse, "Ethics in action: ethical principles for doing qualitative health research," *Qualitative Health Research*, vol. 17, no. 8, pp. 1003–1005, 2007.

[65] B. A. Bronken, M. Kirkevold, R. Martinsen, and K. Kvigne, "The aphasic storyteller: coconstructing stories to promote psychosocial well-being after stroke," *Qualitative Health Research*. In press.

[66] H. Ellekjær and R. Selmer, "Stroke—similar incidence, better prognosis," *Tidsskrift for den Norske Laegeforening*, vol. 127, no. 6, pp. 740–743, 2007.

[67] A. L. Holland, A. S. Halper, and L. R. Cherney, "Tell me your story: analysis of script topics selected by persons with aphasia," *American Journal of Speech-Language Pathology*, vol. 19, no. 3, pp. 198–203, 2010.

[68] A. Kagan, N. Simmons-Mackie, A. Rowland et al., "Counting what counts: a framework for capturing real-life outcomes of aphasia intervention," *Aphasiology*, vol. 22, no. 3, pp. 258–280, 2008.

[69] L. Worrall, K. Brown, M. Cruice et al., "The evidence for a life-coaching approach to aphasia," *Aphasiology*, vol. 24, no. 4, pp. 497–514, 2010.

[70] J. Bruner, "The narrative construction of reality," *Critical Inquiry*, vol. 18, no. 1, pp. 1–21, 1991.

[71] P. Atkinson, "The life story interview," in *Institutional Ethnography Using Interviews to Investigate Ruling Relation*, M. I. Devault and L. McCoy, Eds., Sage, London, UK, 2003.

[72] A. W. Frank, *The Wounded Storyteller: Body, Illness, and Ethics*, University of Chicago Press, Chicago, Ill, USA, 1995.

[73] C. A. Faircloth, M. Rittman, C. Boylstein, M. E. Young, and M. Van Puymbroeck, "Energizing the ordinary: biographical work and the future in stroke recovery narratives," *Journal of Aging Studies*, vol. 18, no. 4, pp. 399–413, 2004.

[74] C. A. Faircloth, C. Boylstein, M. Rittman, M. E. Young, and J. Gubrium, "Sudden illness and biographical flow in narratives of stroke recovery," *Sociology of Health and Illness*, vol. 26, no. 2, pp. 242–261, 2004.

[75] C. A. Faircloth, C. Boylstein, M. Rittman, and J. F. Gubrium, "Constructing the stroke: sudden-onset narratives of stroke survivors," *Qualitative Health Research*, vol. 15, no. 7, pp. 928–941, 2005.

[76] S. Kaufman, "Illness, biography, and the interpretation of self following a stroke," *Journal of Aging Studies*, vol. 2, no. 3, pp. 217–227, 1988.

[77] A. W. Frank, "The standpoint of storyteller," *Qualitative Health Research*, vol. 10, no. 3, pp. 354–365, 2000.

[78] B. B. Shadden and F. Hagstrom, "The role of narrative in the life participation approach to aphasia," *Topics in Language Disorders*, vol. 27, no. 4, pp. 324–338, 2007.

[79] J. Hinckley, "Hope for happy endings: stories of clients and clinicians," *Topics in Stroke Rehabilitation*, vol. 17, no. 1, pp. 1–5, 2010.

[80] N. Simmons-Mackie, A. Raymer, E. Armstrong, A. Holland, and L. R. Cherney, "Communication partner training in Aphasia: a systematic review," *Archives of Physical Medicine and Rehabilitation*, vol. 91, no. 12, pp. 1814–1837, 2010.

[81] K. Sundin, A. Norberg, and L. Jansson, "The meaning of skilled care providers' relationships with stroke and aphasia patients," *Qualitative Health Research*, vol. 11, no. 3, pp. 308–321, 2001.

[82] K. Sundin, L. Jansson, and A. Norberg, "Understanding between care providers and patients with stroke and aphasia: a phenomenological hermeneutic inquiry," *Nursing Inquiry*, vol. 9, no. 2, pp. 93–103, 2002.

[83] K. Sundin and L. Jansson, ""Understanding and being understood" as a creative caring phenomenon—in care of patients with stroke and aphasia," *Journal of Clinical Nursing*, vol. 12, no. 1, pp. 107–116, 2003.

[84] K. Hilari, S. Northcott, P. Roy et al., "Psychological distress after stroke and aphasia: the first six months," *Clinical Rehabilitation*, vol. 24, no. 2, pp. 181–190, 2010.

[85] R. MacKay, ""Tell them who i was" [1]: the social construction of aphasia," *Disability and Society*, vol. 18, no. 6, pp. 811–826, 2003.

[86] J. J. Hinckley, "Finding messages in bottles: living successfully with stroke and aphasia," *Topics in Stroke Rehabilitation*, vol. 13, no. 1, pp. 25–36, 2006.

[87] K. Hilari, "The impact of stroke: are people with aphasia different to those without?" *Disability and Rehabilitation*, vol. 33, no. 3, pp. 211–218, 2011.

[88] N. Simmons-Mackie, T. T. Threats, and A. Kagan, "Outcome assessment in aphasia: a survey," *Journal of Communication Disorders*, vol. 38, no. 1, pp. 1–27, 2005.

11

Associations between Upper Extremity Motor Function and Aphasia after Stroke

Shuo Xu [ID],[1] Zhijie Yan,[1,2] Yongquan Pan,[1] Qing Yang,[1] Zhilan Liu,[3] Jiajia Gao,[4] Yanhui Yang,[5] Yufen Wu,[6] Yanan Zhang,[7] Jianhui Wang,[8] Ren Zhuang,[9] Chong Li [ID],[1,10] Yongli Zhang,[1,11] and Jie Jia [ID][1,12,13]

[1]Department of Rehabilitation Medicine, Huashan Hospital, Fudan University, Shanghai, China
[2]Xinxiang Medical University, Xinxiang, China
[3]Department of Rehabilitation Medicine, Shanghai Fourth Rehabilitation Hospital, Shanghai, China
[4]Department of Neurorehabilitation, The Shanghai Third Rehabilitation Hospital, Shanghai, China
[5]Department of Rehabilitation Medicine, Shaanxi Provincial Rehabilitation Hospital, Shaanxi, China
[6]Department of Rehabilitation Medicine, Liuzhou Traditional Chinese Medicine Hospital, Guangxi, China
[7]Department of Rehabilitation Medicine, The Third Affiliated Clinical Hospital of Changchun University of Chinese Medicine, Jilin, China
[8]Department of Rehabilitation Medicine, Nanshi Hospital Affiliated to Henan University, Henan, China
[9]Department of Rehabilitation Medicine, Changzhou Dean Hospital, Jiangsu, China
[10]Shanghai University of Sport, Shanghai, China
[11]Fujian University of Traditional Chinese Medicine, Fujian, China
[12]National Clinical Research Center for Aging and Medicine, Huashan Hospital, Fudan University, China
[13]National Center for Neurological Disorders, Shanghai, China

Correspondence should be addressed to Jie Jia; shannonjj@126.com

Academic Editor: Grigorios Nasios

Background and Purpose. Poststroke aphasia (PSA) often coexists with upper extremity (UE) motor dysfunction. However, whether the presence of PSA affects UE motor performance, and if language function associates with UE motor performance, are unclear. This study is aimed at (1) comparing the motor status of UE between patients with PSA and without PSA and (2) investigating the association between language function and UE motor status in patients with PSA. *Methods.* Patients with stroke were compared and correlated from overall and three periods (1-3 months, 4-6 months, and >6 months). Fugl-Meyer assessment for the upper extremity (FMA-UE) and action research and arm test (ARAT) were used to compare the UE motor status between patients with PSA and without PSA through a cross-sectional study among 435 patients. Then, the correlations between the evaluation scale scores of UE motor status and language function of patients with PSA were analyzed in various dimensions, and the language subfunction most closely related to UE motor function was analyzed by multiple linear regression analysis. *Results.* We found that the scores of FMA-UE and ARAT in patients with PSA were 14 points ((CI) 10 to 18, $p < 0.001$) and 11 points lower ((CI) 8 to 13, $p < 0.001$), respectively, than those without PSA. Their FMA-UE ($r = 0.70$, $p < 0.001$) and ARAT ($r = 0.62$, $p < 0.001$) scores were positively correlated with language function. Regression analysis demonstrated that spontaneous speech ability may account for UE motor function ($R^2 = 0.51$, $p < 0.001$; $R^2 = 0.42$, $p < 0.001$). Consistent results were also obtained from the analyses within the three time subgroups. *Conclusion.* Stroke patients with PSA have worse UE motor performance. UE motor status and language function showed positive correlations, in which spontaneous speech ability significantly accounts for the associations.

1. Introduction

Patients after stroke who have both upper extremity (UE) motor impairment and/or language dysfunction are common [1]. These two types of poststroke dysfunction are the most apparent neuropsychological deficits occurring after stroke: UE motor deficit occurs in about 80% of stroke survivors, aphasia in 21%-38%, and cooccurrence in about 24% [2–4]. PSA with UE motor dysfunction impacts social participation and quality of life, and it can also be associated with multiple comorbidities and lead to worse prognosis [5, 6]. Due to the adjacent anatomical location, ischemia or hemorrhage in the middle cerebral artery (MCA) often leads to UE motor dysfunction and nonfluent aphasia. Nevertheless, there are small samples of study that have analyzed the relationship between hand-arm motor dysfunction and aphasia using lesion volume and location as control variables, showing that the association is not determined by anatomical relationships alone. The extents and limitations of UE and language cortical reciprocity remain under debate; it is likely that UE movement and language have shared neural correlates not merely depending on anatomical proximity and vascular factors.

In Huashan Hospital, there is an original operation, a contralateral seventh cervical nerve transfer to improve UE motor function in patients with chronic central injury [7]. After the surgery, we found that patients with PSA not only improved their UE motor status but also their language function. These phenomena suggest a deep neural mechanism relationship between language function and UE motor status after stroke. Several studies [8–11] have focused on the potential relationship between UE motor status and language function. From a human evolution perspective, language was spurred by freedom of hand movement as an additional consequence of this upright posture. Gestures are a combination of UE movements and language [12]. A retrospective cohort study addressed the possible interaction between motor impairment and aphasia recovery after stroke. Motor responders showed better linguistic performances at the final aphasia assessment than motor nonresponders, while language responders reached a higher level of motor functioning than language nonresponders [8]. Meanwhile, a significant response in one domain was not associated with any deterioration in the other. Furthermore, Harnish et al. examined five patients with aphasia and hemiparesis poststroke during six weeks of UE therapy but not receiving speech therapy. Patients were assessed not only for the UE motor recovery but also for changes in their language abilities. fMRI data demonstrated shifts in increased blood oxygen improvements in both UE motor status and language function scores [13]. However, current studies rarely focus on simultaneous UE motor dysfunction with language deficits and even less on both functions' concurrent recovery during stroke recovery. Most studies only unexpectedly found this phenomenon or were mostly exploratory paradigm intervention studies [1, 14–16]. Few studies have focused on the difference in UE motor function status between patients with PSA and nonphasic poststroke patients. Moreover, no study provides evidence on the correlation between UE motor status and language function after stroke [8, 9], which leads to low attention to UE-language correlation so that UE and speech-language therapies are completely separated during UE motor and (or) speech rehabilitation.

To cover this gap, the present study investigated the UE motor status and language function of stroke patients by a cross-sectional investigation. We hypothesized that there were differences in motor status between stroke patients with PSA and without PSA and that there were some relationships between the speech-language function and UE motor status in patients with PSA.

Therefore, the objectives of this study were (1) to compare the UE motor status between patients with PSA and without PSA, (2) to investigate the association between language function and UE motor status in patients with PSA, and (3) based on (2), to determine which dimension of PSA evaluation is most closely related to the UE motor status.

2. Methods

2.1. Study Population and Design. This study was conducted between May 2020 and June 2021 in the departments of rehabilitation medicine of six hospitals from different regions in China. Patients were consecutively screened for the following criteria: (1) aged 18 years or older; (2) native Chinese speaker, (3) stroke onset > 1 week, (4) with a primary diagnosis of acute cerebrovascular accident according to the WHO diagnostic criteria confirmed by computed tomography (CT) or magnetic resonance imaging (MRI), (5) underwent rehabilitation assessed by a team of specialists (physicians, speech therapists, and occupational therapists), and (6) had ability to complete all the assessment. However, individuals were excluded if the consent of the patient's family could not be obtained; if there was no imaging available; if they had a previous history of stroke; if they had a severe hearing impairment or visual impairment; if they had other primary medical conditions that could influence language and motor function; such as a brain tumor, Parkinson's disease, severe poststroke depression, and Alzheimer's disease; or if they had undergone surgical evacuation.

Patients were evaluated in a single test session performed by speech therapists and occupational therapists who had received consistency training. One trained researcher performed the data collection. Patients' baseline characteristics were evaluated, including age at stroke onset, gender, comorbidities, hand dominance, time poststroke, lateralization, and stroke type. After 2326 patients were screened, those who met the above conditions participated in this study, 214 among whom with PSA were in the observational PSA group. A group of 221 patients without PSA after stroke matched for age and sex participated and were distributed into the non-PSA group as controls. The sample sizes were estimated referring to other similar studies [8, 17, 18]. As an important outcome, the UE motor impairment and function between the two groups were compared. Further evaluation was done in the observational PSA group to see the association between UE motor status and language function evaluation scores. For further validation purposes, the relationships between them were analyzed by multiple linear regression. Then, to observe the difference between different time periods from stroke onset, subsequent stratification analyses by time (1-3 months, 4-6 months, and >6 months) were performed. Our study used a cross-sectional observational design. The ethics committee approved the study protocol of Huashan Hospital of Fudan University and all participating centers according to the 1964 Declaration of Helsinki's ethical standards and its later amendments. This trial is registered with ChiCTR2000033792. All patients or their families provided written informed consent before study enrollment.

2.2. Measurement Instruments and Evaluation

2.2.1. Evaluation of PSA: Aphasia Quotient of Western Aphasia Battery-Revised (WAB-AQ) and Boston Diagnostic Aphasia Examination (BDAE). PSA was evaluated using the Chinese version of WAB-AQ, a commonly used clinical evaluation of PSA that assesses the presence, type, and severity of aphasia with a 0-100 scale (score < 93.8 are indicative of aphasia). The WAB-AQ elaborately evaluates the domains of expression and comprehension, yielding summary scores for the following four domains: spontaneous speech, auditory verbal comprehension, repetition, and naming. The four dimensions of scores were recorded and counted. AQ, the weighted composite of these four scores, was used as the independent variable of interest in this study and is indicative of the overall severity of the patients' PSA. On the other hand, for easy screening and observation, the BDAE severity grading standard was chosen to classify the severity of patient language dysfunction with grade criteria of 0, 1, 2, 3, 4, and 5 [19]. Grade 0 is meaningless language or auditory comprehension, while grade 5 is a barely recognizable language disorder, and the patient may have some subjective difficulties, but it is not easy for the listener to detect. All patients have to be assessed by BDAE, and only if the grade < 5 will WAB-AQ be evaluated.

2.2.2. Evaluation of UE Motor Impairment: Fugl-Meyer Assessment for the Upper Extremity (FMA-UE). The FMA was used to assess extremity motricity, balance, some sensory details, and joint dysfunction in hemiplegic patients. We evaluated the only motor function of the UE, including measurement of voluntary movement, velocity, coordination, and reflex activity. A total of 33 items are included. A 3-step (0-1-2) ordinal scale is applied to each item (0 = details cannot be performed; 1 = details are performed only partly; 2 = details are performed throughout the full range of motion of the joint). This gives a total maximum score of 66, which defines a normal motor function (42 and 14 for the arm and hand, respectively). FMA-UE mainly aims at evaluating UE motor impairment and dysfunction after stroke.

2.2.3. Evaluation of UE Motor Function: Action Research Arm Test (ARAT). Instruments needed to perform the test are as follows: woodblocks, a ball, a washer and bolt, a stone, two different sizes of alloy tubes, two glasses, a marble, and a

6 mm ball bearing (instrument model: OT-KL-40400). The test is a 4-grade scale ranging from 0 to 3 with a maximum score = 57 (0 = can perform no part of the test; 1 = can perform the test partially; 2 = can complete the test but takes an abnormally long time or has great difficulty; and 3 = can perform test normally). ARAT is a quantitative test for the UE function and includes four subsets: grasp, grip, pinch, and gross movement. Both ARAT and FMA-UE are widely used and are the most recognized methods to evaluate the motor status of UE in patients with stroke. The difference is that ARAT is mainly aimed at motor function assessment and activity measurement, while FMA-UE pays more attention to dysfunction and impairment.

2.3. Statistical Analysis. Data were analyzed with IBM SPSS Statistics version 26.0. Demographics and clinical variables, presented as mean ± standard deviation for continuous variables and proportions for categorical variables, were compared between observation and control groups using the independent sample Student t-test, the Chi test, and the Mann–Whitney U-test, as appropriate. The Spearman correlation analysis between WAB-AQ and FMA-UE scores was made to address the association question. Then, to eliminate the influence of some factors on the correlation analysis, the correlation coefficients between WAB-AQ and FMA-UE are corrected for age, education, and duration poststroke. Similarly, this method is also used between WAB-AQ and ARAT scores and between the four parts of WAB-AQ (spontaneous speech, understanding, repetition, and naming) and FMA-UE as well as ARAT scores. In addition, all patients were stratified according to 3 time periods (1-3 months, 4-6 months, and >6 months) and compared, and correlated analyses were performed within each of the three periods by the same method as the overall analysis. In the end, we performed two multiple linear regression analyses, using the "enter" method, to determine which dimension of WAB-AQ was the most informative in accounting for the UE motor function with WAB-AQ including spontaneous speech, comprehension, repetition, and naming scores as independent variables and ARAT or FMA-UE scores as dependent variables.

3. Results

3.1. Demographics. From a total of 2326 patients, we excluded 1891, leaving 435 patients for analysis (see Figure 1). 435 patients underwent a complete systematic assessment with a median course of 15 weeks (IQR: 7-32). The median age of the patients was 60.6 years (SD = 11.2). A total of 153 were female, and 282 were male. Table 1(a) shows the patient characteristics, presented for the total group and for the patients with PSA ($n = 214$, 49.2%) and without PSA ($n = 221$, 50.8%). 370 patients suffered from ischemic stroke and 65 from hemorrhage. A total of 330 patients showed right-sided hemiparesis, while 105 patients showed left-sided hemiparesis. Stratification according to stroke duration showed 69 in the PSA group and 76 in the non-PSA group for patients stratified according to a period of 1-3 months; 69 in the PSA group and 72 in the non-

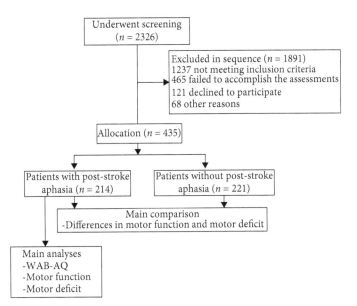

FIGURE 1: Flow chart of the study sample and procedures of the comparison and analyses. WAB-AQ indicates the Western Aphasia Battery-Aphasia Quotient; FMA-UE indicates the Fugl-Meyer assessment for the upper extremity; ARAT indicates the action research and action test.

PSA group for patients stratified according to a period of 4-6 months; and 76 in the PSA group and 73 in the non-PSA group for patients stratified according to a period >6 months. No statistically significant difference was found in age, gender, comorbidities, hand dominance, time poststroke, and type of stroke between groups.

3.2. Comparison between Groups and Distribution of PSA Group.

The FMA-UE and ARAT scores were compared between groups through the Wilcoxon rank sum test. The confidence interval estimation of median difference based on the Wilcoxon rank sum test is obtained by the Hodges-Lehmann method. The contrast revealed a significant difference between groups ($p < 0.001$; Table 1(b)), and it showed that the non-PSA group had significantly higher scores than the PSA group ($p < 0.001$, Figure 2). Detailed scores of the four dimensions in the 214 PSA patients are summarized in Table 1(b). After stratification according to the stroke time, the three comparisons (PSA versus non-PSA) of subgroups (1-3 months, 4-6 months, and >6 months) still obtained consistent results ($p < 0.001$, Figure 2).

3.3. Correlations between PSA and Motor Function and Deficit.

Table 2 illustrates the results of the correlation analyses between language functions (WAB-AQ, spontaneous speech, comprehension, repetition, and naming score) and UE motor status (FMA-UE and ARAT scores) from the overall perspective and from the perspective of the three time periods. We adjusted the correlation coefficients with age, education, and duration poststroke. Overall, moderate to strong positive correlations were found between WAB-AQ and ARAT score ($r = 0.62$, $p < 0.001$, Figure 3(b)). Further, there were stronger correlations between WAB-AQ and FMA-UE score ($r = 0.70$, $p < 0.001$, Figure 3(a)). For all the factors analyzed, their correlation coefficients varied from 0.45 to 0.72, of which the weakest correlation was comprehension, and the strongest was spontaneous speech. All

results of partial correlation analysis, taking age, education, and duration poststroke as covariates, are shown in Table 2. Consistent with overall correlation results, the results of the partial correlation analyses according to the time stratification are shown in Table 2. We found that the highest correlation coefficient was WAB-AQ and FMA-UE in 4-6 months ($r = 0.76$, $p < 0.001$). Overall, the time stratification association trends were consistent with the overall analyses (see Figure 4).

3.4. Factors Associated with Motor Dysfunction.

Two multiple linear regression analyses were performed to identify the most related factors that affect ARAT and FMA-UE scores. In the first regression model between four variables of WAB-AQ (spontaneous speech, comprehension, repetition, and naming score) and ARAT score, the results demonstrated that the four independent variables of WAB-AQ explained 42% of the variance in the ARAT score ($R^2 = 0.42$, $p < 0.001$). However, only the spontaneous speech score was significant ($R^2 = 0.42$, $p < 0.001$, Figure 3(d)). The other three variables had no significant difference ($p > 0.05$). The second regression model also examined the four independent variables with the FMA-UE score. The results demonstrated that the four independent variables of WAB-AQ explained 51% of the variance in the FMA-UE score ($R^2 = 0.51$, $p < 0.001$). Similarly, only the spontaneous speech score was significant ($R^2 = 0.51$, $p < 0.001$, Figure 3(c)); the other three variables had no significant difference ($p > 0.05$).

4. Discussion

Our results demonstrated that the UE motor status of patients without PSA is better than those with PSA, and there are positive relationships between UE motor status and language functions in patients with PSA (see Table 2). Spontaneous speech ability, one of the language functions, is most closely related to UE motor status, which explained

Table 1

(a) Comparisons of demographic data between the PSA group and the non-PSA group

	PSA group ($n = 214$)	Non-PSA group ($n = 221$)	p value
Female, n (%)	82 (38.3)	71 (32.1)	0.176[b]
Age, mean (SD) (y)	61.1 ± 11.9	60.1 ± 10.4	0.340[a]
Education, mean (SD) (y)	10.32 ± 3.7	10.91 ± 5.4	0.184[a]
Duration poststroke, median (IQR) (week)	16 (6-35)	14 (7-32)	0.316[c]
Type of injury, n (%)			0.586[b]
Ischemia	180 (84.1)	190 (86.0)	
Hemorrhage	34 (15.9)	31 (14.0)	
Affected limb, n (%)			0.297[b]
Right	167 (78.0)	163 (73.8)	
Left	47 (22.0)	58 (26.2)	

(b) Comparisons of clinical variables between the PSA group and the non-PSA group

	PSA group ($n = 214$)	Non-PSA group ($n = 221$)	Mean difference (95% CI)	p value
Motor evaluation, median (IQR)				
FMA-UE	20 (7-40)	35 (23-52)	14 (10, 18)	<0.001[c]
ARAT	5.5 (0-30)	21 (11-45)	11 (8, 13)	<0.001[c]
Language evaluation, median (IQR)				
BDAE	1.57 ± 1.18	5	-3.43 (-3.6, -3.3)	<0.001[d]
WAB-AQ	44.6 (18.1-70.6)			
Spontaneous speech	7.0 (2.0-13.0)			
Comprehension	126.0 (60.0-175.0)			
Repetition	50.0 (9.8-80.0)			
Naming	27.0 (0.8-67.3)			

[a]Two independent sample t-test. [b]χ^2 test. [c]Wilcoxon's rank sum test. [d]Single sample t-test. Abbreviations: SD indicates standard error of the mean; IQR indicates interquartile range; CI indicates confidence interval; FMA-UE indicates the Fugl-Meyer assessment of the upper extremity; ARAT indicates the action research and action test; BDAE indicates the Boston Diagnostic Aphasia Examination; WAB-AQ indicates the Western Aphasia Battery-Aphasia Quotient.

51% of the variance in the motor deficit and 42% in motor function, respectively (see Figures 3(c) and 3(d)). Previous studies have mentioned that the recovery of motor and language function is operated in parallel [20–23]. Due to the lack of data demonstrating UE motor status associated with language function, current stroke rehabilitation evaluations and therapies have treated these two symptoms separately [8, 24]. Patients with PSA receiving speech-language therapy are frequently seated during treatment, with UE impassive and motionless [9]. Our results supported the hypothesis that poststroke patients' UE motor status and language function are highly correlated, and UE motor status assessment and therapy should be integrated into the treatment for patients with PSA [9].

Similar to the findings of previous studies [25, 26], after evaluation of FMA-UE, ARAT, and WAB-AQ, we found that the evaluation scores of patients with PSA were significantly lower than those of nonaphasia patients with no difference in age, educational background, and course of stroke between the two groups not only from an overall perspective but also from three time perspectives (see Figure 4).

PSA is independently associated with increased complications and length of stay during the acute stroke admission after controlling for NIHSS score, with an effect comparable to severe hemiparesis, and sometimes greater [26]. Likewise, patients with PSA have lower motor Functional Independence Measures (FIM) and cognitive FIM scores both at admission and at discharge, compared to those without PSA during the subacute and chronic period [25]. Our findings support their findings and provide a supplement and explanation for this phenomenon. FIM is a routine assessment in stroke rehabilitation centers to quantify the ability to perform daily activities after stroke with a 7-point scale for 5 cognitive and 13 motor tasks such as getting dressed, bowel, and grooming control [10]. FMA-UE and ARAT scales are specifically used to evaluate UE motor deficit and motor function for stroke patients [20]. Overall, our results provide preliminary evidence why aphasia patients have worse FIM scores and long hospitalization.

Hybbinette et al. [27] confirmed the common occurrence of apraxia of speech and aphasia in left hemisphere stroke patients with a hand motor impairment through a

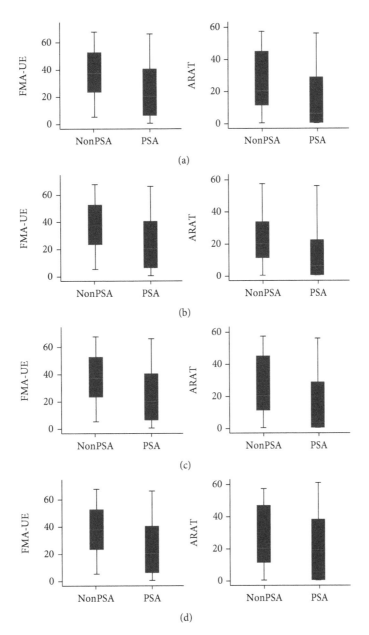

FIGURE 2: Clinical measurement of the FMA-UE and ARAT scores. (a) Comparison of the FMA-UE and ARAT total scores between the non-PSA and PSA groups. (b–d) Comparisons of the FMA-UE and ARAT total scores between the non-PSA and PSA groups in 1-3 months, 4-6 months, and >6 months. Significant differences were observed in both groups. $p < 0.001$. Abbreviation: non-PSA indicates patients without poststroke aphasia; PSA indicates patients with poststroke aphasia; FMA-UE indicates the Fugl-Meyer assessment for the upper extremity; ARAT indicates the action research and action test.

small sample study. Our correlation analyses results show that the four dimensions of language function—spontaneous speech, comprehension, repetition, and naming—were all associated with UE motor status (see Figure 5). The correlation between spontaneous speech and UE motor status is the strongest, while the correlation of comprehension is the weakest among the four dimensions. Because some patients have been paralyzed for a long time, the ARAT scale has basic requirements for the UE function. Some of the patients had low or even zero scores of ARAT, which reduce the correlation coefficient to a great extent (seeing Figure 3(b)). Furthermore, regression analyses show that spontaneous

speech ability can account for UE motor status to some degree. Consistent with previous studies, our results make their conclusions more convincing that the Aachen aphasia test (AAT) is a predictor of functional outcome in patients with aphasia [26]. Its predictive power is like that of other functional tests commonly recognized to predict outcome strongly. Among the language functions in AAT, comprehension seems to be the most important predictive factor of the total and cognitive FIM, while spontaneous speech ability seems to be a motor-FIM predictor. There were unexpected findings in previous studies that in the treatment of UE motor deficits, the patient's language function was

TABLE 2: Pearson's correlation between four parts of WAB-AQ and FMA-UE and ARAT scores.

Language motor	WAB-AQ	Spontaneous speech	Comprehension	Repetition	Naming
			r		
FMA-UE[†]	0.70	0.72	0.53	0.60	0.64
ARAT[†]	0.62	0.66	0.45	0.52	0.57
FMA-UE*	0.59	0.60	0.46	0.52	0.46
ARAT*	0.54	0.60	0.42	0.42	0.45
FMA-UE**	0.76	0.76	0.57	0.65	0.72
ARAT**	0.68	0.68	0.48	0.57	0.67
FMA-UE***	0.71	0.76	0.52	0.62	0.67
ARAT***	0.65	0.70	0.46	0.58	0.61

[†]Correlation analyses of the overall time period. *Correlation analyses of 1-3 months. **Correlation analyses of 4-6 months. ***Correlation analyses of >6 months. FMA-UE indicates the Fugl-Meyer assessment for the upper extremity; ARAT indicates the action research and action test; WAB-AQ indicates the Western Aphasia Battery-Aphasia Quotient. $p < 0.001$. The correlation coefficients are corrected for age, education, and duration poststroke.

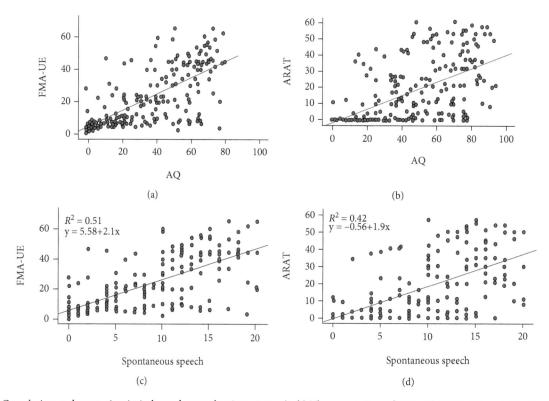

(a)　　　　　　　　　　　　　　　　　(b)

(c)　　　　　　　　　　　　　　　　　(d)

FIGURE 3: Correlation and regression in independent evaluation scores. (a, b) The association of AQ with FMA-UE and ARAT is shown. (c, d) The correlation of spontaneous speech and FMA-UE and ARAT is shown using linear regression equation. $p < 0.001$. FMA-UE indicates the Fugl-Meyer Assessment of the Upper Extremity; ARAT indicates the action research and action test; AQ indicates the Western Aphasia Battery-Aphasia Quotient.

improved, or when the PSA was treated, the UE motor function was improved [15, 28–31]. For example, transcranial direct current stimulation (tDCS) is utilized to stimulate the left primary motor cortex (M1) to study its effect on language function. To explore its clinical effect, some researchers used M1-tDCS to intervene in patients with PSA. The results show that M1-tDCS can improve aphasia patients' motor and communication function in conjunction with enhancing the retrieval ability of action-related words in the long term [16]. Interestingly, studies demonstrated that language function could be improved by asking patients to

watch videos of task-oriented movements of the UE with voice guidance [31]. Similarly, compared with the control group, some movements such as grip without phonetic guidance can also enhance patients' language function with PSA. However, the extent and limitations of UE and speech-language cortical reciprocity remain unclear, and whether the affected anterior brain regions of the language-dominant hemisphere are interwoven with proximate cortical areas supporting UE motor status [24].

Our results provide compelling evidence for the relation between UE motor status and language function in terms of

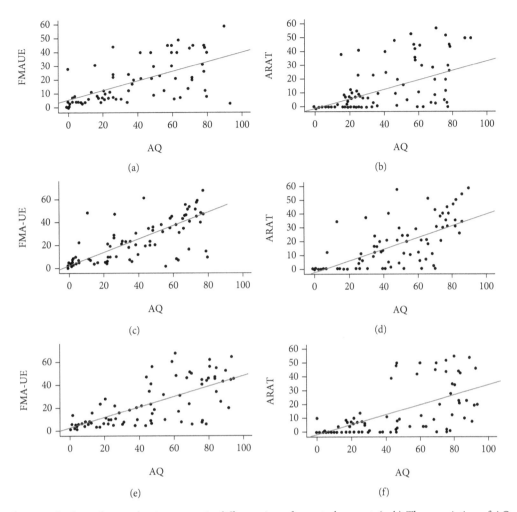

FIGURE 4: Correlations of independent evaluation scores in different times from stroke onset. (a, b) The association of AQ with FMA-UE and ARAT in 1-3 months is shown. (c, d) The association of AQ with FMA-UE and ARAT in 4-6 months is shown. (e, f) The correlation of AQ with FMA-UE and ARAT in >6 months. $p < 0.001$. FMA-UE indicates the Fugl-Meyer assessment of the upper extremity; ARAT indicates the action research and action test; AQ indicates the Western Aphasia Battery-Aphasia Quotient.

behavioral performances and demonstrate that this relationship can be applied to patients' therapy with PSA or UE motor deficit or both after stroke. Patients with PSA have worse hand and UE motor status, which calls for more attention to be given to UE motor rehabilitation in these patients. Interactions between the auditory system and the motor system are related to speech perception. The motor theory of perception has two basic claims: perceiving speech is perceiving gestures and perceiving speech involves the motor system. The mirror neuron system (MNS) is a multimodal system composed of neuronal populations that respond to motor, visual, and auditory stimulation, such as when an action is performed, observed, heard, or read about. In humans, the MNS has been identified using neuroimaging techniques. It reflected the integration of motor-auditory-visual information processing related to aspects of language learning, including action understanding and recognition [32]. Based on MNS, embodied cognition theory believes that various cognitive processes (such as concepts, categories, language, reasoning, and judgment) are closely related to the body's sensorimotor system [33, 34]. Therefore, the

realization of language processing should take advantage of the brain motor network, that is, the interweaving and coupling of language processing and motor execution [35]. These theories can demonstrate our findings from the aspect of neural mechanisms.

Our study has some limitations. We did not classify patients according to recovery stage, severity, and the specific brain damage area in patients. Moreover, our study was performed in the cross-section without longitudinal follow-up; thus, whether the recovery stage affects their correlations is unclear. Furthermore, given the proximity of hand-arm and speech-language neural structures, in many patients with poststroke aphasia, the contralesional UE is often simultaneously impaired so that the association between them seems inevitable [9]. However, we know that the Broca area (BA44,45) is adjacent to the UE motor cortex, which is mainly responsible for spontaneous speech ability. Nevertheless, in addition to spontaneous speech, naming, repetition, and comprehension are also positively associated with UE motor conditions, and there should be a deeper neural mechanism worth exploring. Another limitation is that although our study has a large

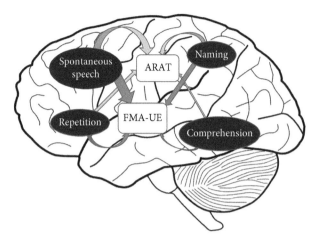

FIGURE 5: The association between UE motor status and language function after PSA. Schematic diagram shows partial correlations in an eight-way analysis of FMA-UE; ARAT; and spontaneous speech, comprehension, repetition, and naming. The degree of the arrow thickness between two modules is proportional to the correlation coefficient. FMA-UE indicates the Fugl-Meyer assessment for the upper extremity; ARAT indicates the action research and action test.

sample size, this also led to a less strict implementation of our inclusion and exclusion criteria, where some of the patients may have been accompanied by other symptoms after stroke. In addition, the fact that the patients were not specifically restricted in terms of damaged brain location and only excluded some patients with large brain lesion only, also diminished the persuasiveness of our findings, and we will go on to restrict these factors in our next study and try to get more rigorous conclusions.

5. Conclusion

To our knowledge, this is the first cross-sectional study to explore the relationship between UE motor status and language function after stroke. Our study demonstrated that patients with PSA tend to be with poorer UE motor status compared to those without PSA, and UE motor status is positively correlated with language function, especially for spontaneous speech ability. Future study should focus more on the deeper mechanisms of the link between UE motor status and language function after strictly controlling the location and severity of brain lesion. In addition, this study provides a new perspective and statistical evidence for a "combined assessment and therapy" approach to UE motor and speech-language rehabilitation, which remains to be demonstrated in future studies.

Abbreviations

UE:	Upper extremity
PSA:	Poststroke aphasia
FMA-UE:	Fugl-Meyer assessment for the upper extremity
ARAT:	Action research and action test
WAB-AQ:	Western Aphasia Battery-Aphasia Quotient
BDAE:	Boston Diagnostic Aphasia Examination.

Authors' Contributions

Shuo Xu and Zhijie Yan contributed equally to this work and are first authors.

Acknowledgments

We would like to thank Dr. Wang Jianhui, Dr. Zhang Yanan, Dr. Wang Jinyu, Dr. Ge Junsheng, and Dr. Yang Yanhui, for their indispensable supports in the implementation of screening and evaluation of patients. This study was supported by the National Key Research & Development Program of the Ministry of Science and Technology of the People's Republic of China (Grant numbers 2018YFC2002300 and 2018YFC2002301), the National Science Foundation of China (Grant number 91948302), and the Foundation for Innovative Research Groups of National Natural Science Foundation of China (Grant number 82021002).

References

[1] A. Primaßin, N. Scholtes, S. Heim et al., "Determinants of concurrent motor and language recovery during intensive therapy in chronic stroke patients: four single-case studies," *Frontiers in Neurology*, vol. 6, p. 215, 2015.

[2] Z. Wu, M. Chen, X. Wu, and L. Li, "Interaction between auditory and motor systems in speech perception," *Neuroscience Bulletin*, vol. 30, no. 3, pp. 490–496, 2014.

[3] J. D. Stefaniak, A. D. Halai, and M. A. Lambon Ralph, "The neural and neurocomputational bases of recovery from post-stroke aphasia," *Nature Reviews Neurology*, vol. 16, no. 1, pp. 43–55, 2020.

[4] R. Palmer, M. Dimairo, C. Cooper et al., "Self-managed, computerised speech and language therapy for patients with chronic aphasia post-stroke compared with usual care or attention control (Big CACTUS): a multicentre, single-blinded, randomised controlled trial," *The Lancet Neurology*, vol. 18, no. 9, pp. 821–833, 2019.

[5] E. De Cock, K. Batens, D. Hemelsoet, P. Boon, K. Oostra, and V. De Herdt, "Dysphagia, dysarthria and aphasia following a first acute ischaemic stroke: incidence and associated factors," *European Journal of Neurology*, vol. 27, no. 10, pp. 2014–2021, 2020.

[6] Q. Fan and J. Jia, "Translating research into clinical practice: importance of improving cardiorespiratory fitness in stroke population," *Stroke*, vol. 51, no. 1, pp. 361–367, 2020.

[7] M. Zheng, X. Hua, J. Feng et al., "Trial of contralateral seventh cervical nerve transfer for spastic arm paralysis," *The New England Journal of Medicine*, vol. 378, no. 1, pp. 22–34, 2018.

[8] V. Ginex, G. Gilardone, M. Viganò et al., "Interaction between recovery of motor and language abilities after stroke," *Archives of physical medicine and rehabilitation*, vol. 101, no. 8, pp. 1367–1376, 2020.

[9] S. Wortman-Jutt and D. Edwards, "Poststroke aphasia rehabilitation: why all talk and no action?," *Neurorehabilitation and neural repair*, vol. 33, no. 4, pp. 235–244, 2019.

[10] R. M. Lazar and A. K. Boehme, "Aphasia as a predictor of stroke outcome," *Current neurology and neuroscience reports*, vol. 17, no. 11, p. 83, 2017.

[11] L. E. Dunn, A. B. Schweber, D. K. Manson et al., "Variability in motor and language recovery during the acute stroke period," *Cerebrovascular diseases extra*, vol. 6, pp. 12–21, 2017.

[12] G. A. Bryant, "The evolution of coordinated vocalizations before language," *Behavioral and Brain sciences*, vol. 37, pp. 549-550, 2014.

[13] S. Harnish, M. Meinzer, J. Trinastic, D. Fitzgerald, and S. Page, "Language changes coincide with motor and fMRI changes following upper extremity motor therapy for hemiparesis: a brief report," *Brain Imaging and Behavior*, vol. 8, no. 3, pp. 370–377, 2014.

[14] M. Meinzer, R. Lindenberg, M. M. Sieg, L. Nachtigall, L. Ulm, and A. Flöel, "Transcranial direct current stimulation of the primary motor cortex improves word-retrieval in older adults," *Frontiers in Aging Neuroscience*, vol. 6, p. 253, 2014.

[15] S. M. Mostafavi, P. Mousavi, S. P. Dukelow, and S. H. Scott, "Robot-based assessment of motor and proprioceptive function identifies biomarkers for prediction of functional independence measures," *Journal of Neuroengineering and Rehabilitation*, vol. 12, no. 1, p. 105, 2015.

[16] A. Buchwald, C. Falconer, A. Rykman-Peltz et al., "Robotic arm rehabilitation in chronic stroke patients with aphasia may promote speech and language recovery (but effect is not enhanced by supplementary tDCS)," *Frontiers in Neurology*, vol. 9, p. 853, 2018.

[17] C. Wu, F. Xue, Y. Lian et al., "Relationship between elevated plasma trimethylamine N-oxide levels and increased stroke injury," *Neurology*, vol. 94, no. 7, pp. e667–e677, 2020.

[18] T. P. Siejka, V. K. Srikanth, R. E. Hubbard et al., "Frailty and cerebral small vessel disease: a cross-sectional analysis of the Tasmanian Study of Cognition and Gait (TASCOG)," *The journals of gerontology. Series A, Biological sciences and medical sciences*, vol. 73, no. 2, pp. 255–260, 2018.

[19] R. M. Lazar, B. Minzer, D. Antoniello, J. R. Festa, J. W. Krakauer, and R. S. Marshall, "Improvement in aphasia scores after stroke is well predicted by initial severity," *Stroke*, vol. 41, no. 7, pp. 1485–1488, 2010.

[20] C. M. Stinear, M. Smith, and W. D. Byblow, "Prediction tools for stroke rehabilitation," *Stroke*, vol. 50, no. 11, pp. 3314–3322, 2019.

[21] R. L. Harvey, "Predictors of functional outcome following stroke," *Physical Medicine and Rehabilitation Clinics*, vol. 26, no. 4, pp. 583–598, 2015.

[22] B. Gialanella, M. Bertolinelli, M. Lissi, and P. Prometti, "Predicting outcome after stroke: the role of aphasia," *Disability and rehabilitation*, vol. 33, no. 2, pp. 122–129, 2011.

[23] E. Moulton, S. Magno, R. Valabregue et al., "Acute diffusivity biomarkers for prediction of motor and language outcome in mild-to-severe stroke patients," *Stroke*, vol. 50, pp. 2050–2056, 2019.

[24] D. Anderlini, G. Wallis, and W. Marinovic, "Language as a predictor of motor recovery: the case for a more global approach to stroke rehabilitation," *Neurorehabilitation and neural repair*, vol. 33, no. 3, pp. 167–178, 2019.

[25] V. Ginex, L. Veronelli, N. Vanacore, E. Lacorte, A. Monti, and M. Corbo, "Motor recovery in post-stroke patients with aphasia: the role of specific linguistic abilities," *Topics in Stroke Rehabilitation*, vol. 24, no. 6, pp. 428–434, 2017.

[26] B. Gialanella, "Aphasia assessment and functional outcome prediction in patients with aphasia after stroke," *Journal of Neurology*, vol. 258, no. 2, pp. 343–349, 2011.

[27] H. Hybbinette, E. Schalling, J. Plantin et al., "Recovery of apraxia of speech and aphasia in patients with hand motor impairment after stroke," *Frontiers in Neurology*, vol. 12, p. 634065, 2021.

[28] I. G. Meister, R. Sparing, H. Foltys et al., "Functional connectivity between cortical hand motor and language areas during recovery from aphasia," *Journal of the neurological sciences*, vol. 247, no. 2, pp. 165–168, 2006.

[29] K. N. Arya and S. Pandian, "Inadvertent recovery in communication deficits following the upper limb mirror therapy in stroke: a case report," *Journal of bodywork and movement therapies*, vol. 18, no. 4, pp. 566–568, 2014.

[30] M. Meinzer, R. Darkow, R. Lindenberg, and A. Flöel, "Electrical stimulation of the motor cortex enhances treatment outcome in post-stroke aphasia," *Brain: A Journal of Neurology*, vol. 139, no. 4, pp. 1152–1163, 2016.

[31] W. Chen, Q. Ye, S. Zhang et al., "Aphasia rehabilitation based on mirror neuron theory: a randomized-block-design study of neuropsychology and functional magnetic resonance imaging," *Neural Regeneration Research*, vol. 14, pp. 1004–1012, 2019.

[32] R. M. Le Bel, J. A. Pineda, and A. Sharma, "Motor-auditory-visual integration: the role of the human mirror neuron system in communication and communication disorders," *Journal of Communication Disorders*, vol. 42, no. 4, pp. 299–304, 2009.

[33] E. Farina, F. Borgnis, and T. Pozzo, "Mirror neurons and their relationship with neurodegenerative disorders," *Journal of Neuroscience Research*, vol. 98, no. 6, pp. 1070–1094, 2020.

[34] D. Jirak, M. M. Menz, G. Buccino, A. M. Borghi, and F. Binkofski, "Grasping language—a short story on embodiment," *Consciousness and Cognition*, vol. 19, no. 3, pp. 711–720, 2010.

[35] C. Cheung, L. S. Hamiton, K. Johnson, and E. F. Chang, "Correction: The auditory representation of speech sounds in human motor cortex," *eLife*, vol. 5, 2016.

12

The Role of the Cognitive Control System in Recovery from Bilingual Aphasia

Narges Radman,[1] **Michael Mouthon,**[1] **Marie Di Pietro,**[2] **Chrisovalandou Gaytanidis,**[2,3] **Beatrice Leemann,**[2] **Jubin Abutalebi,**[4] **and Jean-Marie Annoni**[1]

[1]*Neurology Unit, Department of Medicine, Faculty of Sciences, University of Fribourg, Fribourg, Switzerland*
[2]*Neurorehabilitation Department, University Hospital, University of Geneva, Geneva, Switzerland*
[3]*Neuropsychology Unit, Fribourg Cantonal Hospital, Fribourg, Switzerland*
[4]*Center for Neurolinguistics and Psycholinguistics, San Raffaele University and Scientific Institute San Raffaele, Milan, Italy*

Correspondence should be addressed to Narges Radman; narges.radman@gmail.com

Academic Editor: Swathi Kiran

Aphasia in bilingual patients is a therapeutic challenge since both languages can be impacted by the same lesion. Language control has been suggested to play an important role in the recovery of first (L1) and second (L2) language in bilingual aphasia following stroke. To test this hypothesis, we collected behavioral measures of language production (general aphasia evaluation and picture naming) in each language and language control (linguistic and nonlinguistic switching tasks), as well as fMRI during a naming task at one and four months following stroke in five bilingual patients suffering from poststroke aphasia. We further applied dynamic causal modelling (DCM) analyses to the connections between language and control brain areas. Three patients showed parallel recovery in language production, one patient improved in L1, and one improved in L2 only. Language-control functions improved in two patients. Consistent with the dynamic view of language recovery, DCM analyses showed a higher connectedness between language and control areas in the language with the better recovery. Moreover, similar degrees of connectedness between language and control areas were found in the patients who recovered in both languages. Our data suggest that engagement of the interconnected language-control network is crucial in the recovery of languages.

1. Introduction

Due to the increasing number of multilinguals in modern society, the incidence of language impairments induced by brain lesions (aphasia) in this population is growing rapidly [1, 2]. The rehabilitation of multilingual aphasic patients represents an important challenge for clinicians because (i) since the representation of first (L1) and second (L2) languages partly overlaps in bilinguals' brains, brain lesions do not necessarily affect L1 and L2 equally [3]; and (ii) recovery patterns for each language in multilingual aphasic patients vary considerably and so far are unpredictable [4].

Most of the current literature indicates that language recovery in bilingual aphasic patients depends on the degree of language mastery or language-specific factors [5–7]. For example, similarities in typology, phonological, morphological, lexical, and syntactic aspects between languages are shown to affect the pattern of recovery of languages in bilingual aphasic patients [1, 6]. Such an approach is also supported by evidence that changes in second language expertise and use are associated with an increase of connectivity within the language network of healthy subjects. However, growing evidence suggests that the control system may also play a key role in this process [5, 8, 9]. In healthy bilingual speakers, cognitive control system is strongly involved in language production [10] because language representations must be manipulated and monitored both within the language being spoken and across languages to select the appropriate vocabulary and syntax and to inhibit the nontarget language [11].

Abutalebi and Green [10], for instance, propose a "dynamic view" in which the pattern of language recovery in bilingual aphasia depends on the patient's ability to select and control language activation [10, 12]: (i) a parallel recovery, in which both impaired languages improve to a similar extent, and, concurrently, occurs when both languages are inhibited to the same degree; (ii) an antagonistic recovery, in which the patient is able to speak in one language on one day while on the next day only in the other, occurs when inhibition affects only one language for a period of time and then shifts to the other language (with disinhibition of the previously inhibited language); (iii) a selective recovery, in which one language remains impaired while the other recovers, occurs if the lesion has permanently raised the activation threshold for one language; and (iv) a pathological mixing, in which the elements of the two languages are involuntarily mixed during language production, occurs when languages can no longer be selectively inhibited [9, 10, 13].

While this theory accounts for the large variability in recovery patterns of multilingual aphasia, there is only sparse evidence for any association between control function and language recovery since control functions are rarely specifically assessed in aphasic patients. Aglioti et al. [5] reported the case of a bilingual aphasic patient who showed a greater deficit in her more used L1 than in her less practiced L2, following lesions mainly involving the left basal ganglia. The authors suggest that the patient's deficit in L1 may be considered as a pathological fixation on a foreign language resulting from a deficit in switching between languages. However, the patient had a normal performance in the Wisconsin card-sorting test (WCS), a nonverbal task testing the ability to change from one criterion of choice to another. This result suggested that, in the absence of a remarkable impairment in control functions (shown in WCS which evaluated "shifting," a part of control functions), the patient's fixation behavior was mostly linguistic. Moreover, since the assessment of executive functions was conducted one year after the stroke, anatomo-functional plastic reorganization of the language and control networks could already have taken place and likely confounded the results. An earlier evaluation (e.g., at acute or subacute phase) following the stroke could have better shown whether this so-called pathological fixation on L2 and the L1 impairment has resulted from impairment in cognitive control function. Verreyt et al. [14] reported the case of an early French-Dutch bilingual aphasic who, following a lesion to the left thalamus, presented larger impairment in Dutch. By showing cognate facilitation and cognate interference effects in different lexical decision tasks and an impaired performance in the flanker task, the authors suggested that the differential pattern of impairment in language could be explained by a language-control deficit. In addition, Abutalebi et al. [9], in a longitudinal, single-case study of a chronic bilingual aphasic patient combining fMRI and dynamic causal modelling (DCM), showed an increased connectivity within the control and language networks for the treated and recovered language. In line with the Paradis's activation threshold theory, which holds that lesions that do not completely damage language areas but cause an imbalance in activating and inhibiting languages are responsible for aphasia in bilinguals [12], they found that the engagement of the areas mediating language control played a crucial role in language recovery in bilingual aphasic patients. They showed that connections between language and control areas were stronger in the language that recovered better, probably because it received more resources for its functioning.

The network underlying language control described by Abutalebi and Green [10] and Abutalebi et al. [9] includes the prefrontal cortex (mainly inferior prefrontal cortex including LIFGOrb (left inferior frontal gyrus pars orbitalis, BA47)), the anterior cingulate cortex (ACC) (BAs24, 32, 33), and the basal ganglia. This network is interconnected with language areas involved in word production (LIFGTri: left inferior frontal gyrus pars triangularis, BA45) and "basal temporal language area, BTLA" involved in semantic decoding during picture naming (posterior part of the left inferior temporal gyrus BAs19 and 37). In the bilingual brain, the prefrontal cortex is involved in word production in the less proficient language and in inhibiting responses from the more proficient language. Together with the anterior cingulate that detects response conflicts, it constitutes a control loop in which the identification of conflict triggers a top-down signal from the prefrontal cortex to modulate the nontarget representation (see [10, 15, 16]). The left caudate and the ACC are strongly connected to the prefrontal cortex [17] and work together with this structure to inhibit interferences from the nontarget language. The ACC signals potential response conflicts or errors to the prefrontal cortex (i.e., in the case that an erroneous language has been chosen) and the prefrontal cortex then seeks to avoid incorrect selection. Finally, the basal ganglia may subserve language planning, that is, the activation of a given language as a main function of the left caudate and the control of articulatory processes in the left putamen (see [18, 19]). Using linguistic and nonlinguistic switching tasks, it has been shown that the neuroanatomical bases of language control and domain-general cognitive control share the partially overlapping structures, although their involvement may vary [20, 21]. It is worth noting that understanding neural mechanisms underlying patterns of recovery has many implications for the therapeutic approach.

Based on the hypothesis of a key role for cognitive control in bilingual language production and in the recovery of bilingual aphasia, our study aims to test whether among the different control areas proposed by Abutalebi et al. [9], changes in certain connections between control and language areas influence the recovery of language (namely, between LIFGTri and LIFGOrb and LC and ACC). To this aim, we tested five late bilingual patients who suffered from aphasia following a focal left-hemispheric brain lesion. The patients were evaluated at two time points (subacute and chronic phases, three months apart). Three main analyses were conducted to examine the pattern of changes in patients' language and control functions, connectivity within language-control network, and possible correlation between behavioral performances and connectivity with language-control network.

(A) As a descriptive marker of behavioral improvement/changes in language and control functions, the patients were behaviorally evaluated for their pattern of recovery of language and executive functions using general aphasia evaluation (GAE), picture naming and executive tasks (linguistic and nonlinguistic switching).

(B) In order to investigate the connections within the language-control network, we used fMRI analyses and applied dynamic causal modelling in the fMRI picture naming task in L1 and L2 to examine whole brain activation patterns and the effective connectivity between the control areas (ACC, left caudate nucleus, and LIFGOrb) and the regions involved in language production (especially LIFGTri). We further examined whether global changes in connectedness within language-control network are associated with the recovery of languages.

(C) To directly assess the hypothesis advanced in the language-control model [9], we examined the correlations between the recovery of language functions and the changes in the strength of connections between the above-mentioned areas using group analyses. In fact, as Meier et al. [22] in a DCM study on chronic aphasic patients and a group of controls have found that language network parameters are specifically associated with naming abilities in picture naming task, we consider that there should be a difference in connection strength in L1 and L2 and also according to naming improvement across time.

We chose to evaluate bilingual aphasic patients during the subacute phase since this population has rarely been studied in the acute and subacute phases. This will allow us to better understand the contribution of the control system in the recovery of language in bilingual aphasia, especially during the period when spontaneous recovery process mainly takes place [6, 23]. In addition, in this phase, the spontaneous recovery and neural plasticity processes are ongoing and given that bilingual population is strongly relied on cognitive control system, we assume that the changes in cognitive control system and its interconnection with the language system probably play a role in the recovery of aphasia.

2. Methods

2.1. Participants

2.1.1. Aphasic Patients. We recruited right-handed late (age of acquisition (AoA) of L2 after 6 y/o) bilingual patients aged between 18 and 85 years old, who suffered from aphasia following a focal left-sided ischemic or hemorrhagic stroke. The following languages were included in the study: French (in each case as subjects' L1 or L2) and English, German, Spanish, or Italian. During the recruitment procedure, we excluded patients with a history of premorbid language impairment, several brain lesions, or severe aphasia.

A total of eleven patients were recruited for this project. However, only six patients completed all the steps of the study and, among them, five subjects fulfilled our criteria of the selection of regions of interest (ROIs) for the DCM analyses and therefore are reported in this paper. Five more patients performed the first session of the study and then declined to participate in the second session (see Section 2.3 for details of the steps of the study) and were therefore not included in the analyses. Among the five patients included in this paper

(aged 61.6 (±6.9) years old and including two females), three patients were French (L1) and English (L2) and two patients were Italian (L1) and French (L2). All the patients were late bilinguals (AoA: 16.5 ± 5.1). The lesion of each patient is shown in a figure specifically designed for each of them (Figures 3(a)–7(a)). The study procedure was approved by the local Ethics Committees of Geneva University Hospital (CE 12-274) and Fribourg Cantonal Hospital (018/12-CER-FR).

Case Description

Patient 1. YL is a 61-year-old man who is a French (L1)-English (L2) bilingual. Mr. YL was born in French-speaking part of Switzerland. The language of teaching at school was French. Mr. YL estimates an advanced level of English for reading, speaking, and comprehension (all between 95 and 100% according to the self-evaluation scale of L2 level). Before the stroke, his language usage was mainly in French; he spoke 100% French with his family and 80% with his friends. He followed TV and radio programs only in French. However, his reading was 50% in French and 50% in English (readings in English are mainly work-related books and documents), and he used mainly English at his workplace (80%).

Mr. YL was admitted to Geneva University Hospital (HUG) with right sensorimotor hemiparesis, right facial palsy, and impaired comprehension and language production mainly manifested in L2 following a left frontotemporal ischemic stroke. A secondary hemorrhagic event in the ischemic area was seen three days after the ischemic event (Figure 3(a)). A first language evaluation showed a transcortical sensory aphasia; he presented mainly auditory comprehension problems and produced repeated semantic errors. However, spontaneous speaking was relatively fluent.

Patient 2. MR is a 65-year-old Italian (L1)-French (L2) bilingual woman. She was born in Italy to Italian parents and followed primary school in Italy. She moved to the French-speaking part of Switzerland at the age of 24, and then she has taken some courses to learn French. Before the stroke, she used Italian and French quite equally; she used French at work (100%), and Italian for TV or radio programs (100%). She used 50% in Italian and 50% in French to speak with her family and friends and to read books and journals.

MR was admitted to HUG for resection of a meningioma on the left greater wing of the sphenoid bone. Two days after the resection of the meningioma, she presented a right sensorimotor hemiparesis and a severe language production problem plus a lesser degree of comprehension problems in both languages, caused by an epidural hematoma with pressure over the operation site and ischemic changes in the left frontobasal area (Figure 4(a)). The initial language evaluation showed anomia in both L1 and L2.

Patient 3. CA is a 63-year-old woman who is an Italian (L1)-French (L2) bilingual. She was born in Italy to Italian parents and followed primary school in Italy. She moved to the French-speaking part of Switzerland at the age of 10; thereafter she started to learn French. Mrs. CA followed secondary school in Switzerland where the teaching language was

French. She has also basic knowledge in English and Spanish, which she has learned at school. Before the stroke, the main language of conversation was French with her husband and children (90%) and at work (75%) and she spoke Italian with her parents (100%).

She was admitted to HUG because of right hemiparesis and severe global aphasia due to a left basal ganglia hemorrhagic stroke with no evidence of midline shift (Figure 5(a)). Within a few days, global aphasia developed into severe anomia with hypophonia mainly affecting L2.

Patient 4. RG is a 49-year-old bilingual French (L1)-English (L2) male patient. He finished primary and secondary schools in the French-speaking part of Switzerland. He started to learn English at school at the age of 14. He used English quite frequently in his daily life; he used French and English equally at work (50% French and 50% English for teaching and customer care). He followed TV and radio programs and also read books and journals 50% in French and 50% in English. However, he spoke only in French with his friends and family. According to the self-evaluation questionnaire filled in by his wife, his language abilities were estimated as follows: speaking 50%, comprehension 70%, reading 85%, and writing 30%.

He was admitted to Fribourg Cantonal Hospital with a sudden right hemiparesis and anomia and no other language symptoms due to a left sylvian ischemic stroke (Figure 6(a)).

Patient 5. GH is a 79-year-old bilingual French (L1)-English (L2) male patient. He has learned English around the age of 18 when he first travelled to the US and England. He has then moved to Sweden and started to learn Swedish too. He has been working in Sweden for about 18 years teaching guitar in both English and Swedish. He then moved back to Switzerland at the age of 66. He then continued to teach playing guitar to children. He used both French and English in his teachings (50% French and 50% English). With his family he spoke only in French; however with his friends he spoke 50% in French and 50% in English. He followed TV and radio program mostly in French (75% in French and 25% in English) and he read books and journals only in French.

He was admitted to HUG with a paresthesia in his left arm and global aphasia. GH was a known case of auricular fibrillation before this acute event. The cerebral CT scan after the acute event confirmed an ischemic lesion in the left frontal, insula, and sylvian areas (Figure 7(a)). Within a few days, global aphasia developed into severe anomia and increased switching behavior.

More details of patients can be found in Tables 1 and 2 and Supplementary Data 1 available online at http://dx.doi.org/10.1155/2016/8797086.

2.1.2. Control Subjects. The data and results on the control subjects are presented in Supplementary Data 2 and 3.

2.2. Assessment of Premorbid Language Proficiency. Subjects were assessed using a questionnaire on their immersion in both L1 and L2, AoA, how long they had lived in a region where predominantly the second language was spoken, which language they spoke with their family members, in school,

and in present activities (watching TV/listening to radio, reading books, and mental arithmetic), and if the language was acquired in school or out of school only. In the self-evaluation part, subjects (or their family members) had to indicate in percentages how well they would estimate their reading, speaking, comprehension, and writing skills.

2.3. Study Design. Patients were assessed at subacute (three to five weeks after stroke onset, T1) and chronic (three months after T1 evaluation, T2) phases. In both sessions we used the same procedures, listed as follows: (1) behavioral assessment of the severity of aphasia as well as a combination of language-control function evaluations; (2) in an fMRI recording session, the patients performed a language production task (picture naming) in each language (see Section 2.6.1 for picture naming task).

2.4. Behavioral Tasks. General aphasia evaluation (GAE): global severity of the aphasia and language capacities was assessed using a separate evaluation of language capacities in each language (i.e., L1 and L2 were evaluated separately, one day apart). This evaluation consisted of a brief test of object naming (ten objects to name), automatic speech (series: days of the week, counting from 1 to 25), word and phrase repetition, yes/no questions, object recognition, following oral and written instructions (simple, semicomplex, and complex commands), description, and verbal fluency. All these tests were extracted from the Bilingual Aphasia Test (BAT) [24] except for yes/no questions which were extracted from the Mississippi Aphasia Screening Test (MAST) [25]. This evaluation material has been already used in our previously published works, for example, [26]. As a result, a production index of maximum 52 scores (i.e., the sum of the scores obtained from production tasks including object naming, series, verbal fluency, word and phrase repetition, and description) and a total score (maximum 96 scores) was obtained.

Language-control functions were evaluated using the following:

(a) A linguistic switching task (adapted from Abutalebi et al. 2008 for aphasic patients [27]): forty images (black and white line drawing picture) of Snodgrass and Vanderwart [28] (all noncognate words) were used for each list. Eight pairs of lists were prepared (a combination of French as first or second language and the other four languages). The words of each pair were matched for word frequency. The subjects were asked to name, as quickly as possible, the images in L1 when the image appeared on the upper part and name the image in L2 when the image appeared on the lower part of the screen. After a fixation cross of 500 ms, the images were presented on the screen for 5,000 ms and were followed by a blank screen of variable duration of 3,000–7,000 ms (to provide a random duration of the interstimulus interval). Therefore, the subjects had at most between 8,000 and 12,000 ms to respond. However, only first-attempt correct responses within five seconds of the presentation of the image were scored as correct. Each trial was started manually

TABLE 1: Assessment of premorbid L2 proficiency.

	Subject 1	Subject 2	Subject 3	Subject 4	Subject 5
First language (L1)	French	Italian	Italian	French	French
Second language (L2)	English	French	French	English	English
AoA (y/o)	10	24	10	14	18
Lived in region speaking L2	0	41	53	>1	>1
Family					
First language of mother	French	Italian	Italian	French	Swiss German
Language spoken with mother	French	Italian	Italian	French	French
First language of father	French	Italian	Italian	French	French
Language spoken with father	French	Italian	Italian	French	French
First language of partner	French	French/Italian	Italian	French	—
Language spoken with partner	French	Italian	French	French	—
Childhood (<7 y/o)					
Language taught in school	French	Italian	No info.	French	French
Language spoken with peers at school	French	Italian	No info.	French	French
Language spoken with family	French	Italian	Italian	French	French
Present					
Spoken at work	15% L1, 85% L2	100% L2	75% L2, 25% L1	50% L1, 50% L2	50% L1, 50% L2
Watching TV/listening to radio	100% L1	100% L1	50% L1, 50% L2	50% L1, 50% L2	75% L1, 25% L2
Speaking with friends	90% L1, 10% L2	50% L1, 50% L2	50% L1, 50% L2	L1	50% L1, 50% L2
Reading books	50% L1, 50% L2	50% L1, 50% L2	50% L1, 50% L2	50% L1, 50% L2	100% L1
Mental arithmetic	100% L1	75% L1, 25% L2	50% L1, 50% L2	L1	100% L1
Self-evaluation of L2 (0–100)					
Speaking	100	95	100	55	80
Writing	98	15	100	75	50
Comprehension	100	95	100	80	89
Reading	100	75	100	35	70

by the experimenter when the word "ready?" was presented on the screen. The first six trials of the task were cued with the language in which the image should be named (L1 or L2) written on the left of the image (Figure 1(a)). This task lasted between 10 and 12 minutes depending on patients' response time.

(b) A nonlinguistic switching task: four images (a red or blue circle or square) were presented on the upper or the lower part of the screen. Subjects were instructed to name, as quickly as possible, the color of the image when the image was presented on the upper part of the screen and to say the shape of the image when it was presented on the lower part of the screen. After a fixation cross of 500 ms, the images were presented on the screen for 5,000 ms and were followed by a blank screen of variable duration of 3,000–7,000 ms (to provide a random duration of the interstimulus

interval). Therefore, the subjects had at most between 8,000 and 12,000 ms to respond. However, only first-attempt correct responses within five seconds of the presentation of the image were scored as correct. Each trial was started manually by the experimenter when the word "ready?" was presented on the screen. The first six trials of the task were cued with the category in which the image should be named (color or shape) written on the left of the image (Figure 1(b)). The task lasted around 10–12 minutes depending on patient's response time.

For all the tasks, instructions were given both written on the screen and orally, and the subjects performed a short training session just before starting the task. The evaluation of the language-control function was performed in the more proficient language (usually L1). Moreover, because of slowness of patients and fatigability, for all the tasks we did

TABLE 2: Demographic data.

	Subject 1	Subject 2	Subject 3	Subject 4	Subject 5
Age	61	65	63	49	79
Gender	M	F	F	M	M
Scholarity (years)	16	12	12	18	16
Lesion site	Left frontotemporal	Left frontobasal area	Left basal ganglia	Left sylvian	Left frontal-insula-sylvian
Lesion etiology	Ischemic + hemorrhagic stroke	Epidural hematoma	Hemorrhagic stroke	Ischemic stroke	Ischemic stroke
Time after stroke at T1 (days)	34	21	64	7	21
Time after stroke at T2 (days)	120	118	166	110	135
Language therapy between T1 and T2					
Language of therapy	L1	L2	L2	—	L1
Number & duration of therapy sessions	25 sessions (45 min./session)	1 session (30 min.)	41 sessions (45 min./session)	—	10 sessions (45 min./session)
Type of therapy	CAT CIAT	CAT	CAT	—	CAT

CAT: computer assisted therapy for anomia to improve lexical access.
CIAT: constraint induced aphasia therapy.

not record reaction times, and the analyses were focused on response accuracy.

2.5. Behavioral Data Analyses. Because of the limited number of patients, differences in lesion size and site, and variability of symptoms, we used primarily a multiple single-case approach for our analyses between T1 and T2. For comparison of the patients' scores in the two sessions, a McNemar Chi-squared test is used for each case. GAE, picture naming, and "combined production score" (i.e., the average response accuracy percentage in picture naming and production score of the GAE) are assessed as language performances. Specifically, we focused on the "combined production score" which could better represent language production performance.

2.6. Functional Magnetic Resonance Imaging Task

2.6.1. Picture Naming in L1 and L2

Stimuli. Five lists (one list per language) of 40 noncognate words (black and white line drawing pictures) were selected from Snodgrass and Vanderwart [28]. The words were matched for word frequency across all the lists.

Procedure. Each fMRI session started with a picture naming in L1; in this part, the subjects were instructed to name the pictures that appeared on the screen in their L1. After a fixation cross of 500 ms, the images were presented on the screen for 5,000 ms and were followed by a blank screen of variable duration of 4,100–6,100 ms (to provide a random duration of the interstimulus interval). Therefore, the subjects had at most between 9,100 and 11,100 ms to respond. However, only first-attempt correct responses within five seconds of the

presentation of the image were scored as correct. Each task lasted around 7-8 minutes (a total of around 15 minutes for picture naming in both L1 and L2). After about 30 seconds of rest, the subjects started their second task in which they had to name the pictures in their second language. The first six trials of the task were cued with the language in which the image should be named (L1 or L2) written on the left of the image. For the fMRI tasks, a short training was performed before the subjects entered the scanner. In this training, which contained 10 trials, the subjects were presented with black and white line drawing pictures selected from Snodgrass list and were asked to name the pictures in their L1 or L2 to become familiar with the task.

2.7. FMRI Acquisition. Data of the aphasic patients were acquired using three different 3T scanners on two different sites; Site 1: Fribourg Cantonal Hospital (HFr) and Site 2: University Hospital of Geneva (HUG). The scanners which were used were (1) Discovery MR750; GE Healthcare, Waukesha, Wisconsin, with a 32-channel receive head coil (Site 1), (2) Magneton Trio, Siemens Medical Solutions, Erlangen, Germany, with a 12-channel receive head coil (Site 2), and (3) Magneton Prisma, Siemens Medical Solutions, Erlangen, Germany, with a 20-channel receive head (Site 2). Subjects were in a supine position with their heads stabilized by foam to reduce head movements. They wore headphones (MKII system from MR confon, Magdeburg, Germany) coupled with an MRI-compatible microphone (FOMRI-III system from Optoacoustics, Israel) to record oral response during the experiment. In the first scanner, visual stimuli were presented on an LCD screen (NordicNeuroLab, Bergen, Norway). In the other two scanners, the stimuli were displayed on a screen by a video projector (Hitachi CP-X1200 with long focal distance

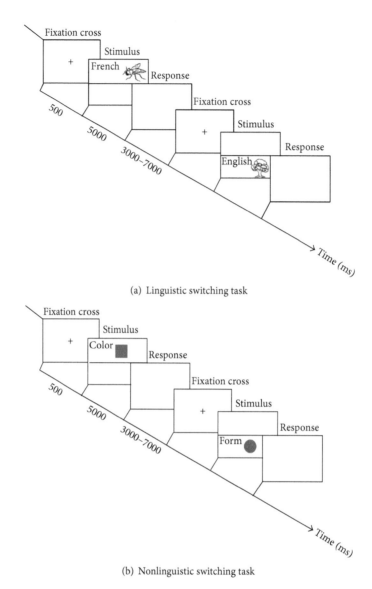

(a) Linguistic switching task

(b) Nonlinguistic switching task

FIGURE 1: (a) Linguistic switching task. This task includes 40 trials. Only the six first trials were cued; the language in which the image should be named (L1 or L2) is written in the left of the image. (b) Nonlinguistic switching task. This task includes 40 trials. Only the six first trials were cued; the category in which the image should be named (color or form) is written in the left of the image.

Hitachi LL-504, Hitachi Ltd., Tokyo, Japan) through a mirror system. In all three cases, the stimuli resolution was 1024 × 768 with a refresh rate of 60 Hz. The E-Prime 2 software (Psychology Software Tools, Pittsburgh, USA) was used to show stimuli and record behavioral data.

2.8. MRI Acquisition. MRI acquisition parameters were optimized for each site. From the first site in Fribourg (Scanner 1), T1-weighted images were acquired with a FSPGR BRAVO sequence, voxel size: $0.86 \times 0.86 \times 1$ mm, field of view (FOV) = 220 mm, number of coronal slices: 276, TR/TE = 7300/2.8 ms, flip angle = 9, phase acceleration factor (PAF) = 1.5, and intensity correction (SCIC). Functional T2* weighted echo planar images (EPI) with blood oxygenation level-dependent (BOLD) contrast were acquired with voxel size: $2.3 \times 2.3 \times 3$ mm, FOV = 220 mm, 37 ascending axial slices, interslice

spacing = 0.2 mm, TR/TE = 2000/30 ms, flip angle = 85, and PIAF: 2. In addition, a B0 field inhomogeneity mapping sequence was acquired to correct for geometrical distortion that occurred along the phase-encoding direction (using a Gradient Echo protocol) with the same scan coverage as the functional scan: number of slices = 37, FOV = 220 mm, TR/TE$_1$/TE$_2$ = 50/4.9/7.3 ms [29]. From the second site (scanners 2 and 3), T1 weighted images were acquired with an MP Rage sequence, voxel size: $0.86 \times 0.86 \times 1.1$ mm, FOV = 220 mm, number of coronal slices: 208, TR/TE = 2500/2.94 ms for scanner 2 and 2500/2.97 for scanner 3, flip angle = 9, and PAF: 2. Functional T2* weighted EPI with BOLD contrast were acquired with voxel size: $2 \times 2 \times 3.5$ mm, FOV = 240 mm, 29 ascending axial slices, interslice spacing = 0.35 mm, TR/TE = 2000/30 ms, flip angle = 85, and PIAF: 2. A B0 field inhomogeneity mapping sequence was also acquired with the same scan coverage as the functional MRI sequences: number of slices = 29, FOV = 240 mm, and $TR/TE_1/TE_2$ = 400/5.19/7.65 ms. On average, a total of 248 volumes were acquired during the picture naming in L1 and picture naming in L2. Each fMRI acquisition session started with six seconds of dummy scans to ensure a steady-state magnetization of the tissues.

2.9. Functional MRI Preprocessing. We used the SPM8 software (Welcome Trust Centre for Neuroimaging, Institute of Neurology, University College London), running on MATLAB 2012b (MathWorks, Inc., MA, USA), to analyze functional MRI data (fMRI). FMRI images were preprocessed following the standard procedure proposed by Friston [30]. Preprocessing steps included a spatial realignment, unwrapping (using the FieldMap 2.1 toolbox [31]), slice timing (with middle temporal slice as reference), coregistration on T1 image, normalization on the Montreal Neurological Institute (MNI) space with $3 \times 3 \times 3$ mm^3 voxel size, and smoothing with a Gaussian kernel of 8 mm full width at half maximum (FWHM). In order to exclude the brain lesion from the analyses, a mask file of the brain lesion of each subject was manually drawn on axial slices of the standard Montreal Neurological Institute's (MNI) brain template using the MRIcron software (https://www.nitrc.org/projects/mricron) and used during the preprocessing of data on SPM. The preprocessed volumes were submitted to fixed effects analyses at the subject level by applying the general linear model to each voxel [32]. Each stimulus onset was modelled as an event encoded in condition-specific "stick-functions" and convolved with a canonical hemodynamic response function. A separate model was built for picture naming in L1 and picture naming in L2. In addition, movement parameters were included as regressors of no interest. Time series from all voxels were submitted to a high-pass filter with a 1/250 Hz threshold, and an autoregressive function (AR (1)) was applied.

2.10. Dynamic Causal Modelling (DCM). DCM is a widely used method for investigating context-dependent causal interactions between brain regions and it describes the architecture of the network (i.e., the ROIs and the connections). In DCM, the brain is treated as a dynamic input-state-output system. A given experiment is considered as a designed perturbation of neuronal dynamics that is propagated throughout a network of interconnected nodes. Three sets of parameters are estimated in DCM: the direct influence of stimuli on regional activity (driving input), the intrinsic connections between regions, and the changes in the intrinsic connectivity between regions induced by adding or removing a modulatory influence (modulatory effect).

We based our analyses on this model, which has been defined by Abutalebi et al. [9]. Because of the variability of lesion site in our patients, in order to be able to compare changes in connectivity with the same model across all subjects/conditions, we have defined this model for all subjects and conditions. We have not selected a fully connected model (i.e., with all possible connections within the network) to avoid having a very complex model and overfitting of the

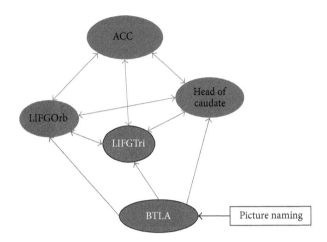

FIGURE 2: The structure of language-control network. This network was proposed by Abutalebi et al. (2009). Connections between brain areas involved in picture naming (in black) and control (in red). The modulatory effect of the experimental task (picture naming in L1 and L2) was added to the model on BTLA. ACC: anterior cingulate cortex, LIFGTri: left inferior frontal gyrus-pars triangularis, LIFGOrb: left inferior frontal gyrus-pars orbitalis, BTLA: basal temporal language area.

data. In addition the structure of this model was designed based on *a priori* hypotheses already tested by previous works. Therefore, the selection of the ROIs and the intrinsic connections was based exactly on the work by this group. Accordingly, the following five ROIs were selected for the network: BTLA, LIFGTri (areas related to language processing), head of left caudate, ACC (areas involved in cognitive control function), and LIFGOrb as a part of both language and cognitive control systems. As per Abutalebi et al. [9], we also included only left-hemispheric regions as our main focus was the effect of control areas on the intrahemispheric reorganization of language areas (see Figure 2 for the model structure). The same model was used for all subjects (patients and controls) and for both testing sessions. Using TD-ICBM-MNI template atlas, we prepared the mask for the ROIs. Individual subject time series data from each subject's individual activation map threshold at $p < 0.05$ uncorrected were extracted from each 7 mm spherical ROI centered at the subject's local maximum inside the ROIs. For the patients, we have verified visually whether the ROIs were affected by the lesion. When the patients or control subjects did not fulfill our criteria (showing activation with threshold < 0.05 uncorrected in all 5 ROIs and/or absence of lesion in the ROIs) they were removed from the analyses. This way, we have removed one patient (as one of the ROIs was inside the lesion) and one control participant (as he did not show activation in one of the ROIs in the desired threshold) [33].

However, in order to take into account the modulatory effect of the language task on the network (which was not included previously in the model by Abutalebi et al.), we inserted the modulatory effect of the task over BTLA (as the sensory input of the network) [33] and LIFGTri as two different models. We compared the three models (two models with modulatory effect of picture naming on LIFGTri or BTLA and a model with no modulatory effect) using a Bayesian model selection with a fixed effect strategy which assumes that the optimal structure is assumed to be identical across subjects, and the model with modulatory effect over the BTLA best explained fMRI activation through the different patients and controls (separately) during the naming in L1 and L2 according to this comparison. We therefore employed this model in all our subjects. The DCM model was deterministic, bilinear with one state per region. The analyses of DCM were performed using SPM12 and using the data preprocessed in SPM8.

2.11. FMRI Data Analyses. Considering the limited number of patients and the effect of the different scanners used in this study, we primarily performed the analyses at a single-case level. Patterns of brain activation in the four different conditions (picture naming in L1 and L2 at T1: subacute phase and T2: chronic phase) for each patient are shown in the figure representing the data related to the patient (Figures 3(b)–7(b)).

Regarding the DCM analyses, in order to investigate how connection strength changes over time for single intrinsic connections within the network, the differences in the strength of connection between L1 and L2 (L2 – L1) at each session are presented in a graph for each patient. These graphs represent the pattern of difference in connection strength in language-control network while performing picture naming in L1 and L2 across time (these graphs are shown in Figures 3(d)–7(d)).

At the group level, correlation analyses were performed with aphasic patients to investigate possible correlations between the changes in connection strength (especially for the connections between control and language areas) and the changes in combined production scores for each language separately.

3. Results

3.1. General Approach. (A) We first conducted McNemar Chi-squared tests comparing language performance (GAE and picture naming scores) in L1 and L2 and control function (linguistic and nonlinguistic switch task scores) across time; (B) using DCM on fMRI, we compared the strength of connectivity within the language-control network between L1 and L2 across time at single subject level; (C) at the group level, we then performed a correlation analysis between the recovery of language production scores and the changes in the strength of connection between language and control areas. A description of the main results of the analyses is provided here, and a complete reporting of the scores and results is provided in Table 3 and Supplementary Data 1.

3.2. Single-Case Analyses

3.2.1. Patient 1

(A) Behavioral Scores. At T2 (chronic phase), the combined production score showed improvement in L1 (χ^2: 12.7, *p*:

0.005) but no changes in L2. In addition, no improvement was found in linguistic and nonlinguistic switching tasks accuracy (Figure 3(c)).

(B) Changes in Connectivity in the Language-Control Network. For each single intrinsic connection within the network, the differences in connection strengths between L1 and L2 (L2 – L1) at each session are shown in Figure 3(d). At T1 (subacute phase), seven connection strengths were greater for L1 and eight connections had greater coupling values for L2. At T2 (chronic phase), however, the majority of connections (10 out of 15) had stronger coupling values for L1 compared to L2 (i.e., the following five connections had higher strength values in L2 at T2 (chronic phase): connections from LC to ACC, LIFGTri, and LIFGOrb, from LIFGTri to LC, and from BTLA to LIFGTri). The rest of the 15 connections had higher strength values in L1 at T2 (chronic phase). These changes in strength values indicated a globally higher connectedness inside the language-control network for L1.

3.2.2. Patient 2

(A) Behavioral Scores. At T2 (chronic phase), the combined production score improved in both L1 (χ^2: 9.09, *p*: 0.002) and L2 (χ^2: 5.14, *p*: 0.023). However, no significant improvement was found in linguistic (χ^2: 3.2, *p*: 0.07) and nonlinguistic switching tasks (χ^2: 0.5, *p*: 0.47) (Figure 4(c)) (see Table 3 for details of the patient's performance).

(B) Changes in Connectivity in the Language-Control Network. Regarding the DCM analyses for each single intrinsic connection within the network, the same approach was used as for patient 1 (Figure 4(d)). Importantly, a notable change was seen in the language-control network in the pattern of differences in connection strengths between L1 and L2 from T1 (subacute phase) and T2 (chronic phase): at T1, five connections had greater strength values for L1 and 10 connections had greater strength for L2. At T2 (chronic phase), seven connections had greater strength values for L1 and eight connections had greater strength values for L2. Across time, eight connections showed different patterns of difference between L1 and L2. In particular, the connections from ACC to LIFGTri, from LIFGOrb to LIFGTri, and from ACC to LC had higher strength values for L2 compared to L1 at T2 (chronic phase), while the connections from LC to ACC, LIFGTri, and LIFGOrb, from ACC to LIFGOrb, and from LIFGTri to AB47 showed greater strength values for L1 compared to L2 at T2 (chronic phase). Although reorganization happened in the connection strengths for L1 and L2 at T2 (chronic phase), there was a similar degree of connectedness within the language-control network for L1 and L2.

3.2.3. Patient 3

(A) Behavioral Scores. At T2 (chronic phase), the combined production score showed improvement in both L1 (χ^2: 25.07, *p* < 0.0001) and L2 (χ^2: 4.16, *p*: 0.041) at T2 (chronic phase). The patient also showed a significant improvement in both

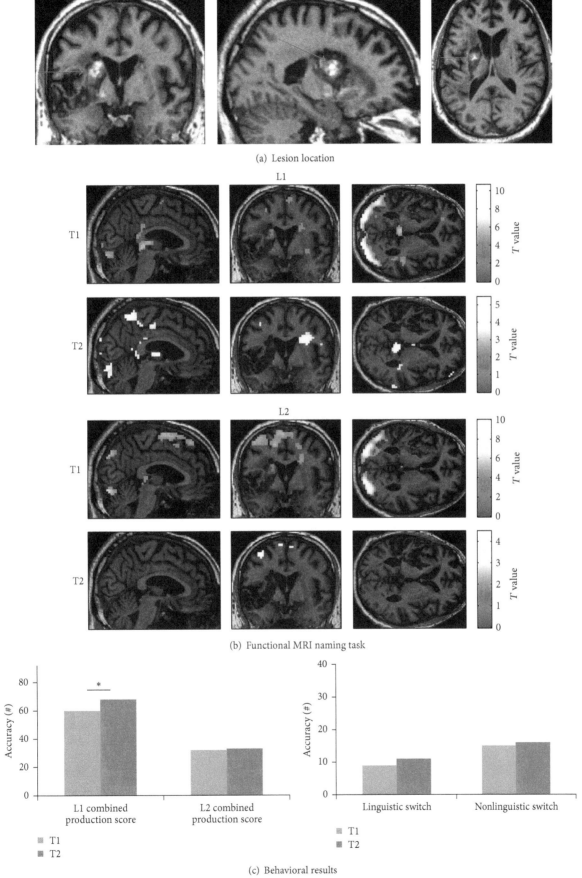

(a) Lesion location

(b) Functional MRI naming task

(c) Behavioral results

FIGURE 3: Continued.

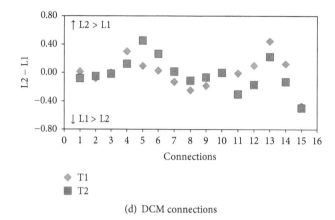

(d) DCM connections

Figure 3: Patient 1. (a) Ischemic stroke in left frontotemporal area in the T1-weighted MRI image at T1. (b) Pattern of brain activation in different conditions while picture naming, with an uncorrected $p < 0.001$ for the main effects. (c) Behavioral results of the combined production scores in both languages, linguistic and nonlinguistic switching scores across sessions. * represents p value < 0.05. (d) Differences between L1 strength values and L2 strength values for each single connection across sessions. (1) ACC to LIFGTri. (2) ACC to LIFGOrb. (3) ACC to LC. (4) LC to ACC. (5) LC to LIFGTri. (6) LC to LIFGOrb. (7) LIFGTri to LC. (8) LIFGTri to ACC. (9) LIFGTri to LC. (10) LIFGOrb to ACC. (11) LIFGTri to LIFGOrb. (12) LIFGOrb to LIFGTri. (13) BTLA to LIFGTri. (14) BTLA to LIFGOrb. (15) BTLA to LC.

linguistic and nonlinguistic switching tasks across time (χ^2: 17.05, $p < 0.0001$ and χ^2: 21.04, $p < 0.0001$, resp.) (Figure 5(c)) (see Table 3 and Supplementary Data 1 for details of the patient's performance).

(B) Changes in Connectivity in the Language-Control Network. The differences between L1 and L2 (L2 − L1) in the strength of single intrinsic connections within the network are shown in Figure 5(d). The raw differences in the strength of connections within the language-control network in this patient also indicated differing patterns in the connection strengths between L1 and L2 from T1 (subacute phase) and T2 (chronic phase) in half of the connections; notably, the connections from ACC to LIFGTri and forward and backward connections between LIFGTri and LIFGOrb showed greater connection strengths for L1 compared to L2 at T2 (chronic phase). However, forward and backward connections between LC and LIFGOrb and the connection from BTLA to LIFGTri and LIFGOrb had higher connection strength values for L2 compared to L1 at T2 (chronic phase). Overall, at T1 (subacute phase), seven connections had higher strength values in L1 while at T2 (chronic phase), nine connections had higher strength values in L1. Altogether, there was a similar degree of connectedness within the language-control network for L1 and L2 at T2 (chronic phase).

3.2.4. Patient 4

(A) Behavioral Scores. At T2 (chronic phase), the combined production score improved in L2 (χ^2: 8.16, p: 0.004) and no improvement was seen in L1 (already spared at T1 (subacute phase)). His performance in the linguistic switching task improved significantly (χ^2: 4.16, p: 0.041) and his nonlinguistic switching performance was spared at T1 (subacute phase) (Figure 6(c)).

(B) Changes in Connectivity in the Language-Control Network. At the single intrinsic connection level, the differences between L1 and L2 (L2 − L1) in strength of single intrinsic connections within the network for each session are shown in Figure 6(d). At T1 (subacute phase), around half of connections had higher strength values for L1 (eight out of 15), while at T2 (chronic phase), only three connections had greater values for L1 (i.e., connection from LIFGTri to LC, LIFGTri to LIFGOrb, and BTLA to LIFGOrb) and the rest of the connections showed higher coupling values for L2. These changes indicated a globally higher connectedness inside the language-control network for L2 at T2 (chronic phase).

3.2.5. Patient 5

(A) Behavioral Scores. The combined production score improved in both L1 (χ^2: 9.09, p: 0.002) and L2 (χ^2: 12.07, p: 0.0005) at T2 (chronic phase), although the patient still made several language switching errors. However, no improvement was seen in the linguistic and nonlinguistic switching task performances (Figure 7(c); more details can be found in Table 3 and Supplementary Data 1).

(B) Changes in Connectivity in the Language-Control Network. At the single intrinsic connection level, the differences between L1 and L2 (L2 − L1) in the strength of single intrinsic connections within the network for each session are shown in Figure 7(d). Importantly, several connections showed inverse patterns between T1 (subacute phase) and T2 (chronic phase); that is, four connections (from ACC to LIFGTri, ACC to LIFGOrb, LIFGTri to ACC, and LIFGTri to LIFGOrb) had higher strength values for L1 at T2 (chronic phase), and four connections (from LC to LIFGTri, LIFGOrb to ACC, LIFGOrb to LIFGTri, and BTLA to LIFGTri) had greater strength values for L2 at T2 (chronic phase). As with the changes

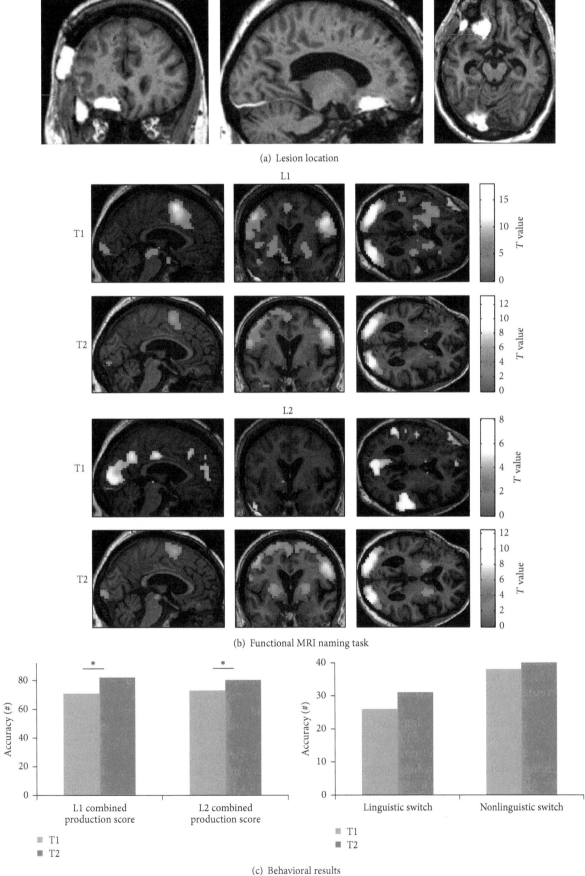

(a) Lesion location

(b) Functional MRI naming task

(c) Behavioral results

FIGURE 4: Continued.

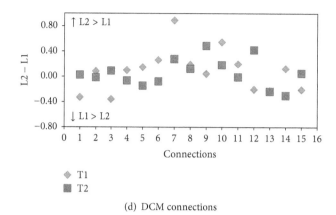

(d) DCM connections

FIGURE 4: Patient 2. (a) The T1-weighted MRI image at T1 shows an epidural hematoma with pressure over the operation site on the left frontobasal area. (b) Pattern of brain activation in different conditions while picture naming, with an uncorrected $p < 0.001$ for the main effects. (c) Behavioral results of the combined production scores in both languages, linguistic and nonlinguistic switching scores across sessions. ∗ represents p value < 0.05. (d) Differences between L1 strength values and L2 strength values for each single connection across sessions. (1) ACC to LIFGTri. (2) ACC to LIFGOrb. (3) ACC to LC. (4) LC to ACC. (5) LC to LIFGTri. (6) LC to LIFGOrb. (7) LIFGTri to LC. (8) LIFGTri to ACC. (9) LIFGOrb to LC. (10) LIFGOrb to ACC. (11) LIFGTri to LIFGOrb. (12) LIFGOrb to LIFGTri. (13) BTLA to LIFGTri. (14) BTLA to LIFGOrb. (15) BTLA to LC.

seen in patients 2 and 3, there was a similar connectedness within the language-control network in L1 and L2 at T2 (chronic phase).

3.3. Group Analyses of fMRI and DCM Analyses

3.3.1. FMRI Results. For the aphasic patients, the patterns of activation at each session of picture naming in L1 and L2 were presented for each patient separately; a threshold of uncorrected $p < 0.001$ was selected to visualize the main effects (Figures 3(b)–7(b)). As our main aim of the fMRI study was to perform DCM analysis based on a previously published model, we did not statistically compare the activations in the different conditions.

3.3.2. DCM Results

(C) Correlation Analysis between Language Production Recovery and Changes in the Strength of Connection. At the group level, in the aphasic patients, the changes in the strength of intrinsic connections between language and control areas (specifically between ACC, LC, and LIFGOrb from control subnetwork to LIFGTri in language subnetwork) were implemented to correlate with the changes in combined production scores.

In the aphasic patients, we found a significant correlation between changes in the combined production scores in L1 and changes in the strength of connection from ACC to LIFGTri (while performing picture naming in L1) (Spearman's rho: 0.921, p: 0.026). Moreover, changes in the combined productions score in L2 were negatively correlated to the changes in the strength of connections from LIFGTri to LIFGOrb (Spearman's rho: −0.900, p: 0.037).

3.4. Supplementary Analyses of DCM. To better compare the changes in the number of connections with higher strength

values between the improved versus unimproved language across time, we concatenated the data of patients 1 and 4 (who improved language production in only one language). This combined analysis showed a higher number of connections in the improved language at T2 (chronic phase) (χ^2: 4.44, p 0.035).

4. Discussion

Using a longitudinal design, we examined language production recovery in five late bilingual patients suffering from poststroke aphasia at subacute and chronic phases following a stroke. From three weeks to four months following a stroke, (A) we monitored modifications in language and control performance to identify whether language recovery was linked with the recovery of control functions. Moreover, (B) using a DCM approach, we examined how the interconnections between language and control areas changed with the recovery of language production, and (C) we then investigated the possible correlation between changes in language production performances and changes in the strength of each single connection within language-control network across time.

Considering the changes in the combined production scores, three of our five patients recovered in both L1 and L2 (patients 2, 3, and 5), one patient recovered in L1 (patient 1), and one (patient 4) in L2 only (the latter patient already had a high accuracy score in L1 at the subacute phase). Two patients (patient 3 with recovery in both languages and patient 4 with recovery in L2) showed improvement in language-control functions (Table 4). No decrease in control functions was observed among the patients.

Descriptive analyses of the DCM suggested a relationship between the pattern of recovery of language production and changes in the strength of connections across time. In patient 1, who recovered only L1 production score across time, the majority of connections within language-control network (10

TABLE 3: General aphasia evaluation, picture naming, and control functions scores at T1 and T2.

| Task | Session | General aphasia evaluation (GAE) | | | | | | | | | | | Picture naming (/40) | Combined production score (/92) | Language control | |
		Object naming (/20)	Series (/6)	Verbal fluency (/3)	Repetition (/13)	Yes/no questions (/20)	Pointing (/5)	Following commands (/8)	Reading commands (/11)	Description (/10)	Production score (GAE) (/52)	Total (/96)			Linguistic switch (/40) (number of switching errors)	Nonlinguistic switch (/40) (number of switching errors)
Subject 1	T1 L1	10	6	0	13	13	4	4	2	10	39	62	20	59	9 (7)	15 (13)
	T1 L2	4	4	0	13	16	4	1	3	10	31	55	1	32		
	T2 L1	13	6	0	13	17	5	6	8	8	40	76	28	68	11 (5)	16 (24)
	T2 L2	4	4	0	13	16	4	1	3	10	31	55	2	33		
Subject 2	T1 L1	16	6	0	13	16	5	4	9	10	45	79	26	71	26 (5)	38 (1)
	T1 L2	19	6	1	9	20	5	5	7	10	45	82	28	73		
	T2 L1	19	6	1	13	18	5	5	9	10	49	86	33	82	31 (4)	40
	T2 L2	20	6	0	13	16	5	5	9	10	49	84	31	80		
Subject 3	T1 L1	18	6	0	13	18	5	8	7	10	47	85	7/14	54/66	14 (11)	4 (15)
	T1 L2	18	6	0	13	20	5	7	4	10	47	83	31	78		
	T2 L1	20	6	1	13	20	5	8	11	10	50	94	31	81	33 (2)	27 (8)
	T2 L2	20	6	0	13	20	5	8	11	10	49	93	35	84		
Subject 4	T1 L1	18	6	2	13	16	5	8	11	10	49	89	39	88	30 (0)	38 (2)
	T1 L2	11	6	0	13	20	4	8	10	6	36	78	27	63		
	T2 L1	20	6	3	13	18	5	8	11	10	59	94	38	90	36 (1)	40 (0)
	T2 L2	12	6	3	13	18	4	8	11	8	42	83	31	73		
Subject 5	T1 L1	18	6	0	13	18	5	2	9	10	47	81	19	66	19 (17)	25 (3)
	T1 L2	12	4	0	13	20	5	4	8	10	39	76	19	58		
	T2 L1	18	6	0	13	18	5	4	11	10	47	85	30	77	19 (13)	29 (4)
	T2 L2	16	6	0	13	16	5	4	11	10	45	81	27	72		

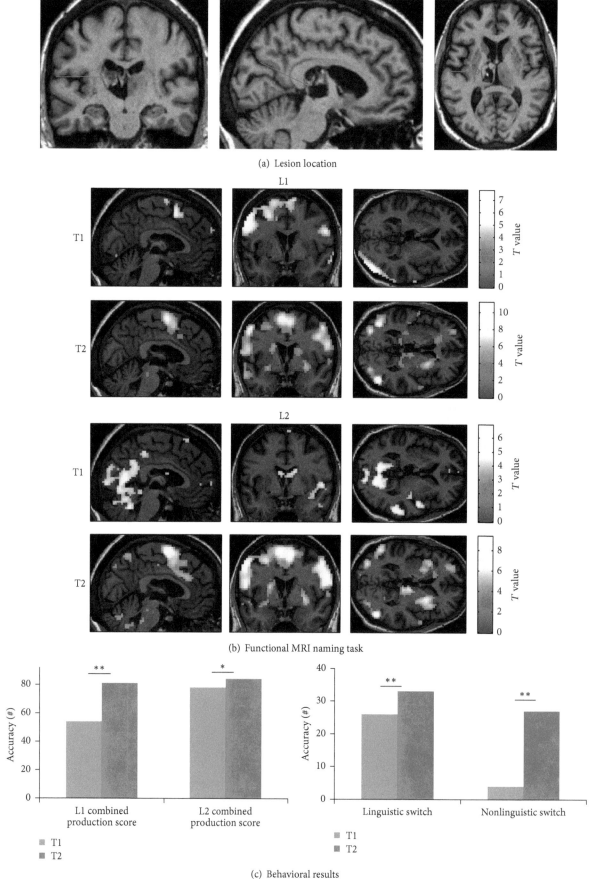

(a) Lesion location

(b) Functional MRI naming task

(c) Behavioral results

FIGURE 5: Continued.

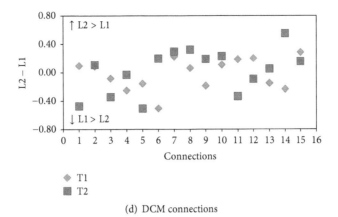

(d) DCM connections

FIGURE 5: Patient 3. (a) The T1-weighted MRI image at T1 shows a hemorrhagic stroke in the left basal ganglia. (b) Pattern of brain activation in different conditions while picture naming, with an uncorrected $p < 0.001$ for the main effects. (c) Behavioral results of the combined production scores in both languages, linguistic and nonlinguistic switching scores across sessions. ∗ represents p value < 0.05 and ∗∗ represents p value < 0.001. (d) Differences between L1 strength values and L2 strength values for each single connection across sessions. (1) ACC to LIFGTri. (2) ACC to LIFGOrb. (3) ACC to LC. (4) LC to ACC. (5) LC to LIFGTri. (6) LC to LIFGOrb. (7) LIFGTri to LC. (8) LIFGTri to ACC. (9) LIFGOrb to LC. (10) LIFGOrb to ACC. (11) LIFGTri to LIFGOrb. (12) LIFGOrb to LIFGTri. (13) BTLA to LIFGTri. (14) BTLA to LIFGOrb. (15) BTLA to LC.

TABLE 4: Summary of the recovery patterns.

Subject	L1-combined production	L2-combined production	Linguistic switch	Nonlinguistic
Patient 1	↑	→	→	→
Patient 2	↑	↑	→	→
Patient 3	↑	↑	↑	↑
Patient 4	→	↑	↑	→
Patient 5	↑	↑	→	→

out of 15 connections) had higher connection strength values at the chronic phase, indicating a higher connectedness within the language-control network while picture naming in L1. The similar pattern of changes in the connectedness within language-control network took place in patient 4 who recovered only L2 (i.e., at the chronic phase he showed higher connectedness within language-control network while picture naming in L2). In these two patients with recovery of only one language, combined analyses revealed that improvement in production score in one language was associated with an increase in the number of connections with higher strength values at T2 (chronic phase) while performing the task in that specific language. In addition, showing a similar pattern of changes in the language-control network connectedness, patients 2 and 5 at T1 (subacute phase) in the majority of connections had higher coupling values for picture naming in L2, while at T2, the coupling values of 7 connections were higher in L1 and 8 connections had higher coupling values in L2 task. Also, patient 3 showed higher coupling values for the majority of connections for L1 picture naming at T1 (subacute phase), while at T2, the coupling values of 7 connections were higher in L1 and 8 connections had higher coupling values in L2 task. Taken together, in patients 2, 3, and 5 who recovered both L1 and L2, a redistribution of the connection strength occurred across

time; the strength of the connections between language and control areas was similarly distributed at T2 (chronic phase) over the network during picture naming in L1 and L2. In the control group with main L2 exposure and usage in daily life, a higher connectedness was seen within the network for L1 compared to L2 (see Supplementary Data 2 and 3). We will discuss each of these results in turn.

Although the role of control functions in the recovery of bilingual aphasia has been suggested in several studies [8, 9], in our patients, at the behavioral level, the improvement in language-control functions alone could not explain their patterns of language recovery. The observed pattern of language and control recovery does not directly support Paradis' statement that when language-control function is intact, one can expect a parallel recovery of languages, and in the presence of language-control problems one may expect the weaker language in the premorbid stage to be impaired [34]. However, Green and Abutalebi [35] suggest that, along with premorbid proficiency, languages that were mostly used following stroke may become more proficient and easily manageable, especially in the case of reduced resources for controlling the use of two languages.

Our findings on the changes in the differences in connectedness between L1 and L2 within the language-control network are in line with the results of Abutalebi et al. [9],

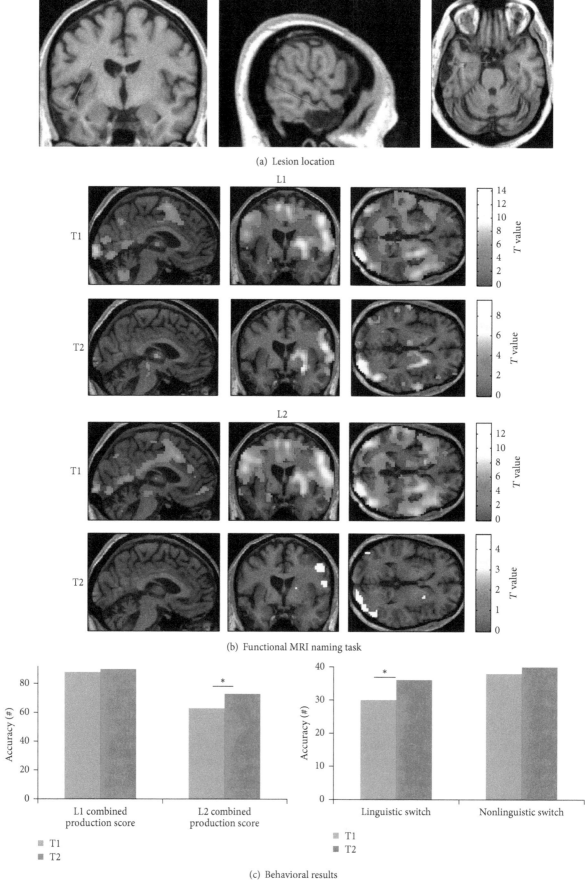

(a) Lesion location

L1

T1

T2

L2

T1

T2

(b) Functional MRI naming task

(c) Behavioral results

FIGURE 6: Continued.

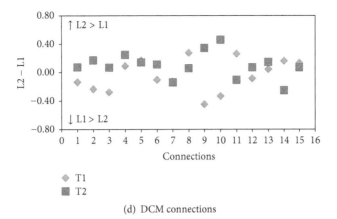

(d) DCM connections

FIGURE 6: Patient 4. (a) The T1-weighted MRI image at T1 shows a left sylvian ischemic stroke. (b) Pattern of brain activation in different conditions while picture naming, with an uncorrected $p < 0.001$ for the main effects. (c) Behavioral results of the combined production scores in both languages, linguistic and nonlinguistic switching scores across sessions. * represents p value < 0.05. (d) Differences between L1 strength values and L2 strength values for each single connection across sessions. (1) ACC to LIFGTri. (2) ACC to LIFGOrb. (3) ACC to LC. (4) LC to ACC. (5) LC to LIFGTri. (6) LC to LIFGOrb. (7) LIFGTri to LC. (8) LIFGTri to ACC. (9) LIFGOrb to LC. (10) LIFGOrb to ACC. (11) LIFGTri to LIFGOrb. (12) LIFGOrb to LIFGTri. (13) BTLA to LIFGTri. (14) BTLA to LIFGOrb. (15) BTLA to LC.

in the case of a bilingual aphasic patient for whom the language which recovered better showed increased connections between language and control networks. Our DCM results support a role for language-control interconnections in language recovery in bilingual aphasic patients [9, 10, 35] and are in line with the "dynamic view" of language production, which posits that patterns of language recovery are related to alterations in language control. Interestingly, for patients in whom both languages recovered (patients 2, 3, and 5), the two languages were connected to the control system to the same extent. Additionally, when one language recovered better, there was a greater engagement of language-control interconnections in this language. Previous studies of the association between global patterns of brain connectivity and the recovery of language functions have suggested that decreased functional connectivity between anterior and posterior areas of the default mode network (DMN) is associated with cognitive impairment. Accordingly, therapy-induced increases in functional connectivity between anterior and posterior areas of the DMN have been reported in a group of chronic monolingual aphasic patients [36]. In a further study, Sebastian and colleagues [37] evaluated the recovery of naming functions from acute to chronic phase and showed that the degree of functional connectivity between language-specific areas in both hemispheres was important for optimal recovery of naming functions.

Furthermore, our results suggest that a change in connection strength from ACC to LIFGTri during picture naming in L1 was associated with L1 recovery; the coupling between these two areas became stronger when L1 recovered. LIFGTri, along with the LIFG pars opercularis (BA44), is known to be involved in different steps of language production [38], namely, in syntactic encoding [39], speech praxis [40], and verb retrieval [41]. ACC is known to be involved in conflict and error monitoring, including domain-general control functions in healthy populations [42]. In the normally

functioning bilingual brain, ACC, in connection with the prefrontal cortex, is a component of the circuit involved in inhibiting interference from the nontarget language [1, 18, 43] while in a healthy brain, this interference is caused mainly by the more proficient language (usually L1); our results could be explained by the fact that in the presence of language and control dysfunction (e.g., following a stroke), conflicts may arise between L1 and L2 even in the case of different proficiencies. Therefore, a higher engagement of the circuit between ACC and LIFGTri could possibly facilitate performance in the recovery of L1 by blocking the interference of information from L2.

Analyses of the changes in connectivity strengths across time suggest that, in patients with L2 recovery (four out of five patients), the connection from LIFGTri to LIFGOrb becomes weaker for L2 compared to L1. This finding is also supported by the result of a correlation analysis showing that the recovery of combined production scores in L2 negatively correlates with changes in the strength of connection from LIFGTri to LIFGOrb. In other words, when L2 recovers, the coupling from LIFGTri to LIFGOrb decreases. These two regions are strongly anatomofunctionally interconnected as subregions of the inferior frontal gyrus [40]. LIFGTri is selected as the main language production area and LIFGOrb is a part of language-control network, which is involved in both language production and language-control processes (lexical semantic processes along with LIFGTri and selecting among lexical competitors) [44, 45]. The reason for the decrease of coupling from LIFGTri to LIFGOrb in L2 production could be explained by the Revised Hierarchical Model of lexical and conceptual representation in the bilingual brain [46, 47]. In this psycholinguistic model the conceptual system is common across languages, even in the less proficient L2. However, L1 is hypothesized to have privileged access to the conceptual system, favored by a strong connection between the areas involved in lexical and semantic processing (resp., LIFGTri

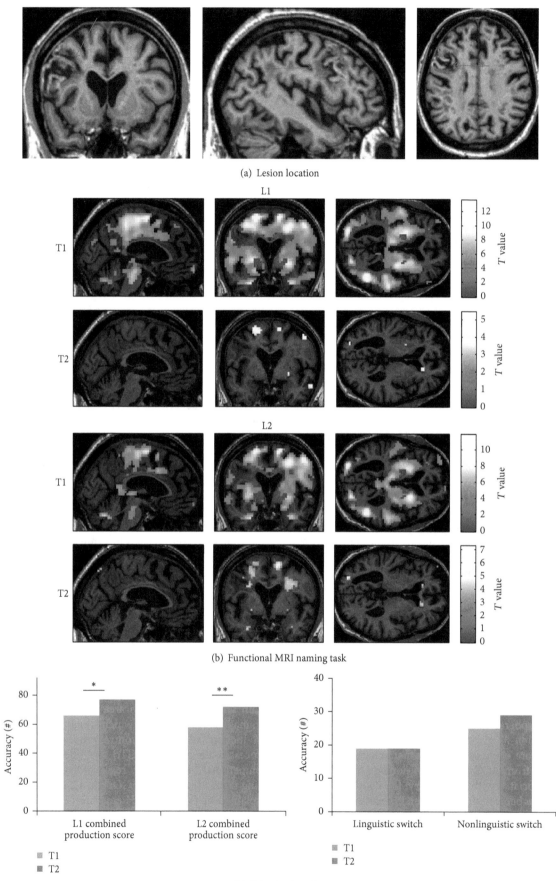

(a) Lesion location

(b) Functional MRI naming task

(c) Behavioral results

FIGURE 7: Continued.

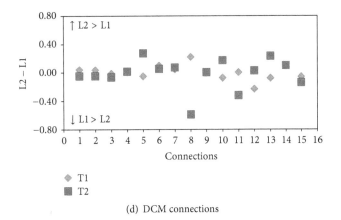

(d) DCM connections

Figure 7: Patient 5. (a) An ischemic lesion in the left frontal, insula, and sylvian areas in the T1-weighted MRI image at T1. (b) Pattern of brain activation in different conditions while picture naming, with an uncorrected $p < 0.001$ for the main effects. (c) Behavioral results of the combined production scores in both languages, linguistic and nonlinguistic switching scores across sessions. ∗ represents p value < 0.05 and ∗∗ represents p value < 0.001. (d) Differences between L1 strength values and L2 strength values for each single connection across sessions. (1) ACC to LIFGTri. (2) ACC to LIFGOrb. (3) ACC to LC. (4) LC to ACC. (5) LC to LIFGTri. (6) LC to LIFGOrb. (7) LIFGTri to LC. (8) LIFGTri to ACC. (9) LIFGOrb to LC. (10) LIFGOrb to ACC. (11) LIFGTri to LIFGOrb. (12) LIFGOrb to LIFGTri. (13) BTLA to LIFGTri. (14) BTLA to LIFGOrb. (15) BTLA to LC.

and LIFGOrb in our study). Hence, a weaker connectivity between these two areas may help in the process of L2 recovery.

The present study suffers from several limitations. First, we could not implement certain language and control tasks since they were too demanding for aphasic patients, especially in the acute and subacute phases. A comprehensive evaluation of language and control would have helped better understand the possible correlation between the recovery of control functions and the recovery of language performance following a stroke. Even though we narrowed our selection of tasks to a limited series of evaluation materials, half of the initially recruited patients dropped out of the second session of the study. Another limitation of this study was the small number of included patients; their results may not be easily applicable to all bilingual aphasic patients. In addition, we could not control the age of the patients in the study (the age of patients ranged from 49 to 79 years old). It is known that the age factor can affect behavioral performance, functional brain activity, and connectivity within brain areas as a result of alteration in neuronal activity and connectivity in aging brain [48, 49]. However, as the design is mainly within-subject the age does not seem to affect importantly the results. In addition, regressing out the effect of age from the analyses would not let any significant results due to the small sample size. Moreover, the use of different MRI scanners in this study restricted us in carrying out a direct group comparison of brain activation in different conditions. Finally, as obtaining an accurate measure of premorbid proficiency following their stroke was impossible, the evaluation of premorbid second language proficiency was restricted to a detailed questionnaire filled in by a family member or the patient himself.

It worth noting that, in the present study, only three patients followed language therapy sessions and the therapy was computer assisted to improve lexical access and in turn improve naming performances. One patient (patient 1)

received therapy in his L1 (French) and he then improved in L1 production. This lack of improvement in L2 could be explained by the very low L2 usage and immersion by this subject. It has been previously suggested by Edmonds and Kiran [50] that the effect of therapy in less mastered language is more likely to transfer to the untreated language as the subject is more relied on borrowing word from the more proficient language. Another explanation of the absence of transfer of the effect of language therapy in L1 to the untreated L2 is the fact that he did not show improvement in control functions across time [8]. Patient 3 received therapy in her L2 (French), which she has been used and was immersed in an equal level as her L1 since 53 years ago. She improved in both L1 (Italian) and L2 across time. Her improvement in both languages can be explained by high immersion in both languages as well as improvement in the cognitive control functions. Patient 5 attended to a limited number of therapy sessions (10 sessions) in his L1 (French) and he improved in both L1 and L2 (English). In this patient, the recovery of both languages cannot be explained by the choice of therapy or the pattern of changes in cognitive control functions. Therefore, no consistent pattern of the effect of therapy and possible cross language transfer of the effect of therapy was found. Therefore, our interpretation of these results is not based on the language therapy. Moreover, because of the timing of the study sessions (at three weeks and around four months following the stroke), the process of spontaneous recovery should be still ongoing [6, 23]. Accordingly, this recovery takes place as the result of a combination of spontaneous recovery and language therapy.

5. Conclusion

Taken together, our findings supply additional evidence that the engagement of the interconnected language-control network is crucial for the recovery of languages. Furthermore, we suggest that L1 recovery is improved by increased connectivity between ACC and LIFGTri, which prevents conflicts from the second language. However, L2 recovery requires a decrease in connectivity from LIFGTri to LIFGOrb in order to decrease the automatic activation of the L1 lexical system, which, according to the Revised Hierarchical Model, has stronger links with the conceptual system.

Competing Interests

The authors declare that there is no conflict of interests regarding the publication of this paper.

Acknowledgments

This work was supported by a grant from the Swiss National Foundation for Science to Jean-Marie Annoni (nos. 32-138497 and 325130-156937). The authors would like to thank Dr. Lucas Spierer, Dr. Ferath Kherif, Professor Dimitri Van de Ville, and Dr. Peter Zeidman for their scientific support and healthcare personnel of Geneva and Fribourg Hospitals.

References

[1] Y. Faroqi-Shah, T. Frymark, R. Mullen, and B. Wang, "Effect of treatment for bilingual individuals with aphasia: a systematic review of the evidence," *Journal of Neurolinguistics*, vol. 23, no. 4, pp. 319–341, 2010.

[2] F. Grosjean, *Bilingual Life and Reality*, Harvard University Press, 2010.

[3] T. H. Lucas II, G. M. McKhann II, and G. A. Ojemann, "Functional separation of languages in the bilingual brain: a comparison of electrical stimulation language mapping in 25 bilingual patients and 117 monolingual control patients," *Journal of Neurosurgery*, vol. 101, no. 3, pp. 449–457, 2004.

[4] A. I. Ansaldo, K. Marcotte, L. Scherer, and G. Raboyeau, "Language therapy and bilingual aphasia: clinical implications of psycholinguistic and neuroimaging research," *Journal of Neurolinguistics*, vol. 21, no. 6, pp. 539–557, 2008.

[5] S. Aglioti, A. Beltramello, F. Girardi, and F. Fabbro, "Neurolinguistic and follow-up study of an unusual pattern of recovery from bilingual subcortical aphasia," *Brain*, vol. 119, no. 5, pp. 1551–1564, 1996.

[6] M. Gil and M. Goral, "Nonparallel recovery in bilingual aphasia: effects of language choice, language proficiency, and treatment," *International Journal of Bilingualism*, vol. 8, no. 2, pp. 191–219, 2004.

[7] N. Radman, L. Spierer, M. Laganaro, J.-M. Annoni, and F. Colombo, "Language specificity of lexical-phonological therapy in bilingual aphasia: a clinical and electrophysiological study," *Neuropsychological Rehabilitation*, vol. 26, no. 4, 2016.

[8] A. I. Ansaldo and L. G. Saidi, "Aphasia therapy in the age of globalization: cross-linguistic therapy effects in bilingual aphasia," *Behavioural Neurology*, vol. 2014, Article ID 603085, 10 pages, 2014.

[9] J. Abutalebi, P. A. D. Rosa, M. Tettamanti, D. W. Green, and S. F. Cappa, "Bilingual aphasia and language control: a follow-up fMRI and intrinsic connectivity study," *Brain and Language*, vol. 109, no. 2-3, pp. 141–156, 2009.

[10] J. Abutalebi and D. Green, "Bilingual language production: the neurocognition of language representation and control," *Journal of Neurolinguistics*, vol. 20, no. 3, pp. 242–275, 2007.

[11] D. Green, *Bilingualism: Language and Cognition*, vol. 1, Cambrdige University Press, Cambrdige, UK, 1998.

[12] D. W. Green and C. J. Price, "Functional imaging in the study of recovery patterns in bilingual aphasia," *Bilingualism: Language and Cognition*, vol. 4, no. 2, pp. 191–201, 2001.

[13] M. Paradis, "Language and communication in multilinguals," in *Handbook of Neurolinguistics*, B. Stemmer and H. Whitaker, Eds., pp. 417–430, Academic Press, San Diego, Calif, USA, 1998.

[14] N. Verreyt, M. De Letter, D. Hemelsoet, P. Santens, and W. Duyck, "Cognate effects and executive control in a patient with differential bilingual aphasia," *Applied Neuropsychology: Adult*, vol. 20, no. 3, pp. 221–230, 2013.

[15] J. G. Kerns, J. D. Cohen, A. W. MacDonald III, R. Y. Cho, V. A. Stenger, and C. S. Carter, "Anterior cingulate conflict monitoring and adjustments in control," *Science*, vol. 303, no. 5660, pp. 1023–1026, 2004.

[16] D. W. Green and J. Abutalebi, "Language control in bilinguals: the adaptive control hypothesis," *Journal of Cognitive Psychology*, vol. 25, no. 5, pp. 515–530, 2013.

[17] L. M. McCormick, S. Ziebell, P. Nopoulos, M. Cassell, N. C. Andreasen, and M. Brumm, "Anterior cingulate cortex: an MRI-based parcellation method," *NeuroImage*, vol. 32, no. 3, pp. 1167–1175, 2006.

[18] J. Abutalebi and D. W. Green, "Neuroimaging of language control in bilinguals: neural adaptation and reserve," *Bilingualism: Language and Cognition*, vol. 19, no. 4, pp. 689–698, 2016.

[19] A. Hervais-Adelman, B. Moser-Mercer, C. M. Michel, and N. Golestani, "fMRI of simultaneous interpretation reveals the neural basis of extreme language control," *Cerebral Cortex*, vol. 25, no. 12, pp. 4727–4739, 2015.

[20] D. A. Magezi, A. Khateb, M. Mouthon, L. Spierer, and J.-M. Annoni, "Cognitive control of language production in bilinguals involves a partly independent process within the domain-general cognitive control network: evidence from task-switching and electrical brain activity," *Brain and Language*, vol. 122, no. 1, pp. 55–63, 2012.

[21] F. M. Branzi, M. Calabria, M. L. Boscarino, and A. Costa, "On the overlap between bilingual language control and domain-general executive control," *Acta Psychologica*, vol. 166, pp. 21–30, 2016.

[22] E. L. Meier, K. J. Kapse, and S. Kiran, "The relationship between frontotemporal effective connectivity during picture naming, behavior, and preserved cortical tissue in chronic aphasia," *Frontiers in Human Neuroscience*, vol. 10, article 109, 2016.

[23] S. F. Cappa, "Spontaneous recovery from aphasia," in *Handbook of Neurolinguistics*, B. Stemmer and H. A. Whitaker, Eds., pp. 536–547, Academic Press, San Diego, Calif, USA, 1998.

[24] M. Paradis and G. Libben, *The Assessment of Bilingual Aphasia*, Lawrence Erlbaum Associates, Hillsdale, NJ, USA, 1987.

[25] R. Nakase-Thompson, *The Mississippi Aphasia Screening Test*, T.C.f.O.M.i.B. Injury, 2004.

[26] M. Tschirren, M. Laganaro, P. Michel et al., "Language and syntactic impairment following stroke in late bilingual aphasics," *Brain and Language*, vol. 119, no. 3, pp. 238–242, 2011.

[27] J. Abutalebi, J.-M. Annoni, I. Zimine et al., "Language control and lexical competition in bilinguals: an event-related fMRI study," *Cerebral Cortex*, vol. 18, no. 7, pp. 1496–1505, 2008.

[28] J. G. Snodgrass and M. Vanderwart, "A standardized set of 260 pictures: norms for name agreement, image agreement, familiarity, and visual complexity," *Journal of Experimental Psychology: Human Learning and Memory*, vol. 6, no. 2, pp. 174–215, 1980.

[29] P. Jezzard and S. Clare, "Sources of distortion in functional MRI data," *Human Brain Mapping*, vol. 8, no. 2-3, pp. 80–85, 1999.

[30] K. Friston, *Statistical Parametric Mapping: The Analysis of Functional Brain Images*, Elsevier, Amsterdam, The Netherlands, 2007.

[31] J. L. R. Andersson, C. Hutton, J. Ashburner, R. Turner, and K. Friston, "Modeling geometric deformations in EPI time series," *NeuroImage*, vol. 13, no. 5, pp. 903–919, 2001.

[32] K. J. Worsley and K. J. Friston, "Analysis of fMRI time-series revisited—again," *NeuroImage*, vol. 2, no. 3, pp. 173–181, 1995.

[33] M. L. Seghier, P. Zeidman, N. H. Neufeld, A. P. Leff, and C. J. Price, "Identifying abnormal connectivity in patients using dynamic causal modeling of fMRI responses," *Frontiers in Systems Neuroscience*, vol. 4, article 142, 2010.

[34] M. Paradis, "Bilingual and polyglot aphasia," in *Handbook of Neuropsychology*, R. S. Berndt, Ed., Elsevier Science, Amsterdam, The Netherlands, 2001.

[35] D. W. Green and J. Abutalebi, "Understanding the link between bilingual aphasia and language control," *Journal of Neurolinguistics*, vol. 21, no. 6, pp. 558–576, 2008.

[36] K. Marcotte, V. Perlbarg, G. Marrelec, H. Benali, and A. I. Ansaldo, "Default-mode network functional connectivity in aphasia: therapy-induced neuroplasticity," *Brain and Language*, vol. 124, no. 1, pp. 45–55, 2013.

[37] R. Sebastian, C. Long, J. J. Purcell et al., "Imaging network level language recovery after left PCA stroke," *Restorative Neurology and Neuroscience*, vol. 34, no. 4, pp. 473–489, 2016.

[38] B. Horwitz, K. Amunts, R. Bhattacharyya et al., "Activation of Broca's area during the production of spoken and signed language: a combined cytoarchitectonic mapping and PET analysis," *Neuropsychologia*, vol. 41, no. 14, pp. 1868–1876, 2003.

[39] S. Haller, E. W. Radue, M. Erb, W. Grodd, and T. Kircher, "Overt sentence production in event-related fMRI," *Neuropsychologia*, vol. 43, no. 5, pp. 807–814, 2005.

[40] A. Ardila, B. Bernal, and M. Rosselli, "How localized are language brain areas? A review of Brodmann areas involvement in oral language," *Archives of Clinical Neuropsychology*, vol. 31, no. 1, pp. 112–122, 2016.

[41] E. Warburton, R. J. S. Wise, C. J. Price et al., "Noun and verb retrieval by normal subjects: studies with PET," *Brain*, vol. 119, no. 1, pp. 159–179, 1996.

[42] M. M. Botvinick, C. S. Carter, T. S. Braver, D. M. Barch, and J. D. Cohen, "Conflict monitoring and cognitive control," *Psychological Review*, vol. 108, no. 3, pp. 624–652, 2001.

[43] C. J. Price, "The anatomy of language: a review of 100 fMRI studies published in 2009," *Annals of the New York Academy of Sciences*, vol. 1191, pp. 62–88, 2010.

[44] S. L. Thompson-Schill, M. D'Esposito, G. K. Aguirre, and M. J. Farah, "Role of left inferior prefrontal cortex in retrieval of semantic knowledge: a reevaluation," *Proceedings of the National Academy of Sciences of the United States of America*, vol. 94, no. 26, pp. 14792–14797, 1997.

[45] J. F. Demonet, G. Thierry, and D. Cardebat, "Renewal of the neurophysiology of language: functional neuroimaging," *Physiological Reviews*, vol. 85, no. 1, pp. 49–95, 2005.

[46] J. F. Kroll and E. Stewart, "Category interference in translation and picture naming: evidence for asymmetric connections between bilingual memory representations," *Journal of Memory and Language*, vol. 33, no. 2, pp. 149–174, 1994.

[47] J. F. Kroll, J. G. Van Hell, N. Tokowicz, and D. W. Green, "The Revised Hierarchical Model: a critical review and assessment," *Bilingualism*, vol. 13, no. 3, pp. 373–381, 2010.

[48] C. La, P. Mossahebi, V. A. Nair et al., "Age-related changes in inter-network connectivity by component analysis," *Frontiers in Aging Neuroscience*, vol. 7, article 237, 2015.

[49] M. Sugiura, "Functional neuroimaging of normal aging: declining brain, adapting brain," *Ageing Research Reviews*, vol. 30, pp. 61–72, 2016.

[50] L. A. Edmonds and S. Kiran, "Effect of semantic naming treatment on crosslinguistic generalization in bilingual aphasia," *Journal of Speech, Language, and Hearing Research*, vol. 49, no. 4, pp. 729–748, 2006.

13

Intrahemispheric Perfusion in Chronic Stroke-Induced Aphasia

Cynthia K. Thompson,[1,2,3] Matthew Walenski,[1,2] YuFen Chen,[1,4]
David Caplan,[1,5] Swathi Kiran,[1,6] Brenda Rapp,[1,7] Kristin Grunewald,[1,8]
Mia Nunez,[1,8] Richard Zinbarg,[1,8] and Todd B. Parrish[1,4]

[1]Center for the Neurobiology of Language Recovery, Northwestern University, Evanston, IL, USA
[2]Department of Communication Sciences and Disorders, School of Communication, Northwestern University, Evanston, IL, USA
[3]Department of Neurology, Feinberg School of Medicine, Northwestern University, Evanston, IL, USA
[4]Department of Radiology, Feinberg School of Medicine, Northwestern University, Evanston, IL, USA
[5]Massachusetts General Hospital, Department of Neurology, Harvard Medical School, Boston, MA, USA
[6]Department of Speech, Language, and Hearing, College of Health & Rehabilitation, Boston University, Boston, MA, USA
[7]Department of Cognitive Science, Krieger School of Arts & Sciences, Johns Hopkins University, Baltimore, MD, USA
[8]Department of Psychology, Weinberg College of Arts and Sciences, Northwestern University, Evanston, IL, USA

Correspondence should be addressed to Cynthia K. Thompson; ckthom@northwestern.edu

Academic Editor: Zygmunt Galdzicki

Stroke-induced alterations in cerebral blood flow (perfusion) may contribute to functional language impairments and recovery in chronic aphasia. Using MRI, we examined perfusion in the right and left hemispheres of 35 aphasic and 16 healthy control participants. Across 76 regions (38 per hemisphere), no significant between-subjects differences were found in the left, whereas blood flow in the right was increased in the aphasic compared to the control participants. Region-of-interest (ROI) analyses showed a varied pattern of hypo- and hyperperfused regions across hemispheres in the aphasic participants; however, there were no significant correlations between perfusion values and language abilities in these regions. These patterns may reflect autoregulatory changes in blood flow following stroke and/or increases in general cognitive effort, rather than maladaptive language processing. We also examined blood flow in perilesional tissue, finding the greatest hypoperfusion close to the lesion (within 0–6 mm), with greater hypoperfusion in this region compared to more distal regions. In addition, hypoperfusion in this region was significantly correlated with language impairment. These findings underscore the need to consider cerebral perfusion as a factor contributing to language deficits in chronic aphasia as well as recovery of language function.

1. Introduction

Recovery of language in chronic stroke-induced aphasia involves recruitment of undamaged tissue in the contralesional (typically right) and/or the ipsilesional hemisphere of the brain [1–4]. Although it has been suggested that ipsilesional, and even perilesional, tissue is best suited to support recovery, there are several factors that influence recruitment of undamaged tissue during functional recovery, including poststroke alterations in vascular physiology.

Emerging evidence from multiple sources suggests that restoration of cerebral blood flow (the rate at which blood perfuses a neural region) is critically associated with functional recovery. Blood delivers oxygen and glucose to the brain that is required for aerobic metabolism supporting neural activity [5]. In hyperacute stages of stroke, cortical spreading depression originating from the infarction site causes the lesion to expand [6], which affects symptom severity [7]. In addition, perilesional tissue becomes inflamed [8]. A settling of these events (e.g., lesion stabilization, reduced inflammation) contributes to recovery of function in acute stroke-induced aphasia, when perfusion is most likely to reverse to prestroke levels, either spontaneously or through pharmacological interventions [9, 10].

Prestroke perfusion levels, however, may not be regained in all regions of the brain, leaving uninfarcted tissue hypoperfused well past the acute stage. Using arterial spin labeling MRI, Richardson et al. [11] found reduced perfusion values in the left (ipsilesional) hemisphere compared to the right hemisphere in 17 patients with chronic aphasia [11, 12] (see Table 1 for a review of studies of perfusion in chronic aphasia). Notably, negative correlations between perfusion and lesion volume were reported, with larger infarcts corresponding to greater interhemispheric differences in perfusion. However, the duration of aphasic symptoms (time since stroke) did not correlate with reduced perfusion, suggesting a stable state of chronic hypoperfusion in chronic aphasia [11].

Regions of hypoperfused but otherwise intact tissue can create what are essentially functional lesions in chronic stroke, where the neurons are viable but unable to sufficiently support processing [13–15]. Evidence from animal models indicates that although neurons survive with perfusion levels greater than about 10% of normal, neuronal function is compromised when perfusion levels are below roughly 30% of normal [13, 16]. In human adults, normal cerebral blood flow in gray matter ranges from 37 to 64 mL/100 g/min, and lower perfusion may preclude normal functioning [14]. Consideration of hypoperfused regions, therefore, offers an important refinement to the traditional lesion method used to make inferences about structure-function correspondences in the brain [17], in that impaired language functioning may result not only from regions directly lesioned by stroke, but also from "hibernating" hypoperfused regions [18–20]. For example, Love et al. [15] reported hypoperfusion of otherwise spared tissue in the left angular and supramarginal gyri associated with impaired reading in a chronic aphasic patient.

Hypoperfused neural tissue also may not be viable for support of language recovery; rather, regions with lesser reductions or uncompromised cerebral blood flow (rCBF) may be better candidates for treatment-induced upregulation of neural activity. For example, Thompson et al. [19] found that baseline perfusion was higher (i.e., nearer normal levels) in regions that showed upregulation of neural activity in patients who underwent treatment for agrammatism. Fridriksson et al. [20] found a similar pattern in 30 patients who received treatment for anomia: pretreatment perfusion levels in undamaged regions within the left hemisphere language network (excluding infarcted and perilesional regions) predicted patients' naming accuracy, suggesting that higher baseline cerebral blood flow may be related to the potential for a better treatment outcome.

Reduction in cerebral blood flow also alters hemodynamic autoregulation aimed at maximizing the delivery of oxygen by increasing the blood volume or oxygen extraction fraction [21]. This has a fundamental effect on the shape and timing of the hemodynamic response used to measure blood oxygenation level-dependent (BOLD) task changes [12]. If not taken into account, an abnormal hemodynamic response may lead to underestimation and/or inaccurate measurement of the BOLD signal in functional magnetic resonance imaging (fMRI) [19, 22, 23]. Bonakdarpour et al. [24] found that three of five individuals with chronic stroke aphasia showed a delayed hemodynamic response (delayed

blood flow) in left perisylvian, relative to the left occipital, cortex during a lexical decision task. No such delay was seen in right perisylvian regions. Likewise, increased time-to-peak was seen in the five patients in left perilesional tissue during an overt naming task, but not in homologous right hemisphere regions. These delays correlated positively with lesion size (longer delays were seen in individuals with larger lesions) and negatively with aphasia severity as estimated using the Western Aphasia Battery-Revised (WAB-R) [25] (longer delays in individuals with more severe aphasia).

One region suggested to be particularly important for recovery of function is perilesional tissue. In rodent models, perilesional tissue undergoes neurophysiological changes, such as vascular proliferation and remodeling (angiogenesis) [26–29], reduced dendritic complexity, spine density, and synapses [26, 28, 30], and elevated rates of axonal sprouting [31, 32]. Hypoperfusion and reduced glucose metabolism also are prevalent in perilesional space [31, 33]. Notably, reversal to more normal neurophysiology within this region has been shown to coincide with recovery of function in animals as well as in acute phases of aphasia recovery in humans [34–37]. Presently, however, few studies have examined perfusion and/or reperfusion in perilesional tissue in chronic aphasia. Furthermore, within the aphasia literature there has been little research focused on what constitutes perilesional tissue and/or its role in recovery of language. In one study, Richardson [22] found reduced perfusion levels in individuals with chronic aphasia in a perilesional region of interest (ROI), defined as tissue from 3 to 8 mm surrounding the lesion, compared to its right hemisphere homologue.

In sum, prior evidence underscores the importance of examining perfusion in individuals with aphasia into the chronic stage, to augment understanding of the neural basis of language processing following stroke, and to determine the relation between perfusion and recovery of function. This paper examined perfusion in a group of individuals with chronic aphasia induced by left hemisphere ischaemic stroke and a cohort of healthy control participants. We tested between-subjects (aphasic versus healthy participants) differences in perfusion values in the left versus right hemisphere as well as in 38 ROIs in each hemisphere of the brain. We also examined perfusion in the patient group in perilesional ROIs, compared both to right hemisphere homologous regions and to remaining gray matter tissue in the left hemisphere (i.e., unlesioned, outside of the perilesional region). Perfusion was also examined in relation to scores on behavioral language tests reflecting overall aphasia severity, single word production (i.e., naming) and comprehension, spelling, and sentence production and comprehension ability. Finally, we examined perfusion in relation to individual and stroke-specific factors, including sex, age, education, lesion age (i.e., time post stroke), and lesion size (volume).

Overall, we expected reduced perfusion values in left hemisphere (ipsilesional) regions, but not in right hemisphere tissue in participants with aphasia relative to healthy controls. Also, based on prior studies with this clinical population, we expected perilesional perfusion to be reduced compared to the remainder of the left hemisphere and to

TABLE 1: Studies of perfusion in chronic aphasia.

Study	Sample size (n)	Time since stroke	Diagnosis	Treatment protocol	MRI method	Task	Key findings
Love et al., 2002	1	16 years	Anomia, difficulty in reading	—	PASL	Resting state	(i) Hypoperfusion in L angular gyrus, L supramarginal gyrus; neither region infarcted
Peck et al., 2004	3	8–48 months	Nonfluent aphasia	2 with intention treatment; 1 with attention treatment	BOLD TTP	Category member generation	(i) From pre- to posttreatment, average difference across patients in TTP between R auditory cortex and R motor cortex decreased, corresponding to shortened posttreatment response times, and approached the average value for controls
Fridriksson et al., 2006	1	18 months	Aphasia (incl. moderate anomia)	—	PWI/BOLD	Overt picture naming	(i) Delayed TTP in resting state PWI in LH versus RH (ii) Abnormal HRF in activated areas during naming
Bonakdarpour et al., 2007	5	>2 years	Agrammatic aphasia	—	BOLD TTP	Lexical decision	(i) Increased TTP in L perisylvian cortex (3 of 5 individuals) relative to healthy controls (ii) No differences in R perisylvian or L or R occipital cortex
Brumm et al., 2010	3	2–11 years	Expressive aphasia	—	PASL	Resting state	(i) Hypoperfusion in L penumbra (2 voxels); noninfarcted regions of L hemisphere
Thompson et al., 2010	6	6–146 months	Agrammatic aphasia	Treatment of Underlying Forms (TUF)	PASL	Resting state	(i) Regions with upregulated BOLD response (auditory sentence-picture verification task) following treatment showed faster TTP (ii) After treatment, 4 patients decreased TTP in L angular gyrus; 3 decreased TTP in L superior parietal cortex; 4 decreased TTP in R superior parietal cortex
Richardson et al., 2011	17	4–246 months	Aphasia (not specified)	—	PASL	Resting state	(i) Hypoperfusion in L penumbra (8 mm); noninfarcted regions of L hemisphere (ii) Larger lesion correlated with reduced perfusion
Fridriksson et al., 2012	30	6–350 months	13 Broca's; 10 anomic; 3 conduction; 2 Wernicke's; 1 Trans-cortical motor; 1 global	Anomia treatment	PASL	Resting state	(i) Pretreatment perfusion levels in residual language network regions, that is, not infarcted and not perilesional (15 mm), predicted posttreatment improvement in picture naming (ii) Pretreatment perfusion levels in infarcted and perilesional tissue did not predict posttreatment improvement
Bonakdarpour et al., 2015	5	6–96 months	2 Broca's aphasia; 3 anomia	—	BOLD TTP	Overt picture naming	(i) Increased TTP in L hemisphere naming regions relative to healthy controls (ii) No difference in percent signal change

PASL: pulsed arterial spin labeling; PWI: perfusion weighted imaging; TTP: time to peak (of the hemodynamic response function (HRF)); SMA: supplementary motor area.

TABLE 2: Participant information (mean and standard deviation).

Group	Age (years)	Sex	Education (years)	Lesion age (months)	WAB-AQ[1]
Aphasia (n = 35)	57.7 (10.5)	21 M/14 F	15.8 (2.1)	59.3 (53.0)	66.2 (22.7)
Controls (n = 16)	32 (8.5)	8 M/8 F	17.7 (1.7)	—	—

[1] WAB-AQ: Western Aphasia Battery-Aphasia Quotient.

correlate with lesion volume and aphasia severity, but not with lesion age, sex, education, or age.

2. Method

2.1. Participants. We tested 35 participants with aphasia subsequent to a single left hemisphere ischaemic stroke and 16 healthy adult controls (see Table 2). Participants with aphasia, presenting with anomia, dysgraphia, and agrammatism, were recruited from three research sites, Northwestern University (n = 9), Boston University and Massachusetts General Hospital (n = 21), and Johns Hopkins University (n = 5), respectively, as part of a large-scale NIDCD funded Clinical Research Center. Healthy controls were recruited from the greater Chicago area and tested at Northwestern University. The study was approved by the Institutional Review Boards of all three universities and all participants provided informed consent.

All participants were right-handed native English speakers. Participants with aphasia were older (range = 41–79 years; M = 57.7 years) than the healthy controls (range = 24–57 years; M = 32.3 years; two-sample, unequal variance t-test: $t(36)$ = 9.19, p < .0001) and had fewer years of education (M = 15.8 versus M = 17.7 years; two-sample unequal variance t-test: $t(32)$ = 3.33, p = .001). Participants with aphasia passed vision and hearing screenings (pure-tone audiometric screening at 40 dB, 1000 Hz) and had no other diagnosed brain disorders and no history of drug or alcohol abuse. Healthy controls had self-reported normal or corrected-to-normal vision and hearing and no history of speech, language, or learning disorders or substance abuse.

Participants with aphasia were all in the chronic stage and were at least twelve months post-stroke-onset (M: 59.3 months, SD: 53.0, range: 12–209 months). The diagnosis and overall severity of aphasia were based on administration of the Western Aphasia Battery-Revised (WAB-R) [25]; WAB-AQ scores ranged from 11.7 to 95.2 (M: 66.2, SD: 22.7). We also characterized each participant's language abilities using a battery of language tests, which included measures of spoken and written comprehension and production of words and sentences. Single word production and comprehension were tested using 26 items from the Confrontation Naming (CN) and Auditory Comprehension (AC) subtests of the Northwestern Naming Battery (NNB) [38] (10 low frequency nouns from the "Other" category on the NNB and 16 verbs). We used the Psycholinguistic Assessments of Language Processing in Aphasia (PALPA) [39] to evaluate spelling-to-dictation of words with high and low frequency (subtest 40). Finally, the Sentence Production Priming Test (SPPT) and the Sentence Comprehension Test (SCT) from the Northwestern Assessment of Verbs and Sentences (NAVS) [40], which include

30 items each to test canonical and noncanonical structures, were used to evaluate production and comprehension of sentences of different syntactic complexity.

These tests provided the basis for five language domain scores that we used in our data analysis: single word production, single word comprehension, spelling, sentence comprehension, and sentence production. To obtain domain-specific severity scores, the proportion correct score for each domain was converted to a z-score based on the group mean and standard deviation, and the five z-scores were averaged to yield a composite language score for each participant. We correlated these domain and composite scores with z-transformed WAB-AQ scores (see Table 3 for scores by participant), with results showing strong correlations between measures: naming: $r(33)$ = .85, p < .0001; word comprehension: $r(33)$ = .77, p < .0001; spelling: $r(31)$ = .71, p < .0001; sentence comprehension: $r(33)$ = .61, p < .0001; sentence production: $r(33)$ = .79, p < .0001; and composite language score: $r(33)$ = .93, p < .0001. Spelling scores were not available for two participants.

2.2. Data Acquisition. Images were collected on four different 3.0T systems: a Siemens TIM Trio with a 32-channel head coil (Northwestern University), a Siemens Prisma with a 64-channel head/neck coil (Northwestern University), a Skyra with 20-channel head/neck coil (Boston University), and a Philips Intera with a 32-channel head coil (Johns Hopkins). Prior to the study, imaging sequences were equated across sites, using the same parameters in all scanners. Resting CBF maps were collected using a pseudo-continuous arterial spin labeling (pCASL) sequence [41] with two-dimensional gradient echo-planar readout (EPI): field of view (FOV) = 220 mm, in-plane resolution = 3.4 × 3.4 mm^2, 25 slices, thickness = 4 mm with 1 mm gap, and TE/TR = 11 ms/4500 ms. The labeling plane was situated 90 mm below the center of the imaging volume, and labeling pulses were applied for 1.5 s. The postlabeling delay was set to 1900 ms to balance between potential slow flow and adequate signal to noise ratio [42]. Sixty pairs of interleaved control and tag images were acquired for signal averaging. In addition to the ASL scan, high resolution T1-weighted anatomical images were acquired using an MPRAGE sequence [43]: FOV = 256 mm, TE/TR/TI = 2.91 ms/2300 ms/900 ms, 176 sagittal slices, and resolution of 1 mm^3.

2.3. Data Processing. Perfusion-weighted images from the pCASL scan were processed using a pipeline incorporating commands from Statistical Parametric Mapping (SPM8, Wellcome Trust Center for Neuroimaging, London, UK), and code developed in-house with Matlab R2013a (Mathworks,

TABLE 3: WAB Aphasia Quotients (AQ), language domain scores, and composite language scores (as z-scores) for each participant with aphasia.

Participant	WAB-AQ[1]	Composite language	Naming	Spelling	Word comprehension	Sentence comprehension	Sentence production
BU01	.92	.74	1.18	.33	.54	.41	1.23
BU02	−1.81	−1.39	−1.64	−1.20	−2.45	−.56	−1.12
BU03	−.63	−.55	−1.19	−.63	.54	−.56	−.93
BU04	.35	.25	.84	1.38	.29	−.75	−.54
BU06	.02	−.35	.39	−.63	.54	−.94	−1.12
BU07	−.80	−1.07	−.74	−1.12	−.46	−1.91	−1.12
BU09	1.28	1.30	1.07	1.78	.54	1.39	1.72
BU10	.63	.61	.73	.89	.29	1.00	.15
BU11	1.14	1.11	.84	−1.20	.29	1.77	1.53
BU12	−1.15	−.99	−.85	−1.20	−1.20	−.56	−1.12
BU13	1.17	1.42	1.18	1.78	.54	1.77	1.82
BU14	−.08	.16	−.40	.97	.54	−.56	.25
BU15	.92	.11	.84	−1.12	.54	.03	.25
BU17	.36	.02	1.07	−.63	.54	−.56	−.34
BU18	.52	.49	.39	.25	.29	1.39	.15
BU20	−2.34	−1.26	−1.64	−1.04	−1.20	−1.31	−1.12
BU21	−2.40	−1.78	−1.64	−1.20	−4.20	−.73	−1.12
BU22	−.04	.14	−.73	.57	−.46	1.19	.14
BUc01	.85	1.08	1.07	1.46	.54	1.58	.74
BUc04	1.11	1.23	1.18	1.05	.54	1.77	1.62
BUc05	−1.49	−1.00	−1.64	−1.12	−.95	−.17	−1.12
JH06	1.00	.46	−1.08	1.46	.29	1.00	.64
JHc04	−1.02	−.46	−1.07	−.47	.54	−.17	−1.12
JHc05	−.38	−.45	−.17	−1.04	.04	.03	−1.12
JHc06	1.03	.48	.05	.17	.54	−.17	1.82
JHc07	.41	.22	.28	1.05	.29	.03	−.54
NU03	.42	.56	.84	.57	.54	.03	.84
NU04	−.56	−.09	−.74	−.39	.29	−.36	.74
NU05	.35	−.10	.39	−.23	.54	−.94	−.24
NU06	1.00	.46	1.29	−.47	.54	.41	.55
NU08	−.59	−.58	−.51	−1.12	.29	−.56	−1.03
NU13	−.29	−.65	−.63	−1.20	−.71	−1.53	.25
NUc01	.44	.41	1.18	−.07	.54	−.17	.55
NUc02	.22	.05	.84	.81	.54	−1.33	−.63
NUc03	−.56	−.48	−.97	−.87	.04	.03	−.63

[1]WAB-AQ: Western Aphasia Battery-Aphasia Quotient.

Natwick, MA) and implemented on the Northwestern University Neuroimaging Data Archive (NUNDA) [44]. Briefly, the raw EPI images were first aligned to the first image of the time-series to extract 6 motion-related measures for the time-series. The motion parameters and signal from voxels containing 99% CSF were regressed out of the time-series to remove motion-related and physiological fluctuations in the signal [45]. Perfusion-weighted time-series were generated using pairwise subtraction, and outliers were removed based on the following criteria [46]: (a) translation greater than 0.8 mm; (b) rotation greater than 0.8°; (c) global signal or noise greater than 2 times the standard deviation. An average of 7 pairs of images was discarded from each ASL scan based on these criteria. The final perfusion-weighted time-series were then converted into quantitative flow (f) maps in units of mL/100 g/min using the following equation:

$$f = \frac{\lambda \cdot \Delta M}{2\alpha M_0 \cdot T_{1b} \cdot \left(e^{-\text{PLD}/T_{1b}} - e^{-(\tau + \text{PLD})/T_{1b}}\right)}, \quad (1)$$

where λ is the blood/tissue partition coefficient = 0.9 mL/g [47], ΔM is the perfusion-weighted signal, α is the inversion efficiency = 0.85 [41], M_0 is the equilibrium signal of tissue, PLD is the post-labeling delay, τ is the labeling duration, and T_{1b} is the T_1 of blood = 1664 ms [48].

Due to the low resolution of CBF maps, partial volume effects are prominent and need to be corrected before any further analysis. This was implemented as another NUNDA

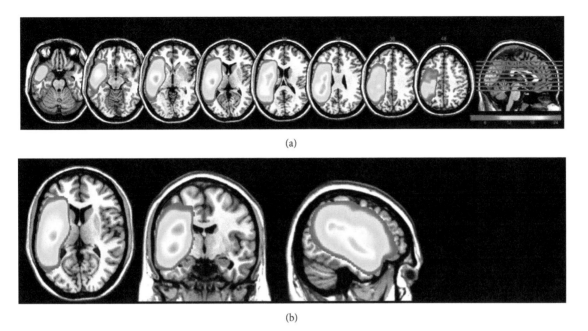

(a)

(b)

FIGURE 1: Lesion overlap map for 35 participants with aphasia, by axial slices (a) and with a three-dimensional view (b), using the neurological convention (left hemisphere is on the left). The color bar indicates the degree of overlap from minimal overlap (violet; N = 2 participants overlapping) to maximum overlap (red; N = 25 participants overlapping). The overlap map was spatially smoothed (3 mm).

pipeline based on the following equation derived from positron emission tomography CBF studies [49]:

$$f_{GM} = \frac{f_{uncorr} - P_{WM} \cdot f_{WM}}{P_{GM}}, \qquad (2)$$

where f_{uncorr} is the uncorrected flow value, P_{GM} and P_{WM} denote gray and white matter probability in the voxel, extracted from tissue segmentation of the high resolution anatomical image, and f_{GM} and f_{WM} are the corresponding tissue-specific flow values. f_{WM} was extracted from voxels containing 99% white matter. To minimize artifactually high CBF due to division by small numbers, the above calculation was limited to voxels containing at least 30% gray matter. The partial volume corrected CBF maps were then spatially normalized to MNI space using the transformation matrix calculated from the high resolution anatomical image.

2.4. Lesion Volume. Lesion volume was derived from lesion maps, developed by manual drawings measured using MRIcron software (http://www.sph.sc.edu/comd/rorden/mri-cron). To delineate the borders of necrotic tissue in each patient, we first determined intensity measures for white and gray matter (WM and GM, resp.) in the contralateral (right) hemisphere for each axial slice. The minimum right hemisphere WM intensity was determined. Left hemisphere lesioned tissue, on each slice, was drawn using the pen tool of MRIcron. Then the minimum WM intensity was applied to the outlined area using the intensity filter function. Additional manual correction was applied using lesion outlines in multiple corresponding coronal and sagittal views. Total lesion volume was calculated by summing the number of lesioned voxels in the left hemisphere for each participant. In

our analyses the size of each voxel was 1 mm^3 and therefore lesion volume is reported in mm^3. Composite axial T1 MR images showing lesion location and overlap for the 35 participants in the study are shown in Figure 1.

2.5. Regions of Interest (ROIs). ROIs were defined based on the Harvard Oxford atlas thresholded at minimum of 25% gray matter, as well as from the Automated Anatomical Labeling (AAL) atlas. The list of ROIs (n = 76, 38 per hemisphere) is given in Table 4. Second, two perilesional ROIs and their right hemisphere homologues were created by dilating the lesion to 6 mm (0–6 mm) and 12 mm (6–12 mm) beyond its boundaries and subtracting the original lesion volume.

Because CBF is a physiological parameter that fluctuates with many factors such as vasoactive agents in food, beverages, and drugs and varies widely between subjects, all CBF values were normalized to the mean CBF of each individual's right occipital lobe ROI, assuming that CBF in this region is not compromised by a left hemisphere stroke resulting in aphasia. Importantly, raw perfusion values in this region did not differ significantly between patients (M = 68.8, SD = 25.5) and controls (M = 77.6, SD = 18.0), based on a one-way ANCOVA adjusting for age ($F(1, 48)$ = 2.55, p = .12).

Mean CBF within each ROI was only computed from voxels with 30% or more gray matter, as these are the only voxels that survived the partial volume correction step detailed above. In addition to correcting for partial volume, the ROIs also accounted for the lesion mask (voxels where the lesion value is set to 1 were excluded) and the field of view of the perfusion scan (an FOV mask was created to exclude all voxels not covered by the perfusion scan). Thus lesions

TABLE 4: (a) Mean raw perfusion values (and standard deviation) for each region of interest (ROI) for patients and healthy controls in the left and right hemisphere. (b) Mean right-occipital-normalized perfusion values (and standard deviation) for each region of interest (ROI) for patients and healthy controls in the left and right hemisphere.

(a)

Region of interest (ROI)	Left hemisphere			Right hemisphere		
	Controls	Patients	% diff	Controls	Patients	% diff
Inferior frontal gyrus, orbital part[1]	74.75 (12.84)	59.98 (23.92)	80%	78.07 (14.77)	71.53 (22.73)	92%
Frontal pole	75.04 (14.11)	68.46 (25.16)	91%	77.08 (16.00)	73.40 (25.03)	95%
Superior frontal gyrus	60.75 (16.51)	67.09 (28.58)	110%	62.66 (17.06)	74.22 (26.20)	118%
Middle frontal gyrus	68.85 (14.09)	62.28 (26.49)	90%	71.39 (16.35)	76.07 (29.97)	107%
IFG, pars triangularis	76.61 (15.53)	58.49 (29.30)	76%	82.37 (20.38)	71.97 (24.18)	87%
IFG, pars opercularis	72.03 (19.32)	50.57 (25.74)	70%	72.87 (19.82)	70.91 (23.61)	97%
Precentral gyrus	62.83 (13.81)	63.10 (22.87)	100%	63.90 (12.72)	77.83 (26.56)	122%
Temporal pole	69.53 (9.78)	51.17 (19.35)	74%	72.23 (10.69)	62.88 (18.99)	87%
Superior temporal Gyrus, anterior	60.67 (19.02)	41.56 (23.52)	69%	62.89 (22.44)	62.60 (23.19)	100%
Superior temporal gyrus, posterior	69.25 (16.40)	45.70 (19.07)	66%	71.41 (17.42)	68.82 (23.58)	96%
Middle temporal gyrus, anterior	65.34 (14.08)	46.73 (25.43)	72%	70.86 (16.02)	61.06 (21.72)	86%
Middle temporal gyrus, posterior	71.00 (14.54)	50.23 (26.53)	71%	73.47 (14.60)	62.30 (24.03)	85%
Inferior temporal gyrus, anterior	53.68 (16.01)	44.55 (26.86)	83%	53.61 (12.95)	45.52 (24.79)	85%
Inferior temporal gyrus, posterior	62.21 (16.40)	48.26 (19.22)	78%	54.44 (10.75)	50.62 (21.34)	93%
Inferior temporal gyrus, temporooccipital part	62.11 (12.94)	47.26 (22.41)	76%	67.39 (16.01)	53.72 (17.41)	80%
Postcentral gyrus	65.27 (14.88)	61.51 (21.92)	94%	65.52 (13.60)	76.04 (23.83)	116%
Superior parietal lobule	64.03 (14.48)	57.39 (22.92)	90%	60.59 (14.89)	69.38 (25.58)	115%
Supramarginal gyrus, anterior	65.10 (16.58)	47.49 (18.24)	73%	63.63 (13.51)	63.00 (21.94)	99%
Supramarginal gyrus, posterior	69.63 (17.40)	48.53 (21.63)	70%	68.57 (12.42)	66.65 (23.02)	97%
Angular gyrus	68.04 (16.70)	46.28 (25.04)	68%	65.94 (11.83)	66.88 (23.02)	101%
Lateral occipital cortex, superior	72.13 (18.07)	60.48 (24.44)	84%	73.05 (14.42)	73.41 (25.21)	100%
Lateral occipital cortex, inferior	77.21 (19.52)	59.67 (36.35)	77%	75.67 (18.08)	70.25 (27.28)	93%
Frontal medial cortex	68.35 (18.82)	57.89 (24.42)	85%	70.51 (18.57)	62.23 (24.21)	88%
Supplementary motor area (SMA)	59.08 (18.25)	62.57 (29.89)	106%	57.70 (16.41)	68.00 (24.91)	118%
Paracingulate gyrus	62.97 (13.94)	55.45 (18.16)	88%	66.20 (15.71)	61.56 (21.89)	93%
Anterior cingulate	61.74 (15.48)	55.41 (18.20)	90%	62.87 (15.38)	59.95 (19.52)	95%
Posterior cingulate	69.11 (16.05)	61.06 (23.29)	88%	70.68 (17.48)	67.99 (23.89)	96%
Precuneus	63.33 (17.26)	57.12 (22.06)	90%	63.91 (18.19)	63.07 (22.55)	99%
Parahippocampal gyrus, posterior	56.73 (24.49)	48.47 (17.98)	85%	56.53 (24.01)	55.70 (19.94)	99%
Temporal fusiform cortex, posterior	46.23 (10.08)	47.19 (18.14)	102%	45.85 (10.27)	46.93 (18.16)	102%
Temporal occipital fusiform cortex	49.67 (15.59)	45.64 (21.72)	92%	49.40 (12.85)	51.23 (21.74)	104%
Occipital fusiform gyrus	61.41 (16.06)	54.07 (29.00)	88%	61.51 (15.54)	58.79 (26.45)	96%
Frontal operculum cortex	60.12 (13.76)	37.58 (25.39)	63%	58.17 (12.15)	58.39 (21.55)	100%
Parietal operculum cortex	63.33 (14.96)	37.37 (16.72)	59%	61.32 (15.02)	59.44 (19.41)	97%
Planum temporale	75.43 (19.61)	50.39 (29.98)	67%	72.83 (19.65)	69.98 (24.90)	96%
Hippocampus	52.66 (10.83)	49.05 (17.47)	93%	54.57 (10.63)	50.49 (18.15)	93%
Cerebellum V	48.40 (19.89)	44.93 (17.66)	93%	50.52 (19.65)	41.83 (17.54)	83%
Cerebellum VI	54.17 (17.05)	47.90 (19.77)	88%	54.07 (15.33)	46.84 (18.76)	87%

(b)

Region of interest (ROI)	Left hemisphere					Right hemisphere				
	Controls	Patients	F	p	% diff	Controls	Patients	F	p	% diff
Inferior frontal gyrus, orbital part[1]	.98 (.15)	.95 (.44)	.40	ns	97%	1.02 (.15)	1.10 (.33)	.85	ns	107%
Frontal pole	.98 (.13)	1.05 (.37)	.21	ns	107%	1.00 (.10)	1.12 (.32)	1.49	ns	112%
Superior frontal gyrus	**.79 (.16)**	**1.03 (.42)**	**4.12**	**.048**	**131%**	**.81 (.16)**	**1.12 (.34)**	**7.91**	**.01**	**138%**
Middle frontal gyrus	.90 (.13)	.95 (.36)	.98	ns	106%	.93 (.14)	1.14 (.34)	3.12	.08	123%
IFG, pars triangularis	1.01 (.20)	.93 (.44)	.00	ns	92%	1.06 (.15)	1.11 (.39)	.93	ns	104%

(b) Continued.

Region of interest (ROI)	Left hemisphere					Right hemisphere				
	Controls	Patients	F	p	% diff	Controls	Patients	F	p	% diff
IFG, pars opercularis	.93 (.16)	.80 (.41)	.16	ns	86%	.94 (.14)	1.08 (.34)	1.89	ns	115%
Precentral gyrus	.82 (.11)	.98 (.37)	1.90	ns	120%	**.83 (.12)**	**1.18 (.33)**	**10.87**	**.002**	**141%**
Temporal pole	**.92 (.17)**	**.78 (.27)**	**5.32**	**.03**	**85%**	.96 (.20)	.97 (.28)	.61	ns	100%
Superior temporal gyrus, anterior	**.78 (.17)**	**.62 (.30)**	**6.74**	**.01**	**80%**	.80 (.19)	.95 (.30)	3.93	.05	118%
Superior temporal gyrus, posterior	**.91 (.17)**	**.71 (.29)**	**8.42**	**.01**	**79%**	.94 (.19)	1.04 (.27)	.84	ns	111%
Middle temporal gyrus, anterior	**.86 (.17)**	**.69 (.28)**	**6.97**	**.01**	**80%**	.93 (.16)	.93 (.28)	.06	ns	100%
Middle temporal gyrus, posterior	**.93 (.15)**	**.75 (.29)**	**7.13**	**.01**	**80%**	.96 (.14)	.93 (.23)	.06	ns	96%
Inferior temporal gyrus, anterior	.71 (.21)	.67 (.36)	.00	ns	94%	.72 (.21)	.67 (.28)	.07	ns	93%
Inferior temporal gyrus, posterior	.81 (.17)	.74 (.29)	.21	ns	91%	.72 (.16)	.77 (.27)	.05	ns	107%
Inferior temporal gyrus, temporooccipital part	.81 (.11)	.71 (.23)	.17	ns	87%	.88 (.13)	.80 (.16)	.00	ns	92%
Postcentral gyrus	.85 (.13)	.97 (.40)	.76	ns	114%	**.86 (.14)**	**1.16 (.34)**	**10.83**	**.002**	**136%**
Superior parietal lobule	.83 (.13)	.89 (.39)	.12	ns	107%	**.78 (.14)**	**1.05 (.35)**	**8.28**	**.01**	**134%**
Supramarginal gyrus, anterior	.84 (.13)	.76 (.34)	.72	ns	90%	.83 (.14)	.95 (.25)	2.61	ns	114%
Supramarginal gyrus, posterior	.90 (.13)	.76 (.33)	3.94	.05	84%	**.90 (.15)**	**1.01 (.26)**	**4.06**	**.049**	**112%**
Angular gyrus	**.88 (.14)**	**.72 (.37)**	**5.29**	**.03**	**81%**	.87 (.13)	1.01 (.28)	1.35	ns	117%
Lateral occipital cortex, superior	.93 (.09)	.93 (.34)	.08	ns	100%	**.95 (.10)**	**1.10 (.26)**	**4.25**	**.045**	**116%**
Lateral occipital cortex, inferior	.99 (.07)	.85 (.30)	3.64	.06	86%	.98 (.07)	1.02 (.14)	.17	ns	105%
Frontal medial cortex	.88 (.18)	.88 (.35)	.05	ns	100%	.91 (.17)	.95 (.31)	.14	ns	104%
Supplementary motor area (SMA)	.77 (.20)	.96 (.44)	2.84	.10	125%	**.75 (.17)**	**1.03 (.34)**	**6.96**	**.01**	**138%**
Paracingulate gyrus	.82 (.13)	.84 (.24)	.97	ns	103%	.86 (.14)	.92 (.23)	1.26	ns	107%
Anterior cingulate	.80 (.12)	.85 (.27)	.61	ns	106%	.82 (.13)	.91 (.25)	2.12	ns	111%
Posterior cingulate	.90 (.13)	.92 (.31)	.03	ns	103%	.91 (.13)	1.02 (.29)	.68	ns	112%
Precuneus	.82 (.12)	.86 (.24)	.38	ns	105%	.82 (.12)	.93 (.20)	1.04	ns	114%
Parahippocampal gyrus, posterior	.73 (.25)	.73 (.21)	.23	ns	100%	.73 (.27)	.84 (.25)	.02	ns	114%
Temporal fusiform cortex, posterior	.60 (.09)	.71 (.20)	1.84	ns	117%	.60 (.09)	.70 (.18)	.01	ns	117%
Temporal occipital fusiform cortex	.64 (.12)	.66 (.20)	.41	ns	104%	.64 (.11)	.74 (.14)	.06	ns	116%
Occipital fusiform gyrus	.79 (.12)	.79 (.28)	.05	ns	99%	.79 (.11)	.85 (.22)	.02	ns	107%
Frontal operculum cortex	.79 (.15)	.60 (.41)	3.91	.05	77%	.76 (.12)	.89 (.26)	3.01	.09	117%
Parietal operculum cortex	**.83 (.16)**	**.61 (.33)**	**6.48**	**.01**	**74%**	.80 (.18)	.91 (.26)	.47	ns	114%
Planum temporale	**.98 (.18)**	**.81 (.53)**	**5.54**	**.02**	**83%**	.95 (.19)	1.06 (.30)	.01	ns	112%
Hippocampus	.70 (.17)	.75 (.27)	.48	ns	106%	.72 (.17)	.76 (.21)	.26	ns	105%
Cerebellum V	.61 (.14)	.66 (.14)	.75	ns	108%	.64 (.15)	.62 (.15)	.36	ns	96%
Cerebellum VI	.69 (.10)	.71 (.18)	.17	ns	103%	.70 (.11)	.70 (.24)	.68	ns	101%

Bold cells: significant group differences ($p < .05$).
[1] Region from Automated Anatomical Labeling (AAL) atlas; all others from Harvard-Oxford Atlas.
% diff: percentage of normal (control participants) perfusion values for people with aphasia by ROI.
Note. Means and standard deviations of normalized perfusion values. F and p values derived from one-way ANCOVA, with age as a covariate.

were excluded from the analysis, as otherwise they might substantially lower the CBF values in the left hemisphere. Indeed, mean CBF across participants in lesioned voxels was substantially lower (M = 17.95, SE = 2.1) than in nonlesioned voxels in the left hemisphere (M = 59.78, SE = 3.1).

2.6. Data Analyses. To test whether perfusion laterality differs broadly between patients and healthy controls, we conducted a 2 (hemisphere: left versus right as a within-subjects factor) × 2 (group: patient versus healthy control as a between-subjects factor) Repeated Measures Analysis of Covariance (RMANCOVA) with age as a covariate. Note that this analysis did not include all voxels from each hemisphere; rather, we included only the data from the 38 regions of interest (ROIs) that were the focus of our investigation. Follow-up tests were one-way ANCOVAs adjusting for age.

The level of statistical significance in all inferential analyses (here and those described below) was $p \leq .05$.

We also tested perfusion values from each of the ROIs (ROI: 76 levels, as a within-subjects factor) with group (patients versus controls) as a between-subjects factor and age as a covariate. Given the large number of ROIs and brain regions included in this analysis, we conducted analogues of protected t-tests to protect against inflated experimentwise Type I error [50]. Simulations have shown that this approach provides adequate Type I error rate protection, while affording better power than other approaches when conducting multiple tests [51]. In the present analysis, this approach consisted of using repeated measures analyses and only testing for group differences within individual regions if there was a significant ROI × group interaction. For the follow-up tests, we used one-way ANCOVA, adjusted for age, comparing patients against controls in each ROI.

2.6.1. Perilesional ROI Analyses. Analyses of perilesional perfusion were also conducted for the patients only, with three RMANOVAs. First, a 2 (perilesional space: 0 to 6 mm versus 6 to 12 mm) × 2 (region: left perilesional versus right homologue) test was performed on data from 35 patients comparing perfusion in the perilesional area of the left hemisphere to a homologous contralateral area in the right hemisphere. A second analysis compared perfusion in perilesional space to that in the remainder of the left hemisphere (i.e., the remainder of the entire hemisphere, not restricted to the 38 ROIs in our other analyses) using a 2 (perilesional space: 0 to 6 mm versus 6 to 12 mm) × 2 (left hemisphere region: perilesional versus the remainder of the left hemisphere) RMANOVA. For the 0–6 mm perilesional space, the remainder of the left hemisphere excluded the lesion and the 0–6 mm space; for the 6–12 mm perilesional space the remainder excluded the lesion and perilesional tissue from 0 to 12 mm. The third analysis examined all three regions across both hemispheres using a 3 (perilesional space: 0–6 mm, 6–12 mm, and 12+ mm) × 2 (left versus right hemisphere) RMANOVA.

2.6.2. Associations between Perfusion and Language and Demographic Variables. First, we computed a difference score for each of the 38 bilateral ROIs as well as perilesional ROIs (i.e., 0–6 mm and 6–12 mm), subtracting left hemisphere perfusion values from right hemisphere perfusion values, such that positive scores indicated lower perfusion in left hemisphere tissue compared to the right. These difference scores then were correlated with composite language scores with partial correlations adjusting for lesion volume. Given that we computed these partial correlations for 38 ROIs, we applied a Holm correction [52] for multiple comparisons. If the partial correlation was significant with the correction applied, we followed up with additional partial correlations between the perfusion difference score and each of the five language domain scores (word production, word comprehension, spelling, sentence comprehension, and sentence production). Finally, we computed partial correlations, adjusting for lesion volume, between mean perfusion values (normalized to the right occipital lobe) for each hemisphere separately

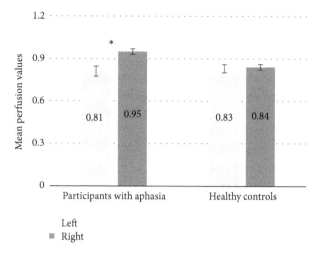

FIGURE 2: Mean right-occipital-normalized perfusion values for participants with aphasia and healthy controls, averaged across the 38 ROIs for the left and right hemispheres. Error bars are standard error. * indicates a significant left versus right difference ($p < .05$).

(excluding the lesion and the 0–6 mm perilesional ROI) with language composite and domain scores and demographic variables (WAB-AQ, age, sex, education, and lesion age), and computed the simple correlation between perfusion and lesion volume itself.

3. Results

The RMANCOVA examining hemisphere by group effects (including age as a covariate) showed a significant group × hemisphere interaction ($F(1, 48) = 11.27$, $p < .01$) (Figure 2). Follow-up RMANOVAs demonstrated no significant difference between the perfusion values (over the 38 ROIs) for the left (M = .83, SD = .08) and right hemispheres (M = .84, SD = .08) in healthy control participants ($F(1, 14) = 1.62$, $p = .22$); however, for the aphasic participants, perfusion values over the 38 ROIs in the right hemisphere (M = .95, SD = .17) were significantly higher than in the left hemisphere (M = .81, SD = .21) ($F(1, 33) = 4.02$, $p = .05$). In addition, one-way ANCOVAs revealed a difference approaching conventional levels of significance with higher perfusion values for the patients compared to the healthy controls in the right ($F(1, 48) = 2.84$, $p < .10$), but not in the left hemisphere ($F(1, 48) = .45$, $p = .51$).

The RMANCOVA examining perfusion differences between participant groups by ROI, with age as a covariate, revealed a significant interaction of group × ROI ($F(75, 3525) = 3.87$, $p < .001$). As mentioned above, we used an analogue of protected t-tests to protect against inflated experimentwise Type I error. That is, for this set of analyses, if the group × ROI interaction had not been significant we would not have tested for group differences in each of the individual ROIs. Given that the interaction was significant, we proceeded by testing for group differences within individual ROIs. As shown in Table 4(b) and Figure 3, the groups differed significantly on 16 of the total 76 ROIs across hemispheres. Age-adjusted perfusion value differences between

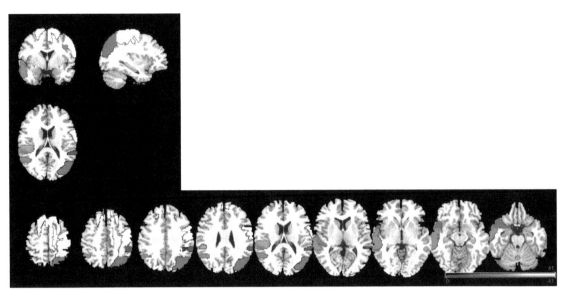

FIGURE 3: ROIs with greater perfusion (hyperperfusion; red-yellow color scale) and lesser perfusion (hypoperfusion; blue-green color scale) in patients relative to control participants, in three-dimensional and axial slice views (left hemisphere is on the left). Only regions that differ significantly across groups (patients versus controls; $p < .05$) are indicated.

the patients and control participants in the left hemisphere were significant in nine ROIs, with lower values for patients in eight of these regions: the anterior and posterior superior and middle temporal gyri, the temporal pole, the angular gyrus, the planum temporale, and the parietal opercular cortex. The superior frontal gyrus showed the opposite pattern with higher values for patients. Age-adjusted perfusion value differences in the right hemisphere were significant in seven ROIs, all in the direction of higher perfusion for the patients: superior frontal gyrus, precentral gyrus, postcentral gyrus, superior parietal lobule, posterior supramarginal gyrus, superior lateral occipital cortex, and supplementary motor area (SMA).

3.1. Perfusion in Perilesional ROIs. The 2 (dilation of perilesional space: 0–6 mm versus 6–12 mm) × 2 (region: left perilesional versus right homologue) RMANOVA revealed a significant dilation × region interaction ($\Gamma(1, 34) = 52.60$, $p < .001$) in the aphasic patient group. For the 0–6 mm dilation there was significantly greater perfusion in the homologous right hemisphere space (M = .99, SD = .23) than the left perilesional hemisphere region (M = .77, SD = .21; $t(34) = 7.64$, $p < .001$). Perfusion was also significantly greater for the 6–12 mm dilation in the homologous right hemisphere space (M = .97, SD = .21) than the left perilesional hemisphere region (M = .92, SD = .23; $t(34) = 2.32$, $p = .027$). The interaction reflects a larger left versus right difference for 0–6 mm than 6–12 mm.

The 2 (dilation of perilesional space: 0–6 mm versus 6–12 mm) × 2 (region: left perilesional versus the rest of the left hemisphere) RMANOVA revealed a significant dilation × region interaction ($F(1, 34) = 53.29$, $p < .001$). Comparisons between the perilesional region and the rest of the left

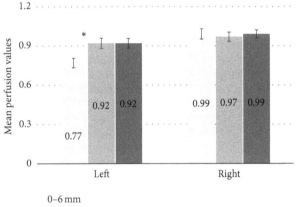

FIGURE 4: Mean right-occipital-normalized perfusion values for participants with aphasia for the left perilesional tissue and the corresponding right homologous regions in the 0–6 mm, 6–12 mm, and remaining (12+ mm) ROIs. Error bars are standard error. ∗ indicates a significant difference ($p < .05$). Significance is not indicated for left versus right differences (all ROIs are significant between hemispheres).

hemisphere (M = .94, SD = .22) was significant for the 0–6 mm ROI (M = .77, SD = .21) ($t(34) = 5.62$, $p < .001$), but not for the 6–12 mm perilesional region (M = .92, SD = .22) ($t(34) = .34$, ns). Perfusion also was significantly lower in the 0–6 mm ROI than in the 6–12 mm ROI ($t(34) = 7.57$, $p < .0001$).

Finally, we conducted an overall 3 (dilation: 0–6 mm, 6–12 mm, rest of hemisphere) × 2 (hemisphere: left versus right) RMANOVA (Figure 4). The interaction between dilation and hemisphere was significant ($F(2, 68) = 34.8$, $p < .0001$). Follow-up t-tests are consistent with the previous analyses, with perfusion in the left hemisphere lower than in the right hemisphere at each dilation (all $ps < .05$). In addition, within the left hemisphere, perfusion in the 0–6 mm region was lower than in the 6–12 mm region ($p < .05$), and perfusion was no different for the 6–12 mm region than the remaining left hemisphere tissue. No within-hemisphere contrasts reached significance in the right hemisphere.

3.2. Relationship between Perfusion, Language Performance, and Patient Variables. Correlational analyses for each ROI difference score (i.e., right minus left hemisphere perfusion values) and composite language scores, adjusting for lesion volume, showed significant negative correlations (i.e., greater difference scores and poorer language performance) in 6 ROIs: anterior inferior temporal gyrus ($r = -.354$, $p = .04$), postcentral gyrus ($r = -.360$, $p = .037$), supplementary motor area (SMA; $r = -.419$, $p = .014$), paracingulate gyrus ($r = -.353$, $p = .04$), anterior cingulate gyrus ($r = -.344$, $p = .046$), and posterior cingulate gyrus ($r = -.360$, $p = .037$). However, no correlation remained significant when the correction for multiple comparisons was applied. Accordingly, we did not follow up on these analyses with correlations between the perfusion difference scores and the five language domain scores.

With respect to the perilesional regions of interest, correlations between the composite language score and perilesional difference scores (i.e., right homologous perilesional ROI minus left perilesional ROI values), with lesion volume included as a covariate, revealed a significant negative correlation for 0–6 mm ($r = -.469$, $p = .007$), but not for 6–12 mm ($r = -.288$, $p = .11$). Thus, we calculated partial correlations with the five language domain scores separately only for the 0–6 mm perilesional ROI, adjusting for lesion volume. Results revealed significant negative associations between perfusion difference scores for the 0–6 mm ROI and single word production ($r = -.354$, $p = .032$), sentence comprehension ($r = -.427$, $p = .015$), and sentence production ($r = -.451$, $p = .01$). No other partial correlations reached significance (all $rs \leq |.30|$, all $ps \geq .097$). These effects are summarized in Table 5.

Finally, partial correlations (adjusting for lesion volume) between average perfusion values in nonperilesional tissue across each hemisphere (in the left, excluding the infarcted region and the 0–6 mm perilesional region; in the right, also excluding regions homologous to the lesion and the 0–6 mm perilesional ROI) and composite language scores for the patient group were not significant for the left hemisphere ($r = .14$, $p = .45$) or the right hemisphere homologous region ($r = .004$, $p = .98$). Likewise, correlations between average perfusion and demographic variables including age, sex, education, and lesion age (in months) revealed no significant correlations or partial correlations (correcting for lesion volume) for either hemisphere (all $rs \leq |.26|$, all $ps \geq .12$). However, a significant negative correlation between perfusion and lesion volume was found for the left ($r = -.37$, $p = .027$) but not the right hemisphere ($r = -.27$, $p = .112$).

4. Discussion

This paper examined perfusion values, normalized to the right occipital lobe, in people with chronic stroke-induced aphasia compared to cognitively healthy, right-handed, non-brain-damaged control participants. We focused our investigation on 38 regions of interest in each hemisphere. Results showed that whereas healthy controls evince no significant between-hemisphere differences in normalized perfusion values, averaged across our ROIs, the aphasic participants' values differ significantly between the left and right hemisphere. However, rather than showing left (ipsilesional) hemisphere hypoperfusion, as predicted, the patients showed normalized perfusion values similar to healthy controls in the left hemisphere, with no significant difference found between the two participant groups. Conversely, the aphasic group showed hyperperfusion in the right (contralesional) hemisphere, with overall perfusion values significantly greater compared to controls. Furthermore, for the aphasic group, right hemisphere perfusion was significantly higher than left hemisphere perfusion. These findings are broadly consistent with those reported by Richardson et al. [11], who found lower perfusion values in the left compared to the right hemisphere in participants with aphasia. However, patient perfusion values were not compared to a healthy control group, precluding the finding that between-hemisphere differences may have resulted from greater than normal right hemisphere perfusion in their patient group rather than lesser than normal left hemisphere perfusion.

Notably, not all regions in the left hemisphere were normally perfused in the patient group, and not all regions in the right hemisphere were hyperperfused. Within the left hemisphere, 8 regions showed a pattern of significant hypoperfusion, and one region showed increased perfusion. The remaining 29 regions did not differ between patients and controls. The lack of an overall effect of left hemisphere hypoperfusion likely reflects this variability, such that focal hypoperfusion was averaged out across the full set of 38 ROIs. In the right hemisphere, perfusion was significantly higher in the patient group compared to healthy controls in 7 regions, but no right hemisphere regions were hypoperfused. The remaining 31 regions did not differ significantly between patients and controls.

Note that this pattern of variable hypo- and hyperperfusion does not appear to be a consequence of our decision to normalize the raw perfusion values to the right occipital lobe. First, the raw perfusion values for the participants with aphasia and the healthy controls did not differ significantly in this region, suggesting that normalization did not introduce a systematic bias across groups.

One interpretation of the unexpected finding of hyperperfused regions in the right hemisphere is that autoregulation of blood flow is adaptive to vascular lesion, with upregulation in undamaged regions. Blood typically directed automatically, for example, to the left hemisphere middle cerebral artery (MCA), is shifted elsewhere, potentially to the left anterior cerebral artery (ACA) or the right MCA. If this were the case, however, we might expect all tissue supplied by these vessels to show equally greater perfusion, and perfusion

TABLE 5: Partial correlations, controlling for lesion volume, between perilesional perfusion and language ability for 35 participants with aphasia.

Difference Right-Left	Partial correlations controlling for lesion volume											
	Composite language		Naming		Spelling		Word comprehen-sion		Sentence comprehen-sion		Sentence production	
	r	p	r	p	r	p	r	p	r	p	r	p
0–6 mm	−.469*	.007	−.354*	.032	−.271	.13	−.299	.097	−.427*	.015	−.451*	.01
6–12 mm	−.288	.11	na		na		na		na		na	

Note. Difference scores were created by subtracting average perfusion in the perilesional area (left hemisphere) from the average perfusion in the analogous right hemisphere area. *p < .05.

in these regions would putatively be higher than that in regions supplied by other sources (e.g., the posterior cerebral artery (PCA)).

Although we did not examine every region supplied by these blood vessels, there may nonetheless be a pattern along these lines. In the left hemisphere, all of the regions found to be significantly hypoperfused are supplied by the MCA: the anterior and posterior superior and middle temporal gyri, temporal pole, angular gyrus, planum temporale, and parietal opercular cortex, whereas one left hemisphere region found to be hyperperfused is supplied by the ACA: the superior frontal gyrus. Regions supplied by the PCA were not abnormally perfused in either hemisphere. Furthermore, there were no hypoperfused regions supplied by the ACA and no hyperperfused regions supplied by the MCA or PCA. Thus, the overall pattern in the left hemisphere seems to be that, among the regions we examined, the regions supplied by the MCA are hypoperfused (or normal) and those supplied by the ACA are hyperperfused or normal, but regions supplied by the PCA show normal perfusion levels.

In the right hemisphere, regions either were normally perfused or showed perfusion levels significantly greater than that of the healthy controls. Of the (significantly) hyperfused regions, one is supplied by the MCA (the posterior supra-marginal gyrus), three are supplied by the ACA (superior frontal gyrus, superior parietal lobule, and supplementary motor area), two are supplied by both the ACA and MCA (precentral and postcentral gyri, which are supplied by the ACA medially and the MCA laterally; our perfusion measures did not distinguish medial versus lateral aspects of these regions), and one is supplied by the PCA (superior lateral occipital cortex). The pattern in the right hemisphere thus appears complementary to the pattern in the left; that is, regions supplied by the MCA are hyperperfused (or normal). Similarly, as in the left hemisphere, hyperperfused regions are supplied by the ACA and regions supplied by the PCA are largely normal.

This appears to be consistent with a compensatory change leading to increased perfusion in regions supplied by the right MCA and bilateral ACA in response to reduced perfusion in regions supplied by the left MCA and may reflect right hemisphere vascular reserve engaged to absorb and distribute additional blood flow. However, this is not clear-cut in that hypoperfused regions in the left were not hyperperfused in the right hemisphere (except for the anterior superior

temporal gyrus, which was significantly hypoperfused in the left hemisphere with hyperperfusion that approached significance in the right).

The functional significance of hyperperfusion in regions within the right hemisphere is also not completely clear. One interpretation is that this reflects maladaptive language processing, although correlations between perfusion difference scores (right-left hemisphere) and language performance (i.e., greater right hemisphere perfusion and poorer language ability) were not significant when corrected for multiple comparisons. Thus, it is unlikely that right hemisphere hyperperfusion alone reflects inefficient language function. Another more likely interpretation is that, because increased perfusion reflects increases in neuronal energy usage, perfusion value increases in our patients may be associated with generally increased cognitive effort. By virtue of a left hemisphere lesion, right hemisphere regions become more actively engaged. This interpretation is also supported by our observed bilateral hyperperfusion in the SMA (though the increased perfusion only approached significance in the left hemisphere). The SMA is one of several domain-general cognitive regions associated with the multiple-demand system in healthy people, which is engaged for language and other cognitive tasks when domain-specific resources are disrupted or unavailable [53, 54]. Notably, the pattern of hyperperfused regions is also in line with the Scaffolding Theory of Cognitive Aging (STAC) [55], which suggests that bilateral frontal regions (i.e., superior frontal and SMA) are engaged as a function of aging to compensate for neurocognitive decline and may also be available when brain damage compromises cognitive ability. Our results encourage further investigation in this direction.

When the brain is divided into regions based on rings of perilesional tissue, the results are less unexpected. Our findings showed that, on average, for perilesional areas, patients had significantly lower perfusion values in the left hemisphere than in homologous regions in the right hemisphere. However, within the left hemisphere, perfusion values became more normal in our participants with increasing distance from the lesion. Thus, even in chronic stages of aphasia a perilesional ring close to the lesion remains substantially hypoperfused. Importantly, relative perfusion values in the 0–6 mm (but not 6–12 mm) perilesional region correlated with language severity, even when accounting for lesion volume. The lesion-adjacent region may therefore not only have a greater reduction in cerebral blood flow, but the extent of reduced blood flow in this region is also predictive of language impairment. For our participant group, perilesional perfusion (0–6 mm only) was significantly correlated with naming, sentence comprehension, and sentence production. We note, however, that this latter finding may reflect the language impairment patterns of our aphasic participants in that the majority of our participants were selected for naming impairments ($n = 21$ from Boston University), with 11 selected for impaired sentence production and comprehension (from Northwestern) and 5 selected for dysgraphia (from Johns Hopkins).

We note, however, that while our results speak to the importance of lesion-adjacent perilesional tissue for impaired language, we did not attempt to determine a precise boundary within which tissue may be underperforming, and beyond which tissue may be functioning normally. There is unfortunately no standard operational definition of what constitutes "perilesional" tissue [20]. Some previous studies have identified hypoperfused tissue in a 3–8 mm ring around the lesion [11], whereas others have reported reduced perfusion as far away as 15 mm from the lesion [20]. The problem here is twofold: an objectively determined anatomical method for determining hypoperfused tissue has not been identified, and any such method needs to account not only for fine-grained differences across brain regions (e.g., at the voxel level), but also for the possibility that perilesional rings may not adequately capture the functional impact of vascular lesions. Depending on the volume and location of the lesion, tissue surrounding it may include both normally perfused and hypoperfused tissue, such that averaging perfusion within the entire ring may lead to spurious results. It is possible, for example, that ribbons of hypoperfused tissue, extending distally from the lesion and including both perilesional and other cortical tissue, may better capture the cognitive effects of brain damage. In addition, lesion-adjacent rings may often include neural tissue that was involved in language processing prior to stroke as well as tissue that was not, thus, precluding determination of a clear relation between perfusion and language impairment. Further research is needed to identify the functional significance of reduced perfusion at various distances from the lesion, in particular regions within lesion-adjacent tissue, and in pathways following the vasculature.

Finally, we note that the only nonlanguage measure that correlated with perfusion in the remaining (undamaged and nonperilesional) portion of the left hemisphere was lesion volume. However, no correlation between lesion volume and perfusion in the right hemisphere region was found. Likewise, no correlations were found between perfusion (in either hemisphere) and lesion age (months after onset of stroke), chronological age, education, or sex. These results are consistent with prior findings in the literature and suggest that perfusion levels reach a stable steady state in individuals with chronic stage aphasia and are also not associated with general demographic variables.

While our results showed patterns of both hypoperfusion and hyperperfusion in chronic aphasia and link some of these perfusion changes to impaired language, questions remain. We did not address what this means for recovery of language in chronic stages of aphasia. With respect to hypoperfusion, the point at which reduced cerebral blood flow results in functional deficiencies or is indicative of a nonreversible state is unknown. Although animal models suggest that perfusion levels below 30% of normal constitute hibernating, nonfunctional tissue, we found correlations between perfusion and language impairment in the 0–6 mm perilesional ROI, where the mean normalized perfusion value was just below 80%. Correspondingly, we also do not know if hyperperfusion reflects language inefficiency, or what levels of perfusion impair (or improve) cognitive function. The regions with the greatest levels of right hemisphere perfusion were not consistently or significantly associated with language disability, and none of the right-occipital-normalized values within the ROIs we examined were more than 40% above those of the normal control participants. The time course by which certain regions of the brain become hyperperfused also is not known. It is possible that heightened perfusion levels in contralesional regions are an immediate consequence of stroke, though it could also be the case that such changes develop slowly over time, possibly reflecting attempts to compensate for left hemisphere brain damage.

5. Conclusions

In summary, we report two key findings regarding perfusion in chronic aphasia. First, we found a varied pattern of hypoperfused and hyperperfused regions across both the left and right hemispheres of the brain. These patterns suggest that autoregulatory shifts in blood flow in response to lesions within the distribution of the left middle cerebral artery may be associated with the abnormal perfusion patterns we observed; however this possibility requires further investigation. Notably, our findings do not strongly support the idea that perfusion changes (in particular right hemisphere hyperperfusion) reflect maladaptive language processing. Rather, we suggest that regions of increased perfusion reflect changes in domain-general cognitive effort. Secondly, we found that perilesional tissue within 6 mm of the lesion is particularly hypoperfused compared to regions more distal to the lesion. Importantly, the degree of hypoperfusion in this perilesional region correlates with performance on standard measures of language ability, when adjusting for lesion volume, with reduced perfusion corresponding to more impaired language. Critically, however, we suggest that perilesional rings may only crudely capture the effects of vascular lesions on perfusion due to heterogeneity of lesion location and volume as well as variability in the properties of lesion-adjacent tissue. Finally, the present results underscore the need to consider chronically altered cerebral blood flow as a contributing factor to the persistent language deficits in chronic aphasia, which might also serve as an additional avenue for targeted recovery of language function.

Competing Interests

The authors declare that they have no competing interests.

Acknowledgments

This work was supported by the NIH-NIDCD, Clinical Research Center Grant, P50DC012283 (PI: C. K. Thompson). The authors wish to thank Xue Wang, Elena Barbieri, Sladjana Lukic, and Brianne Dougherty for assistance with data collection and analysis.

References

[1] R. Mielke and B. Szelies, "Neuronal plasticity in post-stroke aphasia: insights by quantitative electroencephalography," *Expert Review of Neurotherapeutics*, vol. 3, no. 3, pp. 373–380, 2003.

[2] S. C. Cramer, "Repairing the human brain after stroke: I. Mechanisms of spontaneous recovery," *Annals of Neurology*, vol. 63, no. 3, pp. 272–287, 2008.

[3] C. K. Thompson and D.-B. D. Ouden, "Neuroimaging and recovery of language in aphasia," *Current Neurology and Neuroscience Reports*, vol. 8, no. 6, pp. 475–483, 2008.

[4] S. Kiran, "What is the nature of poststroke language recovery and reorganization?" *ISRN Neurology*, vol. 2012, Article ID 786872, 13 pages, 2012.

[5] R. B. Buxton, K. Uludag, D. J. Dubowitz, and T. T. Liu, "Modeling the hemodynamic response to brain activation," *NeuroImage*, vol. 23, no. 1, pp. S220–S233, 2004.

[6] O. W. Witte and G. Stoll, "Delayed and remote effects of focal cortical infarctions: secondary damage and reactive plasticity," *Advances in neurology*, vol. 73, pp. 207–227, 1997.

[7] A. B. Singhal, E. H. Lo, T. Dalkara, and M. A. Moskowitz, "Advances in stroke neuroprotection: hyperoxia and beyond," *Neuroimaging Clinics of North America*, vol. 15, no. 3, pp. 697–720, 2005.

[8] T. Schormann and M. Kraemer, "Voxel-guided morphometry ("VGM") and application to stroke," *IEEE Transactions on Medical Imaging*, vol. 22, no. 1, pp. 62–74, 2003.

[9] R. H. Hamilton, E. G. Chrysikou, and B. Coslett, "Mechanisms of aphasia recovery after stroke and the role of noninvasive brain stimulation," *Brain and Language*, vol. 118, no. 1-2, pp. 40–50, 2011.

[10] D. Saur, R. Lange, A. Baumgaertner et al., "Dynamics of language reorganization after stroke," *Brain: A Journal of Neurology*, vol. 129, no. 6, pp. 1371–1384, 2006.

[11] J. D. Richardson, J. M. Baker, P. S. Morgan, C. Rorden, L. Bonilha, and J. Fridriksson, "Cerebral perfusion in chronic stroke: implications for lesion-symptom mapping and functional MRI," *Behavioural Neurology*, vol. 24, no. 2, pp. 117–122, 2011.

[12] K. P. Brumm, J. E. Perthen, T. T. Liu, F. Haist, L. Ayalon, and T. Love, "An arterial spin labeling investigation of cerebral blood flow deficits in chronic stroke survivors," *NeuroImage*, vol. 51, no. 3, pp. 995–1005, 2010.

[13] J. Astrup, L. Symon, N. M. Branston, and N. A. Lassen, "Cortical evoked potential and extracellular K$^+$ and H$^+$ at critical levels of brain ischemia," *Stroke*, vol. 8, no. 1, pp. 51–57, 1977.

[14] W. J. Powers, G. A. Press, R. L. Grubb Jr., M. Gado, and M. E. Raichle, "The effect of hemodynamically significant carotid artery disease on the hemodynamic status of the cerebral circulation," *Annals of Internal Medicine*, vol. 106, no. 1, pp. 27–35, 1987.

[15] T. Love, D. Swinney, E. Wong, and R. Buxton, "Perfusion imaging and stroke: a more sensitive measure of the brain bases of cognitive deficits," *Aphasiology*, vol. 16, no. 9, pp. 873–883, 2002.

[16] A. E. Hillis, "Magnetic resonance perfusion imaging in the study of language," *Brain and Language*, vol. 102, no. 2, pp. 165–175, 2007.

[17] C. Rorden and H.-O. Karnath, "Using human brain lesions to infer function: a relic from a past era in the fMRI age?" *Nature Reviews Neuroscience*, vol. 5, no. 10, pp. 812–819, 2004.

[18] K. K. Peck, A. B. Moore, B. A. Crosson et al., "Functional magnetic resonance imaging before and after aphasia therapy: shifts in hemodynamic time to peak during an overt language task," *Stroke*, vol. 35, no. 2, pp. 554–559, 2004.

[19] C. K. Thompson, D.-B. den Ouden, B. Bonakdarpour, K. Garibaldi, and T. B. Parrish, "Neural plasticity and treatment-induced recovery of sentence processing in agrammatism," *Neuropsychologia*, vol. 48, no. 11, pp. 3211–3227, 2010.

[20] J. Fridriksson, J. D. Richardson, P. Fillmore, and B. Cai, "Left hemisphere plasticity and aphasia recovery," *NeuroImage*, vol. 60, no. 2, pp. 854–863, 2012.

[21] M. Vergara-Martínez, M. Perea, P. Gómez, and T. Y. Swaab, "ERP correlates of letter identity and letter position are modulated by lexical frequency," *Brain and Language*, vol. 125, no. 1, pp. 11–27, 2013.

[22] M. Veldsman, T. Cumming, and A. Brodtmann, "Beyond BOLD: optimizing functional imaging in stroke populations," *Human Brain Mapping*, vol. 36, no. 4, pp. 1620–1636, 2015.

[23] B. Bonakdarpour, T. B. Parrish, and C. K. Thompson, "Hemodynamic response function in patients with stroke-induced aphasia: implications for fMRI data analysis," *NeuroImage*, vol. 36, no. 2, pp. 322–331, 2007.

[24] B. Bonakdarpour, P. M. Beeson, A. T. Demarco, and S. Z. Rapcsak, "Variability in blood oxygen level dependent (BOLD) signal in patients with stroke-induced and primary progressive aphasia," *NeuroImage: Clinical*, vol. 8, article no. 471, pp. 88–94, 2015.

[25] A. Kertesz, *Western Aphasia Battery-Revised (WAB-R)*, Pearson, San Antonio, Tex, USA, 2006.

[26] C. E. Brown, P. Li, J. D. Boyd, K. R. Delaney, and T. H. Murphy, "Extensive turnover of dendritic spines and vascular remodeling in cortical tissues recovering from stroke," *Journal of Neuroscience*, vol. 27, no. 15, pp. 4101–4109, 2007.

[27] T.-N. Lin, S.-W. Sun, W.-M. Cheung, F. Li, and C. Chang, "Dynamic changes in cerebral blood flow and angiogenesis after transient focal cerebral ischemia in rats: evaluation with serial magnetic resonance imaging," *Stroke*, vol. 33, no. 12, pp. 2985–2991, 2002.

[28] E. V. Shanina, T. Schallert, O. W. Witte, and C. Redecker, "Behavioral recovery from unilateral photothrombotic infarcts of the forelimb sensorimotor cortex in rats: role of the contralateral cortex," *Neuroscience*, vol. 139, no. 4, pp. 1495–1506, 2006.

[29] L. Wei, J. P. Erinjeri, C. M. Rovainen, and T. A. Woolsey, "Collateral growth and angiogenesis around cortical stroke," *Stroke*, vol. 32, no. 9, pp. 2179–2184, 2001.

[30] C. L. R. Gonzalez and B. Kolb, "A comparison of different models of stroke on behaviour and brain morphology," *European Journal of Neuroscience*, vol. 18, no. 7, pp. 1950–1962, 2003.

[31] S. T. Carmichael, K. Tatsukawa, D. Katsman, N. Tsuyuguchi, and H. I. Kornblum, "Evolution of diaschisis in a focal stroke model," *Stroke*, vol. 35, no. 3, pp. 758–763, 2004.

[32] R. P. Stroemer, T. A. Kent, and C. E. Hulsebosch, "Neocortical neural sprouting, synaptogenesis, and behavioral recovery after neocortical infarction in rats," *Stroke*, vol. 26, no. 11, pp. 2135–2144, 1995.

[33] S. T. Carmichael, "Plasticity of cortical projections after stroke," *Neuroscientist*, vol. 9, no. 1, pp. 64–75, 2003.

[34] F. Chollet, V. Dipiero, R. J. S. Wise, D. J. Brooks, R. J. Dolan, and R. S. J. Frackowiak, "The functional anatomy of motor recovery after stroke in humans: A Study with Positron Emission Tomography," *Annals of Neurology*, vol. 29, no. 1, pp. 63–71, 1991.

[35] A. E. Hillis, "Brain/language relationships identified with diffusion and perfusion MRI: clinical applications in neurology and neurosurgery," *Annals of the New York Academy of Sciences*, vol. 1064, pp. 149–161, 2005.

[36] R. G. Lee and P. V. Donkelaar, "Mechanisms underlying functional recovery following stroke," *Canadian Journal of Neurological Sciences*, vol. 22, no. 4, pp. 257–263, 1995.

[37] R. J. Nudo, "Recovery after damage to motor cortical areas," *Current Opinion in Neurobiology*, vol. 9, no. 6, pp. 740–747, 1999.

[38] C. K. Thompson and S. Weintraub, *Northwestern Naming Battery*, Northwestern University, Evanston, Ill, USA, 2014.

[39] J. Kay, R. Lesser, and M. Coltheart, "Psycholinguistic assessments of language processing in aphasia (PALPA): an introduction," *Aphasiology*, vol. 10, no. 2, pp. 159–180, 1996.

[40] C. K. Thompson, *Northwestern Assessment of Verbs and Sentences*, Northwestern University, Evanston, Ill, USA, 2011.

[41] W. Dai, D. Garcia, C. De Bazelaire, and D. C. Alsop, "Continuous flow-driven inversion for arterial spin labeling using pulsed radio frequency and gradient fields," *Magnetic Resonance in Medicine*, vol. 60, no. 6, pp. 1488–1497, 2008.

[42] D. C. Alsop, J. A. Detre, X. Golay et al., "Recommended implementation of arterial spin-labeled perfusion MRI for clinical applications: a consensus of the ISMRM Perfusion Study group and the European consortium for ASL in dementia," *Magnetic Resonance in Medicine*, vol. 73, no. 1, pp. 102–116, 2015.

[43] J. P. Mugler and J. R. Brookeman, "Three–dimensional magnetization–prepared rapid gradient–echo imaging (3D MP RAGE)," *Magnetic Resonance in Medicine*, vol. 15, no. 1, pp. 152–157, 1990.

[44] K. Alpert, A. Kogan, T. Parrish, D. Marcus, and L. Wang, "The northwestern university neuroimaging data archive (NUNDA)," *NeuroImage*, vol. 124, pp. 1131–1136, 2016.

[45] Z. Wang, "Improving cerebral blood flow quantification for arterial spin labeled perfusion MRI by removing residual motion artifacts and global signal fluctuations," *Magnetic Resonance Imaging*, vol. 30, no. 10, pp. 1409–1415, 2012.

[46] Z. Wang, G. K. Aguirre, H. Rao et al., "Empirical optimization of ASL data analysis using an ASL data processing toolbox: ASLtbx," *Magnetic Resonance Imaging*, vol. 26, no. 2, pp. 261–269, 2008.

[47] P. Herscovitch and M. E. Raichle, "What is the correct value for the brain—blood partition coefficient for water?" *Journal of Cerebral Blood Flow and Metabolism*, vol. 5, no. 1, pp. 65–69, 1985.

[48] H. Lu, C. Clingman, X. Golay, and P. C. M. Van Zijl, "Determining the longitudinal relaxation time (T1) of blood at 3.0 tesla," *Magnetic Resonance in Medicine*, vol. 52, no. 3, pp. 679–682, 2004.

[49] A. T. Du, G. H. Jahng, S. Hayasaka et al., "Hypoperfusion in frontotemporal dementia and Alzheimer disease by arterial spin labeling MRI," *Neurology*, vol. 67, no. 7, pp. 1215–1220, 2006.

[50] J. Cohen, P. Cohen, S. G. West, and L. S. Aiken, *Applied Multiple Regression/Correlation Analysis for the Behavioral Sciences*, Lawrence Erlbaum Associates, Mahwah, NJ, USA, 3rd edition, 2003.

[51] S. G. Carmer and M. R. Swanson, "An evaluation of ten pairwise multiple comparison procedures by Monte Carlo methods," *Journal of the American Statistical Association*, vol. 68, no. 341, pp. 66–74, 1973.

[52] S. Holm, "A simple sequentially rejective multiple test procedure," *Scandinavian Journal of Statistics*, vol. 6, no. 2, pp. 65–70, 1979.

[53] F. Geranmayeh, S. L. E. Brownsett, and R. J. S. Wise, "Task-induced brain activity in aphasic stroke patients: what is driving recovery?" *Brain: A Journal of Neurology*, vol. 137, no. 10, pp. 2632–2648, 2014.

[54] A. Hampshire, B. L. Parkin, R. Cusack et al., "Assessing residual reasoning ability in overtly non-communicative patients using fMRI," *NeuroImage: Clinical*, vol. 2, no. 1, pp. 174–183, 2013.

[55] D. C. Park and P. Reuter-Lorenz, "The adaptive brain: aging and neurocognitive scaffolding," *Annual Review of Psychology*, vol. 60, pp. 173–196, 2009.

14

Nao-Xue-Shu Oral Liquid Improves Aphasia of Mixed Stroke

Yuping Yan,[1] Mingzhe Wang,[2] Liang Zhang,[3] Zhenwei Qiu,[4] Wenfei Jiang,[2] Men Xu,[2] Weidong Pan,[2] and Xiangjun Chen[5]

[1]Shanghai Business School, Room 612, Administrative Building, No. 123, Fengpu Avenue, Fengxian District, Shanghai 201400, China
[2]Department of Neurology, Shuguang Hospital Affiliated to Shanghai University of TCM, No. 528, Zhang-Heng Road, Pu-Dong New Area, Shanghai 201203, China
[3]Department of Neurology, Shanghai Seventh Hospital, Shanghai University of Traditional Chinese Medicine, Shanghai 200137, China
[4]Department of Emergency, Shuguang Hospital Affiliated to Shanghai University of TCM, No. 528, Zhang-Heng Road, Pu-Dong New Area, Shanghai 201203, China
[5]Department of Neurology, Hua Shan Hospital Affiliated to Fu Dan University, No. 12, Wu Lu Mu Qi Zhong Road, Shanghai 200040, China

Correspondence should be addressed to Weidong Pan; panwd@medmail.com.cn and Xiangjun Chen; xiangjunchen@hotmail.com

Academic Editor: Zhang Tan

Objective. The objective is to observe whether the traditional Chinese medicine (TCM) *Nao-Xue-Shu* oral liquid improves aphasia of mixed stroke. *Methods.* A total of 102 patients with aphasia of mixed stroke were divided into two groups by a single blind random method. The patients treated by standard Western medicine plus *Nao-Xue-Shu* oral liquid ($n = 58$) were assigned to the treatment group while the remaining patients treated only by standard Western medicine ($n = 58$) constituted the control group. Changes in the Western Aphasia Battery (WAB), Modified Rankin Scale (mRS), National Institutes of Health Stroke Scale (NIHSS), and hemorheology parameters were assessed to evaluate the effects of the treatments. *Results.* Excluding the patients who dropped out, 54 patients in the treatment group and 51 patients in the control group were used to evaluate the effects. Significant and persistent improvements in the WAB score, specifically comprehension, repetition, naming, and calculating, were found in the treatment group when the effects were evaluated at the end of week 2 and week 4, respectively, compared with baseline. The naming and writing scores were also improved at the end of week 4 in this group. The comprehension and reading scores were improved at the end of week 4 in the control group compared with the baseline, but the improvements were smaller than those in the treatment group. The percentages of patients at the 0-1 range of mRS were increased at the end of week 2 and week 4 in both groups, but the improvements in the treatment group were much larger than those in the control group. Greater improvements in the NIHSS scores and the hemorheology parameters in the treatment group were also observed compared with the control group at the end of week 2 and week 4. *Conclusion.* Nao-Xue-Shu oral liquid formulation improved aphasia in mixed stroke patients and thus might be a potentially effective drug for treating stroke aphasia.

1. Introduction

Mixed stroke, also known as hemorrhagic infarction or infarction with hemorrhage, presents as a cerebral infarction combined with intracerebral hemorrhage on computed tomography (CT) brain scans [1, 2]. Current clinical cases of mixed stroke are caused by middle cerebral artery territory and lead to massive temporal infarction with hemorrhage.

Mixed stroke patients with brain infarction and hemorrhage have mutual promoting and mutual transforming characteristics that often appear as epilepsy, dementia, aphasia, and other kinds of advanced neural function damage. Also, there is a higher proportion of patients with mixed apoplexy aphasia, including aphasia and dysarthria, or both kinds of symptoms coexisting in patients that result in communication difficulties, and loss of the ability to communicate socially has a serious impact on the patient's quality of life [3]. Western medicine treatment that consists of decreasing intracranial pressure and adjusting blood pressure and blood density and hemostatic measures can produce contradictory effects and, in other words, may lead to the development of ischemia and at the same time increase bleeding, and vice versa, causing contradiction to treat it [4]. In the theory of traditional Chinese medicine (TCM), one of the integrative medicines [5] has shown that *Nao-Xue-Shu* oral liquid may raise *Qi* and remove blood stasis, clear pathogenic "heat" and "cool" blood (make the abnormal activity of the blood quiet stop bleeding), and eliminate phlegm [6]. In Western medicine, the oral liquid can increase cerebral blood flow, improve microcirculation, prolong thrombus formation, bleeding, and clotting times, and inhibit platelet aggregation, so it can promote phagocytic function and accelerate the absorption of blood swollen in cerebral [6] and might be an effective prescription in the treatment of mixed stroke [7]. For these reasons, the aim of the present investigation was to evaluate whether *Nao-Xue-Shu* oral liquid can improve the aphasia of mixed stroke. We enrolled mixed stroke aphasia patients from the Department of Neurology of Shuguang Hospital affiliated to Shanghai University of Traditional Chinese Medicine and the Department of Neurology of Hua Shan Hospital affiliated to Fu Dan University based on whether or not they were taking *Nao-Xue-Shu* oral liquid in order to identify a reliable treatment for improving the prognosis of the patients.

2. Subjects and Methods

2.1. Subjects. A total of 116 mixed stroke patients with aphasia from our two hospitals were divided into a treatment group (treatment plus *Nao-Xue-Shu* oral liquid, $n = 58$) and a control group (treatment without *Nao-Xue-Shu* oral liquid, $n = 58$) in a single blind fashion. Inclusion criteria for the patients with aphasia of mixed stroke were (1) acute onset, neural function defect syndrome caused by a local brain blood circulation disorder, and duration of symptoms of at least 24 hours [8]; (2) diagnosis by CT and/or magnetic resonance imaging (MRI) of the brain clearly showing cerebral infarction accompanied by cerebral hemorrhage; (3) the patient in a conscious state and with the ability to speak and no comprehension difficulties, with or without dysarthria; and (4) the patient or their guardians providing signed informed consent. Exclusion criteria for those meeting the above inclusion criteria were (1) a patient with an existing consciousness disorder; (2) cerebral hemorrhage caused by another reason such as a tumor or brain trauma caused by cerebral infarction; (3) the existence of serious gastrointestinal bleeding, hemoptysis, or bloody urine; (4) the presence of other diseases caused by vascular dementia, frontotemporal dementia, Parkinson's disease (PD), Alzheimer's disease (AD), or a central nervous system disease such as a brain tumor, multiple sclerosis, encephalitis, epilepsy, normal pressure hydrocephalus (NPH), or other types of dementia; (5) alcohol and/or drug abuse or other known kinds of aphasia or dementia which prohibit the patient from cooperating with the examiner.

The mixed stroke patients with aphasia selected included 83 males and 33 females (age range, 39–87 y; mean ± SD, 64.28 ± 4.74 y), and time from onset to admission was 0.5~2.5 d (0.75 ± 1.08 d). There were 34 cases of left temporal infarction with hemorrhage, 23 cases of right temporal leaf infarction with hemorrhage, 14 cases of left putamen hemorrhage with right basal ganglia infarction, 12 cases of left putamen hemorrhage with right brain stem infarction, 11 cases of right basal ganglia infarction with hemorrhage in the left caudate nucleus, 9 cases of left cerebellar hemorrhage with right basal ganglia infarction, 8 cases of left thalamus hemorrhage with infarction in the right side of the basal ganglia area, and 5 cases of left basal ganglia infarction with right basal ganglia hemorrhage. No significant differences in gender, age, number of cases, duration, or types of diseases between the two groups were found, and the 2 groups were comparable (Table 1).

2.2. Treatment Methods. The control group underwent routine clinical treatments and measures according to the guidelines of Western medicine [9], including monitoring fluctuations in the electrocardiograph (ECG) and blood pressure. To control blood pressure and intracranial pressure, *mannitol* and/or *furosemidum* and *citicoline* were administered by intravenous infusion according to the patient's situation. The patients in the treatment group were treated using the same routine treatments as the control group and were also administered 10 mL of *Nao-Xue-Shu* oral liquid [6, 7] three times per day (Shandong *Wohua* Pharmaceutical Polytron Technologies Inc.), which consists of *Astragalus root, Hirudo, Acorus gramineus, Radix Achyranthis bidentatae, tree Peony bark, Rheum officinale,* and *Ligusticum wallichii* (batch numbers 5040504 and 5040708). The ratio formula of each herb or insect and the craftsmanship are protected by Chinese patent, but the effective elements could pass through the blood brain barrier to modify cerebral hemorrhage by study of cerebral hemorrhage model [10]. Patients who could not ingest the liquid orally were given it by nasal feeding. The patients in the treatment group took *Nao-Xue-Shu* oral liquid for 4 consecutive weeks. The clinical and laboratory parameters were measured before treatment (baseline), at the end of week 2, and at the end of week 4 to evaluate the effects of treatment in the two groups.

2.3. Assessments. (1) Western Aphasia Battery (WAB) [11] is the main outcome measure of aphasia. The examination not only detects fluctuations in aphasia but also assesses the use of visual spatial function, nonlinguistic intelligence abilities, spatial structure ability, ability to perform calculations, and other nonlinguistic function examinations. The WAB test has been used as a common tool in evaluating aphasia and is minimally influenced by race and cultural background in Western countries [12]. The six quotients developed by weighting WAB scores are as follows: comprehension, repetition, naming, reading, calculating, and writing, with the highest score being 100%.

(2) The Modified Rankin Scale (mRS) [13] is a simplification of the overall assessment of the patient's neurological function scale. The higher the score for neural function

TABLE 1: Background characteristics of the patients of mixed stroke with aphasia.

Group	n	Gender		Age (y)	Educational level (n)			Handedness (n)		Aphasia type (n)		
		M	F		Primary	Middle	College or more	L	R	Motor	Receptive	Mixed
Treatment group	54	38	16	63.32 ± 5.1	13	24	17	5	49	23	19	12
Control group	51	37	14	64.6 ± 4.9	11	23	17	4	47	21	17	13

TABLE 2: Quantitative changes of Western aphasia battery (WAB) between before and after the additional treatments in the treatment and control groups.

	Comprehension	Repetition	Naming	Reading	Calculating	Writing
Treatment group						
Before	0.68 ± 0.22	0.53 ± 0.17	0.46 ± 0.31	0.57 ± 0.26	0.43 ± 0.37	0.62 ± 0.25
Week 2	$0.76 \pm 0.17^*$	$0.70 \pm 0.32^*$	0.52 ± 0.28	$0.67 \pm 0.25^*$	$0.56 \pm 0.28^*$	0.67 ± 0.21
Week 4	$0.87 \pm 0.12^{***\#}$	$0.75 \pm 0.21^{***\#}$	$0.62 \pm 0.24^{*\#}$	$0.77 \pm 0.18^{***\#}$	$0.67 \pm 0.22^{***\#}$	$0.77 \pm 0.12^{*\#}$
Control group						
Before	0.69 ± 0.23	0.54 ± 0.12	0.46 ± 0.25	0.56 ± 0.21	0.45 ± 0.29	0.63 ± 0.28
Week 2	0.70 ± 0.21	0.60 ± 0.19	0.49 ± 0.21	0.58 ± 0.24	0.48 ± 0.27	0.65 ± 0.25
Week 4	$0.77 \pm 0.19^*$	0.63 ± 0.25	0.52 ± 0.17	$0.65 \pm 0.22^*$	0.53 ± 0.33	0.68 ± 0.19

Note: $^*p < 0.05$ and $^{**}p < 0.01$ compared with before for the same group; $^{\#}p < 0.05$ compared with control group at the same time.

defect, the more serious the condition; 0 means no movement dysfunction and 6 means death. After 2 and 4 weeks of treatment, an increased percentage in the range of 0-1 of mRS will be used as the main determinant of improvement for movement dysfunction.

(3) The National Institutes of Health Stroke Scale (NIHSS) [14] as the reference index of curative effect include consciousness, gaze, facial paralysis, limb activities, and so on for a total of 11 scoring categories, with 0 points being normal. The higher the score of NIHSS, the more serious the neurologic deficit, NIHSS as a predictor of acute onset for stroke.

(4) Blood hemorheology as a reference index of the curative effect include whole blood viscosity low shear (WBVLS), whole blood viscosity high shear (WBVHS), plasma viscosity (PV), erythrocyte sedimentation rate equation K value (ESRE K value), fibrinogen, and erythrocyte aggregation index (EA index).

2.4. *Statistics.* SPSS17.0 software package was used for statistical analysis of the data. Data are presented as the mean and standard deviation ($-x + s$) or percentage (%). Repeated-measure ANOVA was conducted to test the differences among changes in outcomes at baseline and at the end of week 2 and week 4 for both groups. Differences at baseline between the treatment group and control group were analyzed. A $p < 0.05$ was considered to indicate a statistically significant difference.

3. Results

No significant differences in age, sex, educational level, handedness, aphasia type, baseline WAB score, mRS score, or NIHSS score, or blood parameters of hemorheology were observed between the treatment and control groups (Tables 1

and 2). After two weeks of treatment, there was one death in the treatment group due to severe lung infection, while three subjects died in the control group (one due to acute heart failure, one due to cerebral herniation, and one due to severe pulmonary infection). After 4 weeks of treatment, contact with three subjects in the treatment group was lost after they left the hospital. In the control group, two patients died and contact with two subjects was lost. Fifty-four patients in the treatment group and 51 patients in the control group were ultimately included in the statistical analyses.

The WAB scores in both groups at the end of week 2 and week 4 were better than their baseline scores. The scores for comprehension, repetition, reading, and calculation at the end of week 2 and week 4 in the treatment group were significantly improved compared with before treatment (baseline) ($p < 0.05$ or $p < 0.01$). These scores were much better at the end of week 4 in the treatment group than in the control group ($p < 0.05$). At the end of week 4, the WAB scores for naming and writing were better in the treatment group compared with baseline ($p < 0.05$), while only the comprehension and reading scores in the control group were significantly improved at the end of week 4. The levels of improvement at the end of week 4 were worse in the control group than in the treatment group ($p < 0.05$, Table 2).

The mRS score was significantly improved at the end of week 2 and week 4 in the treatment group ($p < 0.05$ and $p < 0.01$) compared with baseline, and the improvements were markedly better than those in the control group at the end of week 4 ($p < 0.01$). The mRS score only improved at the end of week 4 in the control group ($p < 0.05$) compared with baseline (Figure 1, left). The number of patients with an mRS score in the 0-1 range increased in both groups at the end of week 2 and week 4 (Figure 1, right), although the change was significantly greater in the treatment group.

TABLE 3: Changes in hemorheology between before and after the additional treatments in the treatment and control groups.

	WBVLS (mPa·s)	WBVHS (mPa·s)	PV (mPa·s)	ESRE K value	Fibrinogen (g/L)	EA index
Treatment group ($n = 54$)						
Before	18.83 ± 4.36	3.82 ± 0.57	1.81 ± 0.52	68.27 ± 39.25	4.82 ± 1.25	4.72 ± 0.81
Week 2	17.96 ± 4.09	3.72 ± 0.35	1.68 ± 0.32	59.19 ± 41.62	4.19 ± 1.02	3.96 ± 0.63
Week 4	$16.65 \pm 3.74^{*\#}$	$3.53 \pm 0.32^{*\#}$	$1.47 \pm 0.44^{**\#}$	$53.56 \pm 40.69^{*\#}$	$3.47 \pm 0.72^{*\#}$	$3.25 \pm 0.52^{*\#}$
Control group ($n = 51$)						
Before	18.74 ± 5.05	3.82 ± 0.35	1.81 ± 0.37	67.82 ± 41.25	4.79 ± 1.46	4.70 ± 0.65
Week 2	18.38 ± 5.23	3.79 ± 0.62	1.76 ± 0.42	64.99 ± 39.02	4.02 ± 1.33	4.65 ± 0.92
Week 4	17.99 ± 4.59	3.77 ± 0.53	1.71 ± 0.38	63.47 ± 44.72	3.95 ± 1.49	3.97 ± 0.59

Note. WBVLS: whole blood viscosity low shear; WBVHS: whole blood viscosity high shear; PV: plasma viscosity; ESRE K value: erythrocyte sedimentation rate equation K value; and EA index: erythrocyte aggregation index. $^*p < 0.05$ and $^{**}p < 0.01$ compared with before for the same group; $^\#p < 0.05$ compared with control group at the same duration.

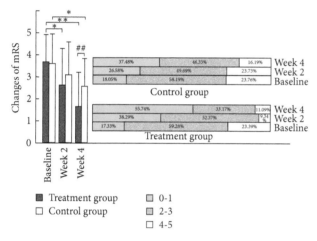

FIGURE 1: Changes in the modified Rankin score (mRS) between before and after the additional treatments in the treatment and control groups. Note: $^*p < 0.05$ and $^{**}p < 0.01$ compared with before for the same group; $^{\#\#}p < 0.01$ compared with control group at the same time.

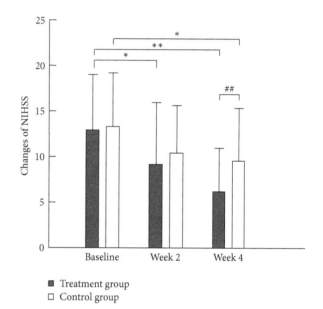

FIGURE 2: Changes in the National Institutes of Health Stroke Scale (NIHSS) scores between before and after the additional treatments in the treatment and control groups. Note: $^*p < 0.05$ and $^{**}p < 0.01$ compared with before for the same group; $^{\#\#}p < 0.01$ compared with control group at the same duration.

The NIHSS scores were improved at the end of week 2 and week 4 in both groups compared with their respective baselines, although the levels were markedly better in the treatment group than in the control group at the end of week 2 and week 4 (Figure 2).

The changes in most parameters in the blood hemorheology index in the treatment group at the end of week 4 were significantly different compared with baseline. The changes observed in all six parameters of the index in the treatment group were different compared with the control group at the end of week 4 (Table 3).

4. Discussion

There were more dropouts and deaths in the control group compared to the treatment group at the end of the study. Our results indicate that compared with baseline the treatment group (*Nao-Xue-Shu* oral liquid) had improved comprehension, repetition, reading, and calculating scores for aphasia parameters at the end of week 2 and the scores for these factors all had improved significantly at the end of week

4 compared with the control group and their baselines (Table 2). The treatment group exhibited improvements not only in the aphasia parameters but also in limb function, indicating that *Nao-Xue-Shu* oral liquid also can be used for treating patients with mixed stroke. After 4 weeks of treatment, the hemodynamic level of the treatment group improved compared with the control group, making it more close to the normal range (Table 3).

Mixed stroke is a common clinical cerebrovascular disease, and the patients experience acute onset and rapid progression. The cause of the disease is often an arterial lesion in the carotid artery system of the brain region, and the infarction area is large and often accompanied by damage to advanced brain function as the result of coma, aphasia, dementia, and epilepsy [15]. These have a serious impact on the quality of life and safety of the patient. Explaining the mechanism of action of *Nao-Xue-Shu* oral liquid in terms of traditional Chinese medicine (TCM) theory may be difficult to understand for most Western doctors. Mixed stroke in TCM is explained as "apoplexia" and an "attack on the viscera and bowels" [16], caused by a *Qi* deficiency, blood stasis, and phlegm. Due to the *Qi* deficiency, the blood stasis and phlegm obstruct the internal structure of blood vessel then intertwist each other, causing the blood stasis with phlegm to insert the vessel in the brain, leading to infarction. The abnormal blood causes intervessel high blood pressure, and forcing the blood stasis with phlegm out of the blood vessel may break the vessel, leading to hemorrhage [17, 18]. In TCM theory, if blood stasis is accompanied by phlegm, it can lead to a more significantly damaged lesion in the brain [19]. This is the mechanism that explains why mixed stroke patients often also have advanced neuronal damage, including aphasia, and the two pathological phenomenons of infarction and hemorrhage can be caused simultaneously. Physiologically, cleaning and powerful *Qi* (*Qing-yang Qi*) can supply energy to the brain to maintain its function and collect and modulate the blood and force it to circulate in correct way in brain blood vessels [17, 18]. If the circulation has been obstructed by the blood stasis with phlegm, the occlusion of blood vessel orifices will occur and the power of *Qi* will decrease; *Qing-yang Qi* is also like nutrition for the brain; if it cannot rise, it can lead to the brain lack of power to speak and understand the language and then can cause dysarthria and dysphagia. When treating this disease, we should consider three TCM pathogenic matters: *Qi*, blood stasis, and phlegm. First, we should eliminate *Qing-yang Qi*, which can modulate blood circulation and control or decrease bleeding. *Astragalus root* as a major component in *Nao-Xue-Shu* oral liquid can provide a stronger *Qing-yang Qi* [19]. The *Qi* also provides energy to raise the nutrient level in blood to the brain when treating the infarction and improves the aphasia. In TCM, *Qi* can improve circulation throughout the entire system and excrete metabolin. The other main component in the oral liquid is *hirudo,* a type of earthworm that has been used for more than one thousand years in China, which can rapidly eliminate blood stasis and treat the second pathogenic condition, that of blood stasis [20, 21], without side effect as bleeding. Other than these two components, the *Nao-Xue-Shu* oral liquid formulation contains 5 other TCM herbs that can help increase *Qi*, remove blood stasis and phlegm, and assist the body to excrete the pathogenic metabolites of blood stasis and phlegm. In fact, *Nao-Xue-Shu* oral liquid contains two famous prescriptions of TCM; one is *Bu-Yang-Huan-Wu decoction*, which originated in the Qing Dynasty (about 185 years ago) and has been used frequently to treat stroke in China and Asia [22, 23]. The other is *Da-Huang-Shu-Chong pill*, which comes from the very famous TCM text *Jin-Gui-Yao-Lue* (By Zhang Zhongjing, about 1700 years ago) and has been used to remove blood stasis from the body [24]. The combination of these 2 prescriptions is the most effective treatments in treating for mixed stroke with aphasia. Clinical pharmacological studies have confirmed that *Nao-Xue-Shu* oral liquid accelerates the absorption of hematoma in the brain of rats, reduces edema around the hematoma accelerating fibrinolysis and inhibiting thrombosis, increases cerebral blood flow, and improves brain blood and oxygen supply, thereby improving blood circulation and promoting the absorption of hematoma [25].

In this study on treating mixed stroke with aphasia, we believe the disease is caused by 3 pathogenetic mechanisms: a deficiency of *Qi*, blood stasis, and phlegm. The sample size of this study is relatively small and a single blind random method was used, so the treatment group might have experienced placebo effects and we therefore cannot draw any definite conclusion. In TCM theory, each Chinese medicine has its own function to modulate the body or deal with diseases, including treating brain problems, but doctors in China are still unable to demonstrate how the medicine passes through the blood brain barrier (BBB). Including TCM herbs [26, 27], many integrative medicines such as Ayurveda medicine [28], electric stimulation [29], and Tai Chi quan [30] cannot confirm that they influence the nerve system directly by Western medical technology, but they have been used in many countries for treating many diseases [5]. *Nao-Xue-Shu* oral liquid contains a type of worm and this is another problem since, according to ethics, it is difficult to introduce such a treatment into foreign countries, although worms are frequently used in TCM treatments and TCM researchers in China have demonstrated they are harmless and safe. In order to validate the causes of the disease based on clinical data, large-scale, multicenter, double-blind randomized control studies will be needed to verify the effectiveness of *Nao-Xue-Shu* oral liquid in the treatment of mixed stroke aphasia.

Acknowledgment

This study was sponsored and supported by the National Natural Science Foundation of China (81373619).

References

[1] T. Ogawa and K. Uemura, "CT and MRI diagnosis of hemorrhagic infarction," *Nippon Rinsho,* vol. 51, supplement, pp. 800–805, 1993 (Japanese).

[2] B. R. Ott, A. Zamani, J. Kleefield, and H. H. Funkenstein, "The clinical spectrum of hemorrhagic infarction," *Stroke,* vol. 17, no. 4, pp. 630–637, 1986.

[3] P. F. Finelli and F. J. DiMario Jr., "Hemorrhagic infarction in white matter following acute carbon monoxide poisoning," *Neurology,* vol. 63, no. 6, pp. 1102–1104, 2004.

[4] M. S. Pessin, C. J. Estol, F. Lafranchise, and L. R. Caplan, "Safety of anticoagulation after hemorrhagic infarction," *Neurology,* vol. 43, no. 7, pp. 1298–1303, 1993.

[5] W. Pan and H. Zhou, "Inclusion of integrative medicine in clinical practice," *Integrative Medicine International,* vol. 1, no. 1, pp. 1–4, 2014.

[6] D. Xue, B. Suo, Y. Sun et al., "Nao-Xue-Shu liquid for hemorrhagic stroke," *Zhong Xi Yi Jie He Xin Nao Xue Guan Bing Za Zhi,* vol. 5, no. 8, pp. 690–691, 2007.

[7] S. Wang, R. Song, Z. Wang et al., "The clinical study for Nao-Xue-Shu liquid absorb hematoma of hemorrhagic stroke," *Zhong Xi Yi Jie He Xin Nao Xue Guan Bing Za Zhi*, vol. 12, no. 4, pp. 452–453, 2014.

[8] E. C. Jauch, J. L. Saver, H. P. Adams et al., "Guidelines for the early management of patients with acute ischemic stroke: a guideline for healthcare professionals from the American Heart Association/American Stroke Association," *Stroke*, vol. 44, no. 3, pp. 870–947, 2013.

[9] J. L. Saver and L. B. Goldstein, "The new standing guideline committee policy of the american stroke association stroke council," *Stroke*, vol. 37, no. 3, p. 753, 2006.

[10] L. Xiaoping, "The laboratory research and clinical study of Nao-Xue-Shu oral liquid," *China Journal of Pharmaceutical Economics*, vol. 6, pp. 128–130, 2012.

[11] C. M. Shewan and A. Kertesz, "Reliability and validity characteristics of the Western Aphasia Battery (WAB)," *Journal of Speech and Hearing Disorders*, vol. 45, no. 3, pp. 308–324, 1980.

[12] J. Horner, D. V. Dawson, A. Heyman, and A. M. Fish, "The usefulness of the Western Aphasia Battery for differential diagnosis of Alzheimer dementia and focal stroke syndromes: preliminary evidence," *Brain and Language*, vol. 42, no. 1, pp. 77–88, 1992.

[13] G. Sulter, C. Steen, and J. De Keyser, "Use of the Barthel index and modified Rankin scale in acute stroke trials," *Stroke*, vol. 30, no. 8, pp. 1538–1541, 1999.

[14] T. Brott, H. P. Adams Jr., C. P. Olinger et al., "Measurements of acute cerebral infarction: a clinical examination scale," *Stroke*, vol. 20, no. 7, pp. 864–870, 1989.

[15] P. M. Pedersen, H. S. Jørgensen, H. Nakayama, H. O. Raaschou, and T. S. Olsen, "Aphasia in acute stroke: incidence, determinants, and recovery," *Annals of Neurology*, vol. 38, no. 4, pp. 659–666, 1995.

[16] D. H. Yi, Y. Li, S. X. Shao, Y. M. Xie, and Y. Yuwen, "Evaluation of the conjoint efficacy in Chinese medicine with the longitudinal latent variable linear mixed model," *Chinese Journal of Integrative Medicine*, vol. 19, no. 8, pp. 629–635, 2013.

[17] L. M. Yang, "[Medico-psychology in Huang di nei jing (Yellow Emperor's Inner Canon)]," *Zhonghua Yi Shi Za Zhi*, vol. 34, no. 1, pp. 21–26, 2004 (Chinese).

[18] J. Zhu, "Textual research and explanation of "Qi-Huang"," *Zhonghua Yi Shi Za Zhi*, vol. 32, no. 4, pp. 200–204, 2002.

[19] Z. Chen, L. Yuan, and G. Zhang, "The clinical and laboratory research of Nao-Xue-Shu liquid in treating for vascular diseases," *Zhong Xi Yi Jie He Xin Nao Xue Guan Bing Za Zhi*, vol. 12, no. 8, pp. 1005–1006, 2014.

[20] F. von Rheinbaben, O. Riebe, J. Koehnlein, and S. Werner, "Viral infection risks for patients using the finished product *Hirudo verbana* (medicinal leech)," *Parasitology Research*, vol. 113, no. 11, pp. 4199–4205, 2014.

[21] F. Le Marrec-Croq, A. Bocquet-Garcon, J. Vizioli et al., "Calreticulin contributes to C1q-dependent recruitment of microglia in the leech Hirudo medicinalis following a CNS injury," *Medical Science Monitor*, vol. 20, pp. 644–653, 2014.

[22] L. H. Shaw, L. C. Lin, and T. H. Tsai, "HPLC-MS/MS analysis of a traditional Chinese medical formulation of Bu-Yang-Huan-Wu-Tang and its pharmacokinetics after oral administration to rats," *PLoS ONE*, vol. 7, no. 8, Article ID e43848, 2012.

[23] Z. Lai, S. Y. Wang, X. Y. Geng, C. Q. Deng, and R. Z. Zhang, "Effects of bu yang huan wu decoction on astrocytes after cerebral ischemia and reperfusion," *Zhongguo Zhong Yao Za Zhi*, vol. 27, no. 10, pp. 763–765, 2002 (Chinese).

[24] T. Jiang and H. Fu, "Progress of experimental studies on prescriptions designed by Zhang Zhongjing," *Journal of Traditional Chinese Medicine*, vol. 16, no. 1, pp. 55–64, 1996.

[25] X. Ai and C. Liu, "The study of cleaning volume of hematoma and protecting neuron function of hemorrhagic rat model by Nao-Xue-Shu liquid," *Zhong Guo Zhong Xi Yi Jie He Xin Nao Xue Guan Bing Za Zhi*, vol. 11, no. 7, pp. 859–861, 2014.

[26] W. Pan, Q. Wang, S. Kwak et al., "Shen-zhi-ling oral liquid improves behavioral and psychological symptoms of dementia in Alzheimer's disease," *Evidence-Based Complementary and Alternative Medicine*, vol. 2014, Article ID 913687, 6 pages, 2014.

[27] J. Shen, X. Chen, X. Chen, and R. Deng, "Targeting neurogenesis: a promising therapeutic strategy for post-stroke treatment with Chinese herbal medicine," *Integrative Medicine International*, vol. 1, no. 1, pp. 5–18, 2014.

[28] P. Santiago Lloret, M. Verónica Rey, and O. Rascol, "Ayurveda medicine for the treatment of Parkinson's disease," *International Journal of Integrative Medicine*, vol. 1, article 6, 2013.

[29] J. Lee, J. Y. Cho, and K. W. Kim, "Rapid treatment of waist pain by nanoscale electric stimulation," *Integrative Medicine International*, vol. 1, no. 1, pp. 19–24, 2014.

[30] F. Li, "Tai Ji Quan exercise for people with Parkinson's disease and other neurodegenerative movement disorders," *International Journal of Integrative Medicine*, vol. 1, no. 4, 2013.

15

105 Inappropriate ICD Shocks in a Patient with Dilated Cardiomyopathy and Broca's Aphasia

Christian Georgi ⓘ, Michael Neuß, Viviane Möller, Martin Seifert, and Christian Butter

Heart Center Brandenburg-Department of Cardiology and Medical School Brandenburg Theodor Fontane, Bernau bei Berlin, Germany

Correspondence should be addressed to Christian Georgi; c.georgi@immanuel.de

Academic Editor: Hajime Kataoka

With a growing number of ICD recipients, device complications are seen more frequently in the clinical setting and outpatient departments. Among the most severe are ICD infections and inappropriate therapies caused by oversensing of atrial tachycardias or lead fracture. We report on a 76-year-old female patient with dilative cardiomyopathy and Broca's aphasia after stroke, who experienced 105 consecutive inappropriate ICD shocks due to cluster missensing of her fractured ICD lead. The diagnosis was complicated and delayed by patient's aphasia emphasizing the need for intensified remote monitoring along with regular in-person visits, especially in people with intellectual or communication disabilities.

1. Introduction

The implantable cardioverter-defibrillator (ICD) has been proven to be an effective therapy in the primary and secondary prevention of sudden cardiac death [1].

Yet inappropriate ICD therapies, mainly due to oversensing or SVTs, remain a great problem in device therapy. A lately published meta-analysis reports of inappropriate therapies in around 10% of patients with ICDs within the first year after implantation [2]. It is well known that ICD shocks, both appropriate and inappropriate, have a negative impact on morbidity and mortality [3, 4].

Beyond mortality rates, ICD shocks, especially inappropriate therapies, are found to cause a decline in the quality of life and reduced daily activity and increased general anxiety in postshock patients [5].

A reduction of inappropriate therapies therefore should be achieved by intensive treatment of the underlying disease, optimal ICD programming, and close monitoring of patients at high risk.

In this context, remote monitoring (RM) is a promising complement to conventional in-clinic follow-ups with the potential to dramatically reduce inappropriate therapies [6], although structural deficits concerning data overload, functional responsibility, and imprecise workflows need to be improved. In particular, for people in rural areas, in patients with impaired mobility or mental status, RM offers the chance for improved safety and quality of life. So far, remote control has not been fully implemented in the follow-up of ICD patients in Northern America and Europe, though [7].

We report on an aphasic patient with more than one hundred inappropriate shocks within a few hours that could have been prevented by more frequent expert consultations and connecting her to a remote monitoring program.

2. Case Report

A 76-year-old female patient was admitted to our emergency department early in the morning with suspected acute coronary syndrome. The patient had suffered from a major stroke causing Broca's aphasia three months prior to this admission and was referred to us from a nearby neurorehabilitation clinic. Initial ECG showed no signs of acute ischemia, but troponin I levels were about 1000-fold elevated. History taking was complicated by patient's aphasia, but she did not appear to be in acute pain at the time of admission.

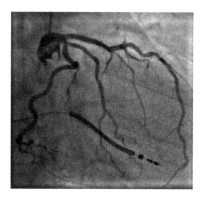

FIGURE 1: Angiogram of the patient coronaries showing no culprit lesion or significant stenosis.

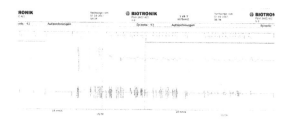

FIGURE 3: Inappropriate shock. Typical high-frequency signals (cluster) in the PS channel indicating a lead insulation problem.

FIGURE 2: Last page of the ICD memory showing 54 shocks in 1:15 h.

With a history of heart failure and an implanted single-chamber ICD, the patient was brought to the catheter lab to undergo coronary angiogram, where no culprit lesion could be detected (Figure 1).

In a phone consultation with the rehab clinic's doctor in charge, he described how the patient had multiple episodes of acute chest and back pain with "electrical twitches" for the course of several hours during the past night. Pain medication was administered and the pain interpreted as musculoskeletal but no other diagnostic or therapeutic steps were taken. Eventually, in the morning, a troponin test was done and found positive, so the patient was referred.

Subsequently, we performed an ICD interrogation, which revealed an EOS (end of service) status and multiple inappropriate ICD therapies in the time between 00:07 AM and 03:46 AM until the battery of the Biotronik ICD was depleted and the device eventually stopped antitachycardia therapy. In summary, the patient suffered 105 consecutive inappropriate ICD shocks within 219 minutes (Figure 2), to our knowledge, the highest shock incidence in such a short period of time. The shocks were caused by cluster missensing on her right ventricular lead (Figure 3), presumably resulting from an insulation defect near the header. Further episodes of oversensing due to clusters could be seen over the preceding five months, occasionally followed by antitachycardia pacing but no shock therapy.

The ICD was implanted in 2008 and exchanged for EOL (end of life) in 2015. The last ambulatory interrogation was in September 2016, just before the first episodes of cluster missensing occurred. The next appointment was scheduled for March 2017 but postponed due to the prolonged hospital stay after apoplexy. The technical analysis of the explanted ICD did not show any technical abnormalities; the chest X-ray revealed no sign of lead fracture.

After discussing the case with patient's family, the defective lead was disconnected, and at the request of the patient and her family, a new ICD and lead were implanted and the patient enrolled in our remote monitoring program.

3. Discussion

Since the first transvenous ICD was implanted in 1980 [8], there is a steadily growing number of ICD implantations and patients with long-lasting devices [9]. In the year 2023, there is an estimated 1.4 million pacemaker and ICD implantations worldwide [10]. Simultaneously, the lead- and generator-associated complications increased over the last years. Lead-associated complications include thrombosis and infection as well as fracture and insulation problems with the risk of inappropriate therapies. From large clinical trials, we know that about 5-20% of patients with ICDs receive inappropriate therapy, mainly due to the missensing of supraventricular arrhythmias, oversensing of external noise, or lead fracture/insulation defects [4]. The psychological impact of inappropriate ICD shocks was investigated in several studies. Among the most frequent side effects are anxiety disorders, posttraumatic stress disorders, panic attacks, depression, nightmare, and insomnia [11].

This case demonstrates possible pitfalls of ICD supply in elderly or handicapped people. The inability of the patient to communicate properly and missing awareness of the staff led to the dreadful course of events. The suspected short circuit between the lead and the scorched battery (Figure 4) might have reduced the current delivered to the whole body and weakened the pain; still the delay in therapy was unnecessary and avoidable. Immediate ECG monitoring would have helped to discover the cause for shock delivery and could have led to shock suppression by simply applying a magnet.

Retrospectively, the earlier access to remote monitoring could have prevented the massive amount of shocks, since the first asymptomatic cluster episodes could be detected

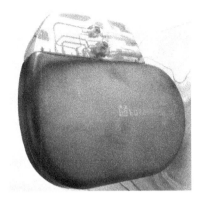

FIGURE 4: Scorched battery of the Biotronik ICD (Iforia 3 VR and Linox SD lead) due to an assumed lead insulation defect near the header.

already some months before the incident described. A significant reduction of the "first-incidence-to-action time" through remote monitoring has been described by many authors [12–14]. The TRUST study demonstrated a median delay of 1 day from occurrence of the event to physician evaluation, compared to 1 month with conventional follow-up [15]. They also confirmed a cost benefit from an economical perspective. Still the need for additional manpower to analyze the huge amount of data, legal issues, and lack of standardization remain open problems [16].

4. Conclusion

Regular in-person visits with cardiologists remain the foundation of appropriate ICD follow-up. Remote monitoring programs, though, are a very useful tool to supplement conventional follow-up and should be established whenever suitable. The transmission of technical data to experts is known to be very effective to detect early malfunctions of implantable devices as ICDs and pacemakers. This clearly helps to avoid inappropriate therapies, detects lead and battery problems, and discovers atrial fibrillation or other arrhythmias.

An increasing number of patients with ICDs, pacemakers, and CRTs require sufficient manpower and technical resources to guarantee high-quality monitoring. Moreover, further training programs for outpatient departments and GPs should be installed since there is a significant lack of knowledge concerning ICD function and troubleshooting.

References

[1] C. M. Tracy, A. E. Epstein, D. Darbar et al., "2012 ACCF/AHA/HRS focused update of the 2008 guidelines for device-based therapy of cardiac rhythm abnormalities: a report of the American College of Cardiology Foundation/American Heart Association Task Force on Practice Guidelines," *Heart rhythm*, vol. 9, no. 10, pp. 1737–1753, 2012.

[2] I. Basu-Ray, J. Liu, X. Jia et al., "Subcutaneous versus transvenous implantable defibrillator therapy: a meta-analysis of case-control studies," *JACC: Clinical Electrophysiology*, vol. 3, no. 13, pp. 1475–1483, 2017.

[3] J. E. Poole, G. W. Johnson, A. S. Hellkamp et al., "Prognostic importance of defibrillator shocks in patients with heart failure," *The New England Journal of Medicine*, vol. 359, no. 10, pp. 1009–1017, 2008.

[4] A. J. Moss, C. Schuger, C. A. Beck et al., "Reduction in inappropriate therapy and mortality through ICD programming," *The New England Journal of Medicine*, vol. 367, no. 24, pp. 2275–2283, 2012.

[5] S. F. Sears, L. Rosman, S. Sasaki et al., "Defibrillator shocks and their effect on objective and subjective patient outcomes: results of the PainFree SST clinical trial," *Heart rhythm*, vol. 15, no. 5, pp. 734–740, 2018.

[6] S. Ploux, C. D. Swerdlow, M. Strik et al., "Towards eradication of inappropriate therapies for ICD lead failure by combining comprehensive remote monitoring and lead noise alerts," *Journal of cardiovascular electrophysiology*, vol. 29, no. 8, pp. 1125–1134, 2018.

[7] R. Ganeshan, A. D. Enriquez, and J. V. Freeman, "Remote monitoring of implantable cardiac devices: current state and future directions," *Current opinion in cardiology*, vol. 33, no. 1, pp. 20–30, 2018.

[8] M. Mirowski, P. R. Reid, M. M. Mower et al., "Termination of malignant ventricular arrhythmias with an implanted automatic defibrillator in human beings," *The New England Journal of Medicine*, vol. 303, no. 6, pp. 322–324, 1980.

[9] M. J. Raatikainen, D. O. Arnar, K. Zeppenfeld et al., "Statistics on the use of cardiac electronic devices and electrophysiological procedures in the European Society of Cardiology countries: 2014 report from the European Heart Rhythm Association," *EP Europace*, vol. 17, Supplement 1, pp. i1–75, 2015.

[10] M. Jager, C. Jordan, A. Theilmeier et al., "Lumbar-load analysis of manual patient-handling activities for biomechanical overload prevention among healthcare workers," *The Annals of occupational hygiene*, vol. 57, no. 4, pp. 528–544, 2013.

[11] J. Jordan, G. Titscher, L. Peregrinova, and H. Kirsch, "Manual for the psychotherapeutic treatment of acute and post-traumatic stress disorders following multiple shocks from implantable cardioverter defibrillator (ICD)," *GMS Psycho-Social-Medicine*, vol. 10, article Doc09, 2013.

[12] A. Lazarus, "Remote, wireless, ambulatory monitoring of implantable pacemakers, cardioverter defibrillators, and cardiac resynchronization therapy systems: analysis of a worldwide database," *Pacing and clinical electrophysiology*, vol. 30, Supplement 1, pp. S2–S12, 2007.

[13] S. Spencker, N. Coban, L. Koch, A. Schirdewan, and D. Muller, "Potential role of home monitoring to reduce inappropriate shocks in implantable cardioverter-defibrillator patients due to lead failure," *EP Europace*, vol. 11, no. 4, pp. 483–488, 2009.

[14] L. Guedon-Moreau, D. Lacroix, N. Sadoul et al., "A randomized study of remote follow-up of implantable cardioverter defibrillators: safety and efficacy report of the ECOST trial," *European Heart Journal*, vol. 34, no. 8, pp. 605–614, 2013.

[15] N. Varma, A. E. Epstein, A. Irimpen, R. Schweikert, C. Love, and TRUST Investigators, "Efficacy and safety of automatic remote monitoring for implantable cardioverter-defibrillator follow-up: the Lumos-T Safely Reduces Routine Office Device Follow-up (TRUST) trial," *Circulation*, vol. 122, no. 4, pp. 325–332, 2010.

[16] M. Bertini, L. Marcantoni, T. Toselli, and R. Ferrari, "Remote monitoring of implantable devices: should we continue to ignore it?," *International Journal of Cardiology*, vol. 202, pp. 368–377, 2016.

16

Aphasia Therapy in the Age of Globalization: Cross-Linguistic Therapy Effects in Bilingual Aphasia

Ana Inés Ansaldo[1,2] and Ladan Ghazi Saidi[1]

[1] Centre de Recherché de l'Institut Universitaire de Gériatrie de Montréal, 4565 Queen Mary Road, Montréal, QC, Canada H3W 1W5
[2] Speech-Language Pathology and Audiology Department, Faculty of Medicine, University of Montreal, Pavillon 7077 Avenue du Parc, local 3001-1, Montréal, QC, Canada H3N 1X7

Correspondence should be addressed to Ana Inés Ansaldo; ana.ines.ansaldo@umontreal.ca

Academic Editor: Jubin Abutalebi

Introduction. Globalization imposes challenges to the field of behavioural neurology, among which is an increase in the prevalence of bilingual aphasia. Thus, aphasiologists have increasingly focused on bilingual aphasia therapy and, more recently, on the identification of the most efficient procedures for triggering language recovery in bilinguals with aphasia. Therapy in both languages is often not available, and, thus, researchers have focused on the transfer of therapy effects from the treated language to the untreated one. *Aim.* This paper discusses the literature on bilingual aphasia therapy, with a focus on cross-linguistic therapy effects from the language in which therapy is provided to the untreated language. *Methods.* Fifteen articles including two systematic reviews, providing details on pre- and posttherapy in the adult bilingual population with poststroke aphasia and anomia are discussed with regard to variables that can influence the presence or absence of cross-linguistic transfer of therapy effects. *Results and Discussion.* The potential for CLT of therapy effects from the treated to the untreated language depends on the word type, the degree of structural overlap between languages, the type of therapy approach, the pre- and postmorbid language proficiency profiles, and the status of the cognitive control circuit.

1. Introduction

1.1. Bilingualism Is a Distinctive Feature of Globalization. Contemporary society is characterized by a bilingual or multilingual mode of communication. Whether for historic, economic, or migration reasons, bilingualism is no longer exceptional, but most often the rule. Whereas some countries have a history of bilingual and polyglot modes of communication, the era of globalization has contributed to the promotion of bilingualism around the world. Nowadays, bilingualism provides better career opportunities in all sectors of the economy and human activity, a fact that has motivated a wider interest in second language learning. Parents are increasingly choosing bilingual education as a result of evidence suggesting that bilingual children may develop specific cognitive advantages [1, 2], including enhanced intellectual development, greater creativity and flexibility, and openness to cultural diversity. For all of these

reasons, social, educational, healthcare, and political policies are expected to adapt to such multilingual and multicultural societies.

1.2. Bilingual Aphasia. Aphasia is an acquired language disorder resulting from brain damage. It refers to a breakdown in the ability to formulate, retrieve, or decode the arbitrary symbols of language. It is usually acquired in adulthood [3].

The bilingual population is large and growing worldwide; therefore, bilingual aphasia is becoming more and more frequent. The complexity of the behavioural patterns observed in bilingual aphasia is big, since it concerns two (or more) languages, whose recovery does not always follow equivalent patterns. Moreover, given the almost endless possible combinations of language pairs, the issue of bilingual aphasia therapy is a big challenge. Thus, even the most avant-garde educational policies aimed at training bilingual speech-language pathologists are likely to provide only partial solutions to the clinical management of this population [4, 5]. Consequently, the study of cross-linguistic-language-therapy effects is likely to become an unavoidable topic in the field of aphasiology in the years to come.

From a neurorehabilitative perspective, bilingualism imposes a certain number of challenges regarding the assessment and intervention provided to bilingual clinical populations, particularly, those that suffer from cognitive impairment. The complexity of this issue extends well beyond the linguistic knowledge required to interact with the patient so as to detect impaired language abilities. Beyond language, there is communication, that is, the ability to decode the pragmatics that characterize a specific linguistic community. This is essential for the proper understanding of communicative behavior, meaning, what is normal, and what is not, in the context of a given culture.

The issue of language impairment in bilinguals has interested cognitive neuroscientists for more than a century. In particular, the study of bilingual aphasia first focused on the variety of aphasia patterns characterizing bilingual clinical populations [5–8]. Furthermore, the development of testing procedures that take into consideration the linguistic particularities gave raise to bilingual aphasia tests for a variety of language pairs, among which the BAT [9, 10] developed for more than 59 languages and the Multilingual Aphaisa Examination developed in six languages [11], along with tests normalized in several languages, such as the Aachen Aphasia [12–14], and the Boston Diagnostic Aphasia Examination [15–18]. These tests provide a linguistically valid assessment of bilingual aphasia.

More recently, aphasiologists have focused on the complex issue of bilingual aphasia language therapy, with the purpose of developing the most efficient procedures for triggering language recovery in this population. This is a relatively new field, and a complex one, given that it requires juggling the complexities of bilingual language processing, which amounts to more than simply the additive processing of two languages.

2. Aims

The purpose of this paper is to discuss the literature on bilingual aphasia therapy, with a focus on the cross-linguistic effects that language therapy provided in one of the two languages of the patient may (or may not) have on the untreated language.

This paper will discuss a number of factors with CLT potential: (a) word category (cognates versus non-cognates), (b) language distance (same versus distant language families), (c) pre and post morbid proficiency in either language, and (d) the impact of cognitive control issues on transfer of therapy effects. Finally, the main clinical implications of research findings on cross-linguistic transfer of therapy effects (CLTE) in bilingual aphasia therapy will be discussed, with the purpose of proving intervention efficacy in bilingual populations with language impairment, while optimizing health care efficiency in terms of resource training and allocation. This research will contribute to intervention efficacy

in bilingual populations with language impairment, while optimizing health care efficiency in terms of resource training and allocation.

3. Methods

The evidence discussed in this paper was collected from the following databases: Medline, ASHA, Cochrane, Aphasiology Archive, Evidence-Based Medicine Guidelines, NHS Evidence, and PsycBite et Speechbite. The key words bilingual, aphasia, cross-language, generalization, cognates, naming treatment, and transfer guided the search. This resulted in fifteen articles, two of which received the largest weight in the analysis, since they were systematic reviews [19, 20] with an A-level recommendation that witnesses for good quality patient-oriented research, according to the AFF taxonomy [21]. The remaining articles report case series, or single-case design studies whose level of evidence is much lower; however, all of these were selected because they respected a number of criteria that allowed some degree of generalization of the reported findings. Specifically, the inclusion criteria consisted the following:

(a) provide details on pre- and posttherapy bilingual aphasia profiles,

(b) describe therapy procedures in sufficient detail to make them replicable,

(c) provide information on therapy frequency,

(d) discuss a number of variables that may have influenced the presence or absence of cross-linguistic transfer effects,

(e) reported evidence which concerns the adult population with acquired language impairment,

(f) reported that patient speaks at least two Indo-European languages with different degrees of proficiency across languages before brain damage,

(g) focused mostly on therapy for word-retrieval deficits, namely, anomia, which constitutes the most widespread aphasia symptom across all aphasia types.

4. Results

4.1. Cross-Linguistic Effects in Bilingual, Healthy, and Brain Damaged Populations. Understanding the mechanisms that rule cross-linguistic transfer in bilingual healthy populations highlights the functioning of the bilingual language system.

There is convergent evidence on the fact that the speech of a bilingual person reflects the influence of one language on the other [22, page 5]. This influence, which results from similarities and differences between the target language and any other previously acquired language, is referred to as *cross-linguistic influence* or *cross-linguistic transfer* (CLT) [22, page 27]. Similarities and differences can be observed at different levels of language processing, namely, the word level, the syntax, and phonology levels, as well as the proficiency level. Thus, the study of CLT effects among healthy bilinguals provides clues about the mechanisms that rule CLTE, some of which have been exploited in bilingual aphasia therapy.

4.1.1. Word Type: Cognates, Clangs, and Noncognates. There is extensive evidence on CLT effects with cognates and clangs, as opposed to noncognates [23, 24]. Cognates are formally equivalent words whose meanings may be identical or almost so [25, page 73] (e.g., "tiger" (/ˈtaɪɡər/) and *"tigre"* (/tigr/)), whereas clangs (or homophones) are phonologically similar words with different meanings (e.g., "bell" /bɛl/; metal object that makes a ringing sound when struck; Sonnette in French) in English and *"belle"* in French (/bɛl/; meaning beautiful). Finally, noncognates are translation equivalents that share semantics but not phonology, such as "butterfly" in English and its Spanish equivalent, *"mariposa"*.

Evidence for the effects of CLT is reflected in faster response times for cognates as compared to noncognates in picture naming [23, 26–31], as well as in word recognition and word translation [30, 32–34]. It has also been argued that cognates are processed as efficiently as monolinguals process mother tongue [35, 36]. Accordingly, cross-linguistic therapy effects with cognates in cases of bilingual aphasia have been examined. Roberts and Deslauriers [30] showed that highly proficient bilinguals with aphasia could better name cognates than non-cognates, and they also produced distinct error types for each target. Specifically, errors with cognates were no response and target description—the latter having a communicative value—whereas noncognates resulted in semantic errors as well as language switching errors [30].

Finally, although the evidence of a cognate effect in bilingual aphasia therapy is not unanimous [30, 37, 38], a generalization of therapy effects with cognates has been reported in a case of Spanish-English bilingual aphasia. Thus, Kohnert [37] reported cross-linguistic generalization of therapy effects from treated L1 (Spanish) to untreated L2 (English) for cognates only. Language treatment consisted of lexical semantic retrieval strategies such as word recognition, semantic association, and cueing [37]. Conversely, Kurland and Falcon [38] report an interference effect with cognates, following intensive language therapy with a semantic approach, in a case of a Spanish-English bilingual with chronic and severe expressive aphasia. This interference effect can be explained by reference to Abutalebi and Green's model [39]. The patient presented a lesion in the basal ganglia, a component of the corticosubcortical network sustaining the inhibition of the nontarget language; this network includes the left precentral cortex, the anterior cingulate, the inferior parietal lobule, and the basal ganglia [39].

Clangs, or homophones, also share phonological similarities with mother tongue words, but, unlike cognates, clangs refer to different concepts. The evidence of a clang effect in bilinguals is not convergent; thus, some authors argue that both orthographic and phonological similarity are required to facilitate word recognition [40, 41], whereas others claim that processing clangs imposed an extra cognitive load resulting from the inhibition of the nontarget semantic representation [42, 43]. In line with this claim, a recent functional connectivity study shows that healthy adults recruit a cognitive control network to process clangs [44]. The extent to which clangs may facilitate cross-linguistic therapy effects in bilinguals with aphasia has not yet been tested; however, the findings within healthy populations [42–45] suggest that clangs may become particularly difficult in cases of bilingual aphasia, given that brain damage entails decreased cognitive resources [46].

There is also a lack of convergence regarding CLTE with noncognates. Kurland and Falcon [38] reported successful CLTE for noncognates only, after therapy with a semantic approach. However, with a similar therapy approach, Kohnert [37] failed to report such an effect and instead found one with cognates. It is not easy to draw any conclusions given that such a small number of studies have compared cognates and noncognates, particularly because factors other than word type may have influenced therapy results in either language, including lesion location and extension as well as cross-linguistic similarities and differences.

4.1.2. Structural Similarities and Differences across Languages. The degree of structural overlap across languages plays a major role in the potential for CLTE [19, 20]. For example, Goral et al. [47] described the case of a trilingual speaker with mild chronic aphasia, who was treated in English, (L2), first on morphosyntactic skills (i.e., pronoun and gender agreement) and then on language production rate. Measurements in the treated language (English) as well as in the two nontreated languages (Hebrew (L1), and French (L3)) were collected after each treatment block.

An improvement in pronoun and gender agreement in the treated language (L2) as well as in the nontreated L3 was observed following the treatment block on morphosyntactic skills in English. Also, there was an improvement in speech rate in English and in French following the second block, but no changes were observed in Hebrew. The authors concluded that selective CLT from L2 to L3 resulted from the structural similarities between English and French, as compared to a lack of similarity between English and Hebrew.

Similarly, Miertsch [48] administered semantic therapy in French (L3) to a trilingual participant with Wernicke's aphasia. Transfer was observed from L3 (French) to L2 (English), but not to L1 (German). These findings were interpreted as the result of structural similarities between French and English, as compared to French and German. However, there is also the possibility that the results in German reflect a plateau effect resulting from the fact that poststroke proficiency in German was higher than in the other two languages [48]. As discussed by Faroqui et al. [19], the years to come will yield more studies on the impact of cross-linguistic structural similarities and differences on CLTE.

4.1.3. Pre-Morbid and Post-Morbid Proficiency in Either Language. A number of studies provide evidence for cross-linguistic transfer of therapy effects (CLTE) from the treated, less proficient second language, to the untreated and better preserved mother tongue. Kiran and Iakupova [49] administered semantic therapy in L2 (English) and measured naming on trained and untrained words both in L2 and L1

(Russian). Following therapy, the participant showed 100% accuracy in both treated and untreated items, thus reflecting successful CLTE. The authors [49] suggest that CLTE reflects the strengthened connections between the weaker (English) language and the stronger (Russian) language.

Likewise, CLTE was reported following intensive semantic therapy in L2 (English) in the case of a native Spanish bilingual individual with chronic, severe expressive aphasia [38], particularly on naming tasks. The authors argued that although CLTE from premorbid less proficient language (L2) to premorbid more proficient language (L1) had been successful, all gains considered that the patient benefited more from therapy in L1 than from therapy in L2.

There is evidence that balanced bilingualism contributes to CLTE [27, 50, 51], and, in cases of unbalanced bilingualism, transfer is observed from the less proficient language to the dominant language. Specifically, parallel recovery in both languages was observed in a premorbid balanced bilingual woman (Flemish, L1/Italian, L2) suffering from chronic aphasia after 2 weeks of picture-naming training through repetition and reading of names of pictures in L2 [51]. Similarly, Edmonds and Kiran [50] investigated the CLT of gains achieved following therapy with Semantic Feature Analysis to treat naming deficits by examining three English-Spanish bilinguals with aphasia, all of whom received a semantic therapy in Spanish (Participant 1) and in English and Spanish (Participants 2 and 3). Therapy effects were tested on treated items, untreated items, and translations; results showed that both within- and cross-language therapy effects were related to premorbid language proficiency. Specifically, Participant 1, a premorbid balanced bilingual, showed CLTE to the untreated English items, whereas Participants 2 and 3 (who were more proficient in English) showed within-language generalization to semantically related items, but no CLT to the untreated Spanish items. Moreover, though following treatment in Spanish, Participants 2 and 3 did not show any within-language generalization; they did show CLT to English, their dominant language. Thus, this data supports the idea that better CLTE is observed from the less proficient (L2) to the more proficient language (L1).

In another study, the authors [27] provided semantic therapy in Spanish to two Spanish-English bilinguals, one of them English dominant and the other one a balanced bilingual. Therapy in Spanish resulted in CLTE for both participants, whereas therapy in English was followed by CLTE in the balanced Spanish-English participant only.

Thus, some studies [27, 38, 49–51] provide evidence that premorbid proficiency in either language modulates CLTE, arguing that CLTE occurs more easily from a less proficient language to the dominant language in unbalanced bilinguals, whereas balanced bilingualism facilitates CLTE no matter which language is treated. Thus, it has been shown that the less proficient L2 relies upon the stronger L1 lexicon, whereas, at high proficiency levels, L1 and L2 lexicons are mostly overlapping [19, 52]. Nevertheless, it is difficult to draw a final conclusion, as some of these studies did not report poststroke proficiency states [27, 50].

A different point of view on the impact of proficiency is presented by Goral [53], who claims that it is postmorbid proficiency that determines the extent of CLTE. Evidence from four different case studies demonstrating successful CLTE with different patterns in multilingual participants with aphasia, included (a) CLTE in L1 (Hebrew) following treatment of L2 (English), (b) CLTE in L4 (German) following treatment of L5 (English), (c) CLTE in L3 (French) following treatment of the strongest language L2 (English), and (d) CLTE in L2 (German) following treatment of most recovered L3 (English). In all cases, CLTE occurred when the therapy was offered in the language with higher postmorbid proficiency, regardless of premorbid proficiency. This is also the case in the limited (only for cognates) CLTE in an L1 and L2 premorbidly highly proficient Spanish (L1) and English (L2) bilingual suffering from nonfluent aphasia reported by Kohnert [37]. This patient showed improvement after receiving therapy in both languages; however, CLTE was seen only when therapy was administered in the language with higher postmorbid proficiency (L1).

Similarly, Croft et al. [54] examined five English-Bengali bilinguals with aphasia and anomia, who received a phonological approach and a semantic cueing approach, both in L1 and L2. While phonological cueing resulted in no significant CLTE, semantic cueing led to CLTE for three out of five patients. In all cases, CLTE occurred only when therapy was offered in L1 [54]. In observing the data on the participants' aphasia profiles, one notes that, for all cases in which successful CLTE was reported, the language of therapy happened to be the stronger post-morbid language. As this postmorbid more proficient language also happened to be L1, the authors took these results as evidence for successful CLTE from L1 to L2, despite the fact that not all participants who were treated in L1 showed successful CLTE. Another case of unsuccessful CLT despite the balanced proficiency both at premorbid and postmorbid proficiency was reported by Abutalebi and colleagues [55]. Thus, no CLTE was observed following L2 treatment in a case of fluent aphasia. The patient was a highly proficient, balanced Spanish (L1) Italian (L2) bilingual, who had become severely anomic in both languages following aphasia, and involuntary language interference, was observed. Treatment in L2 was successful but did not show any CLTE. Unsuccessful CLTE in this case may result from the therapy approach chosen (phonological approach); however, another possibility is that involuntary language switching and unsuccessful CLTE resulted from damage to areas involved in cognitive control.

4.1.4. Cognitive Control and Transfer of Therapy Effects. It has been shown that damage to the cognitive control circuit can prevent CLTE. However, there is also evidence that choosing an appropriate therapy approach (i.e., Switch Back Through Translation) can result in CLTE even when damage to the cognitive control circuit is observed [56]. This can be accomplished by implementing a strategy of translation of involuntary switches which allows bypassing the effects of impaired inhibitory abilities resulting from damage to the cognitive control circuit.

In the case reported by Abutalebi et al. [55], the Spanish (L1) and Italian (L2) bilingual anomic patient had damage to the left lenticular nucleus and surrounding areas. He showed selective L1 recovery at T0, and, when asked to name pictures in L2, he would unintentionally name in L1. However, after receiving therapy in L2, the selective pattern changed in favor of L2 and, thus, when asked to name in L1, he would unintentionally name in L2.

The change of selective recovery pattern and the fact that EM was unable to translate, together with the presence of a lesion within the cognitive control circuit, lead Abutalebi and colleagues [55] to conclude that EM's behavior supports the Dynamic Model on Recovery Patterns in Bilingual Aphasia, proposed by Green and Abutalebi [57]. According to this model [57], the same neural network supports L1 and L2 processing; however, the processing of the weaker language (usually L2) may as well involve the left prefrontal cortex, the basal ganglia, and the anterior cingulated cortex, as a function of proficiency level.

Based on Green and Abutalebi [57], one can argue that the recovery pattern will depend on the integrity of the circuits normally involved in language control; also, it may be hypothesized that damage to that circuit can affect CLTE. Thus, cognitive control encompasses controlling language selection, and its impairment may result in involuntary language mixing and language switching [56]. However, as previously discussed, the evidence shows that it is possible to compensate for this deficit by choosing an appropriate therapy approach, that can be designed by reference to a comprehensive model of bilingual language processing [56]. Precisely, CLTE can be triggered by stimulating both languages simultaneously in the context of a therapy approach that includes translation tasks, even when therapy is provided primarily in one language. Ansaldo et al. [56] reported the case of a Spanish-English bilingual who suffered from pathological language mixing, which caused alternation between Spanish (L1) and English (L2) utterances, in the context of communicating with monolingual Spanish speakers. The authors [56] analysed this behaviour within the framework of Green's model [46] and developed a procedure called SBTT (Switch Back Through Translation), based on the fact that translation from English to Spanish would provide an economic strategy to switch back to the target language, as opposed to inhibiting the nontarget (English) language, a lost ability resulting from brain damage to the language control circuit [56]. The therapy was primarily administered in Spanish and resulted in significant improvement in naming nouns and verbs in Spanish, but, moreover, CLTE to English was as well observed, both with nouns and verbs. Using translation may favour CLTE by stimulating cognitive processes that are common to the two languages of the bilingual individual (i.e., cognitive control of language selection). Further studies are required to explore this hypothesis in depth.

4.2. Promoting CLTE in Bilingual Aphasia Therapy: Main Clinical Implications of Research Findings.

Despite the fact that more work is needed, research on CLTE in bilingual aphasia provides some cues as to the best approach of this clinical population.

In particular, the evidence suggests that language therapy focused on cognates facilitates CLTE. Thus, forming a list of cognates, consulting dictionaries developed for specific language pairs (e.g., Spanish-English: DOC—Dictionary of Cognates and the RDOC—Reverse Dictionary of Cognates [58, 59]) can help clinicians focus language therapy on stimuli with CLTE potential, communicative, and social relevance for the patients, their families, and caregivers. Furthermore, the MDOC project, which aims at joining the cognate matches for five language pairs (http://www.cognates.org/), will become an important resource in the management of bilinguals with aphasia. As for clangs, the evidence in healthy populations shows that their processing implies complex interactions with distinct semantic representations that share L1-L2 phonological forms, which may become particularly challenging for individuals with brain damage. Further research is required to shed light on this issue.

Regarding pre- or postmorbid proficiency, it is not easy to draw an absolute conclusion. Some studies [27, 38, 49–51] suggest that premorbid proficiency matters and that training the premorbid weaker language appears to facilitate CLTE, given that treating the weaker language has a greater effect on the stronger than the reverse. This has proven to be true for premorbidly unbalanced bilinguals and also for balanced bilinguals, who, after a stroke, showed an unbalanced language profile with distinct degrees of impairment in L1 and L2. On the other hand, other cases suggest that postmorbid proficiency is the determinant factor for successful CLTE [53]. Therefore, both premorbid and postmorbid proficiency should be considered when deciding the language of therapy, and, to do so, a thorough assessment of bilingual aphasia is a must.

Moreover, using translation as a CLT strategy may enhance the effects of therapy provided in one language to the untreated language. Translation equivalents are strongly linked, a factor that may facilitate CLTE. This approach may be particularly useful when damage excludes the cognitive control circuit, which supports the ability to switch between L1 and L2.

With respect to the anomia therapy approach, evidence suggests that Semantic Feature Analysis or a combination of this approach with phonological cueing may contribute to CLTE. Semantic Feature Analysis capitalizes on shared semantic representations across languages, and it has been shown to facilitate CLTE in bilinguals with aphasia [27]. Furthermore, the evidence with monolinguals shows that this approach triggers neuroplasticity in cases of severe anomia resulting from extensive brain damage [60].

Also, the impact of semantic and phonological approaches depending on the degree of L1-L2 cognate and clang density or global structural overlap needs to be explored. Hence, the evidence on healthy populations shows that processing structurally distant (i.e., unsimilar) languages entails greater cognitive demands [45]. Considering this evidence, it is likely that brain damage will hinder CLTE in bilinguals speaking distant languages, who suffer from aphasia.

Table 1 summarizes all studies discussed in Section 4.

TABLE 1

Study	Cognates	L1	L2	L3	Language family L1	Language family L2	Language family L3	Language proficiency L1	Language proficiency L2	Language proficiency L3	Therapy approach	Language of therapy	Successful transfer of therapy to untreated language
Roberts and Deslauriers (1999) [30]	×	French	English	NA	Roman	Germanic	NA	Pre-H	Pre-H	NA	NA	NA	NA
Kohnert (2004) [37]	×	Spanish	English	NA	Roman	Germanic	NA	Pre-H Post-I	Pre-H Post-L	NA	Lexical semantic retrieval strategies	L1	Cognates only
Kurland and Falcon (2011) [38]	×	Spanish	English	NA	Roman	Germanic	NA	Pre-H Post-I	Pre-I Post-L	NA	Semantic	L2	Noncognates, only
Goral et al. (2010) [47]	NA	Hebrew	Englis0068	French	Canaanite	Germanic	Roman	Pre-H Post-H	Pre-H Post-I	Pre-H Post-L	Morpho-syntactic skills and language production rate	L2	L3 only
Miertsch (2009) [48]	NA	German	English	French	German	Germanic	Roman	Pre-H Post-H	Pre-H Post-I	Pre-H Post-I	Semantic	L3	Only L2
Kiran and Iakupova (2011) [49]	NA	Russian	English	NA	Slavic	Germanic	NA	Pre-H Post-H	Pre-I Post-I	NA	Semantic	L2	L1
Marangolo et al. (2009) [51]	NA	Flemish	Italian	NA	Germanic	Roman	NA	Pre-H Post-I	Pre-H Post-I	NA	Picture-naming training	L2	yes
Edmonds and Kiran (2006) [50]/P1	NA	English	Spanish	NA	Germanic	Roman	NA	Pre-H Post-NR	Pre-I Post-NR	NA	Semantic feature analysis	L2	No
Edmonds and Kiran (2006) [50]/P2 and P3	NA	English	Spanish	NA	Germanic	Roman	NA	Pre-H Post-NR	Pre-I Post-NR	NA	Semantic feature analysis	L1 and L2	yes
Edmonds and Kiran (2006) [50], b/p1	NA	English	Spanish	NA	Germanic	Roman	NA	Pre-H Post-NR	Pre-I Post-NR	NA	Semantic feature analysis	L2 and L1	From L1 to L2 only
Edmonds and Kiran (2006) [50], b/p2	NA	Spanish	English	NA	Roman	Germanic	NA	Pre-H Post-NR	Pre-H Post-NR	NA	Semantic feature analysis	L1 and L2	From L1 to L2 only
Goral (2012) [53], P.1	NA	Hebrew	English	French	Canaanite	Germanic	Roman	Pre-H Post-H	Pre-H Post-I	Pre-H Post-L	Modified constraint-induced therapy	L2	L1
Goral (2012) [53], P.2	NA	Persian	German	English	Iranian	Germanic	Germanic	Pre-H Post-L	Pre-H Post-I	Pre-H Post-H	Modified constraint-induced therapy	L3, L1, and L2	From L2 to L3 only

TABLE 1: Continued.

	Cognates	L1	L2	L3	Language family L1	Language family L2	Language family L3	Language proficiency L1	Language proficiency L2	Language proficiency L3	Therapy approach	Language of therapy	Successful transfer of therapy to untreated language
Goral (2012) [53], P.3	NA	English	Hebrew	NA	Germanic	Canaanite	NA	Pre-H Post-H	Pre-I Post-I	NA	Modified constraint-induced therapy	L2	L1 but Negative
Goral (2012) [53], P.4	NA	Catalan	Spanish	French	Roman	Roman	Roman	Pre-H Post-H	Pre-H Post-H	Pre-I Post-I	Modified semantic feature analysis, sentence generate-on	L4: German, Pre-I, Post-I	L5: English Pre-I Post-I
Croft et al. (2011) [54]/P1–5	NA	Bengali	English	NA		Germanic	NA	Post-H for 3 Ps	Post-L for 2 Ps	NA	Phonological and semantic cueing	L1 and L2	For semantic cueing only
Abutalebi et al. (2009) [55]	NA	Spanish	Italian	NA	Roman	Roman	NA	Pre-H Post-L	Pre-H Post-L	NA	Phonological training	L2	No

5. Conclusion

Globalization imposes a number of challenges to the field of neurorehabilitation, including challenges in the clinical management of bilinguals with aphasia. In recent decades, the assessment and intervention techniques available to bilingual clinical populations have become a major clinical and research topic.

The study of intervention with bilingual aphasia populations has evolved from a descriptive perspective, mainly focused on case reports, to a neuropsychological and neurofunctional perspective, aimed at unveiling the cognitive and neural mechanisms underlying the behavioral patterns that characterize bilingual aphasia and its recovery. More and more, this avenue is focusing on disentangling the mechanisms that allow for transferring therapy effects from the treated to the untreated language. Most research has focused on anomia, the most widespread aphasia sign.

The literature suggests that cross-linguistic therapy effects are possible but depend on a number of factors. For example, both pre- and postmorbid proficiency factors can affect CLTE. Thus, while treating the premorbid weaker language can show CLTE benefits [27, 38, 49–51], cross-linguistic transfer of therapy effects are as well reported for eight cases whenever therapy is provided in the postmorbid stronger language or when proficiency after stroke is equivalent in both languages. Regarding therapy approach, the evidence from 16 studies reporting the type of therapy administered suggests that semantic approaches result in better CLTE than phonological approaches [54, 55]. Finally as for word types, cognates have better CLT potential than noncognates [30, 37], but the cognate advantage disappears when cognitive control circuits are damaged [38]. This is the case probably because of reduced excitatory and inhibitory resources secondary to the damage in the cognitive control circuit. This impairment prevents correct selection among highly overlapping and competing lexical units (i.e., cognates). Green's Activation, Control and Resource Model [46, 61] assumes that lexical selection of the target word requires sufficient inhibitory (to suppress the non-target node) and excitatory resources (to activate the target node). Furthermore, 11 studies having reported CLT effects show no evidence suggesting that language distance could play a role on the potential for CLT in bilingual aphasia therapy. Thus, among indo-European languages, therapy effects can transfer across languages regardless of what language family they belong to the Indo-European family of languages [37, 47–49, 51, 53, 54].

Major developments in the field can be expected in the years to come. By combining clinical aphasiology, cognitive models of bilingualism, functional neuroimaging, and functional connectivity analysis it will be possible to better understand the mechanism that subserve CLT of therapy effects, and thus design bilingual aphasia therapy approaches accordingly. This will increase the probability of recovery from bilingual aphasia, while optimizing health care efficiency, in terms of resource allocation and training.

References

[1] E. Bialystok, "Cognitive complexity and attentional control in the bilingual mind," *Child Development*, vol. 70, no. 3, pp. 636–644, 1999.

[2] E. Bialystok, "Cognitive effects of bilingualism across the lifespan," in *BUCLD 32: Proceedings of the 32nd Annual Boston University Conference on Language Development*, H. Chan, H. Jacob, and E. Kapia, Eds., pp. 1–15, Cascadilla Press, Boston, Mass, USA, 2008.

[3] A. L. Holland, "Living successfully with aphasia: three variations on the theme," *Topics in Stroke Rehabilitation*, vol. 13, no. 1, pp. 44–51, 2006.

[4] J. G. Centeno, "Bilingual development and communication: dynamics and implications in clinical language studies," in *Communication Disorders in Spanish Speakers: Theoretical, Research, and Clinical Aspects*, J. G. Centeno, R. T. Anderson, and L. K. Obler, Eds., pp. 46–56, Multilingual Matters, Clevedon, UK, 2007.

[5] J. G. Centeno, "Serving bilingual patients with aphasia: challenges, foundations, and procedures," *Revista de Logopedia, Foniatría y Audiología*, vol. 29, no. 1, pp. 30–36, 2009.

[6] A. I. Ansaldo, K. Marcotte, L. Scherer, and G. Raboyeau, "Language therapy and bilingual aphasia: clinical implications of psycholinguistic and neuroimaging research," *Journal of Neurolinguistics*, vol. 21, no. 6, pp. 539–557, 2008.

[7] F. Fabbro, "The bilingual brain: bilingual aphasia," *Brain and Language*, vol. 79, no. 2, pp. 201–210, 2001.

[8] F. Fabbro, "The bilingual brain: cerebral representation of languages," *Brain and Language*, vol. 79, no. 2, pp. 211–222, 2001.

[9] M. Paradis, "Assessing bilingual aphasia," in *Handbook of Cross-Cultural Neuropsychology*, B. Uzzell and A. Ardila, Eds., Lawrence Erlbaum Associates, Mahwah, NJ, USA, 2001.

[10] M. Paradis and G. Libben, *The Assessment of Bilingual Aphasia*, Lawrence Erlbaum Associates, Hillsdale, NJ, USA, 1987.

[11] A. L. Benton, A. Sivan, K. Hamsher, N. Varney, and O. Spreen, *Contributions to Neuropsychology Assessment: A Clinical Manual*, vol. 2, Oxford University Press, New York, NY, USA, 1994.

[12] P. Graetz, R. de Bleser, and K. Willmes, *Akense Afasia Test*, Swets and Zeitlinger, Liss, UK, 1992.

[13] W. Huber, K. Poeck, and D. Weniger, *Achener Aphasie Test (AAT)*, Hogrefe, Göttingen, Germany, 1983.

[14] N. Miller, K. Willmes, and R. de Bleser, "The psychometric properties of the English language version of the Aachen Aphasia Test (EAAT)," *Aphasiology*, vol. 14, no. 7, pp. 683–722, 2000.

[15] M. Laine, H. Goodglass, J. Niemi, P. Koivuselka-Sallinen, J. Toumainen, and R. Martilla, "Adaptation of the Boston diagnostic aphasia examination and the Boston naming test into Finnish," *Scandinavian Journal of Logopedics and Phoniatrics*, vol. 18, no. 2-3, pp. 83–92, 1993.

[16] I. Reinvang and R. Graves, "A basic aphasia examination: description with discussion of first results," *Scandinavian Journal of Rehabilitation Medicine*, vol. 7, no. 3, pp. 129–135, 1975.

[17] Roberts and P. Kiran S, "Assessment and treatment of bilingual aphasia and bilingual anomia," in *Speech and Language Disorders in Bilinguals*, A. Ardila and E. Ramos, Eds., Nova Science, New York, NY, USA, 2007.

[18] O. Spreen and A. H. Risser, *Assessment of Aphasia*, Oxford University Press, New York, NY, USA, 2003.

[19] Y. Faroqi-Shah, T. Frymark, R. Mullen, and B. Wang, "Effect of treatment for bilingual individuals with aphasia: a systematic review of the evidence," *Journal of Neurolinguistics*, vol. 23, no. 4, pp. 319–341, 2010.

[20] K. Kohnert, "Cross-language generalization following treatment in bilingual speakers with aphasia: a review," *Seminars in Speech and Language*, vol. 30, no. 3, pp. 174–186, 2009.

[21] M. H. Ebell, J. Siwek, B. D. Weiss et al., "Strength of recommendation taxonomy (SORT): a patient-centered approach to grading evidence in the medical literature," *The American Family Physician*, vol. 69, no. 3, pp. 548–556, 2004.

[22] M. L. Albert and L. K. Obler, *Neuropsychological and Neurolinguistic Aspects of Bilingualism*, Academic Press, London, UK, 1978.

[23] A. Costa, M. Santesteban, and A. Caño, "On the facilitatory effects of cognate words in bilingual speech production," *Brain and Language*, vol. 94, no. 1, pp. 94–103, 2005.

[24] D. Singleton and D. Little, "The second language lexicon: some evidence from university-level learners of French and German," *Second Language Research*, vol. 7, no. 1, pp. 61–81, 1991.

[25] T. Odlin, *Language Transfer: Cross-Linguistic Influence in Language Learning*, Cambridge University Press, New York, NY, USA, 1989.

[26] A. M. B. de Groot and G. L. J. Nas, "Lexical representation of cognates and noncognates in compound bilinguals," *Journal of Memory and Language*, vol. 30, no. 1, pp. 90–123, 1991.

[27] L. A. Edmonds and S. Kiran, "Confrontation naming and semantic relatedness judgements in Spanish/English bilinguals," *Aphasiology*, vol. 18, no. 5-7, pp. 567–579, 2004.

[28] S. Kiran and L. A. Edmonds, "Effect of semantic naming treatment on crosslinguistic generalization in bilingual aphasia," *Brain and Language*, vol. 91, no. 1, pp. 75–77, 2004.

[29] M. Meinzer, J. Obleser, T. Flaisch, C. Eulitz, and B. Rockstroh, "Recovery from aphasia as a function of language therapy in an early bilingual patient demonstrated by fMRI," *Neuropsychologia*, vol. 45, no. 6, pp. 1247–1256, 2007.

[30] P. M. Roberts and L. Deslauriers, "Picture naming of cognate and non-cognate nouns in bilingual aphasia," *Journal of Communication Disorders*, vol. 32, no. 1, pp. 1–22, 1999.

[31] J. G. van Hell and A. M. B. de Groot, "Conceptual representation in bilingual memory: effects of concreteness and cognate status in word association," *Bilingualism*, vol. 1, no. 3, pp. 193–211, 1998.

[32] I. K. Christoffels, C. Firk, and N. O. Schiller, "Bilingual language control: an event-related brain potential study," *Brain Research*, vol. 1147, no. 1, pp. 192–208, 2007.

[33] A. Costa, A. Caramazza, and N. Sebastián-Gallés, "The cognate facilitation effect: implications for models of lexical access," *Journal of Experimental Psychology: Learning, Memory, and Cognition*, vol. 265, pp. 1283–1296, 2000.

[34] T. H. Gollan, K. I. Forster, and R. Frost, "Translation priming with different scripts: Masked priming with cognates and noncognates in Hebrew-English bilinguals," *Journal of Experimental Psychology: Learning Memory and Cognition*, vol. 23, no. 5, pp. 1122–1139, 1997.

[35] I. Antón-Méndez and T. H. Gollan, "Not just semantics: strong frequency and weak cognate effects on semantic association in bilinguals," *Memory and Cognition*, vol. 38, no. 6, pp. 723–739, 2010.

[36] J. A. Duñabeitia, M. Perea, and M. Carreiras, "Masked translation priming effects with highly proficient simultaneous bilinguals," *Experimental Psychology*, vol. 57, no. 2, pp. 98–107, 2010.

[37] K. Kohnert, "Cognitive and cognate-based treatments for bilingual aphasia: a case study," *Brain and Language*, vol. 91, no. 3, pp. 294–302, 2004.

[38] J. Kurland and M. Falcon, "Effects of cognate status and language of therapy during intensive semantic naming treatment in a case of severe nonfluent bilingual aphasia," *Clinical Linguistics and Phonetics*, vol. 25, no. 6-7, pp. 584–600, 2011.

[39] J. Abutalebi and D. Green, "Bilingual language production: the neurocognition of language representation and control," *Journal of Neurolinguistics*, vol. 20, no. 3, pp. 242–275, 2007.

[40] J. E. Gracia-Albea and M. L. Sanchez-Bernardos, *Test de Gracia-Para el diagnostic de la afasia: Adaptaion Espanola*, Editorial Medica Panamericana, Madrid, Spain, 2nd edition, 1996.

[41] E. Lalor and K. Kirsner, "The representation of "false cognates" in the bilingual lexicon," *Psychonomic Bulletin and Review*, vol. 8, no. 3, pp. 552–559, 2001.

[42] K. E. Elston-Güttler, T. C. Gunter, and S. A. Kotz, "Zooming into L2: global language context and adjustment affect processing of interlingual homographs in sentences," *Cognitive Brain Research*, vol. 25, no. 1, pp. 57–70, 2005.

[43] J. F. Kroll and E. Stewart, "Category interference in translation and picture naming: evidence for asymmetric connections between bilingual memory representations," *Journal of Memory and Language*, vol. 33, no. 2, pp. 149–174, 1994.

[44] L. G. Saidi, V. Perlbarg, G. Marrelec, M. Pélégrini-Issac, H. Benali, and A. I. Ansaldo, "Second language neural networks at low and high proficiency levels: a functional connectivity study," *Brain and Language*, vol. 124, no. 1, pp. 56–65, 2013.

[45] L. Ghazi-Saidi and A. I. Ansaldo, "The neural correlates of phonological transfer effects across distant languages," in *Proceedings of the 18th Annual Meeting of the Organization for Human Brain Mapping*, Beijing, China, June 2012.

[46] D. W. Green, "Control, activation, and resource: a framework and a model for the control of speech in bilinguals," *Brain and Language*, vol. 27, no. 2, pp. 210–223, 1986.

[47] M. Goral, E. S. Levy, and R. Kastl, "Cross-language treatment generalisation: a case of trilingual aphasia," *Aphasiology*, vol. 24, no. 2, pp. 170–187, 2010.

[48] B. Miertsch, J. M. Meisel, and F. Isel, "Non-treated languages in aphasia therapy of polyglots benefit from improvement in the treated language," *Journal of Neurolinguistics*, vol. 22, no. 2, pp. 135–150, 2009.

[49] S. Kiran and R. Iakupova, "Understanding the relationship between language proficiency, language impairment and rehabilitation: evidence from a case study," *Clinical Linguistics and Phonetics*, vol. 25, no. 6-7, pp. 565–583, 2011.

[50] L. A. Edmonds and S. Kiran, "Effect of semantic naming treatment on crosslinguistic generalization in bilingual aphasia," *Journal of Speech, Language, and Hearing Research*, vol. 49, no. 4, pp. 729–748, 2006.

[51] P. Marangolo, C. Rizzi, P. Peran, F. Piras, and U. Sabatini, "Parallel recovery in a bilingual aphasic: a neurolinguistic and fMRI study," *Neuropsychology*, vol. 23, no. 3, pp. 405–409, 2009.

[52] D. Jared and J. F. Kroll, "Cognitive processes bilingual reading," in *Indyslexia Across Languages: Orthography and the Brain-Gene-Behavior Link*, P. McCardle, J. R. Lee, B. Miller, and O. Tzeng, Eds., pp. 262–280, Brookes Publishing, Baltimore, Md, USA, 2001.

[53] M. Goral, "Cross-language treatment effects in multilingual aphasia," in *Aspects of Multilingual Aphasia*, M. Gitterman, M. Goral, and L. K. Obler, Eds., chapter 7, Multilingual Matters, Bristol, UK, 2012.

[54] S. Croft, J. Marshall, T. Pring, and M. Hardwick, "Therapy for naming difficulties in bilingual aphasia: which language benefits?" *International Journal of Language and Communication Disorders*, vol. 46, no. 1, pp. 48–62, 2011.

[55] J. Abutalebi, P. A. D. Rosa, M. Tettamanti, D. W. Green, and S. F. Cappa, "Bilingual aphasia and language control: a follow-up fMRI and intrinsic connectivity study," *Brain and Language*, vol. 109, no. 2-3, pp. 141–156, 2009.

[56] A. I. Ansaldo, L. G. Saidi, and A. Ruiz, "Model-driven intervention in bilingual aphasia: evidence from a case of pathological language mixing," *Aphasiology*, vol. 24, no. 2, pp. 309–324, 2010.

[57] D. W. Green and J. Abutalebi, "Understanding the link between bilingual aphasia and language control," *Journal of Neurolinguistics*, vol. 21, no. 6, pp. 558–576, 2008.

[58] R. M. Molina, *Cognate Linguistics (Cognates)*, Kindle eBook, 2011.

[59] R. M. Molina, *The Dictionary of Cognates*, Kindle eBook, 2011.

[60] K. Marcotte, D. Adrover-Roig, B. Damien et al., "Therapy-induced neuroplasticity in chronic aphasia," *Neuropsychologia*, vol. 50, no. 8, pp. 1776–1786, 2012.

[61] D. W. Green, "Mental control of the bilingual lexico-semantic system," *Bilingualism: Language and Cognition*, vol. 1, no. 2, pp. 67–81, 1998.

17

Brain-Derived Neurotrophic Factor Polymorphism and Aphasia after Stroke

Nathan T. Lee,[1] Fatimah Ahmedy ⓘ,[1] Natiara Mohamad Hashim ⓘ,[2] Khin Nyein Yin ⓘ,[3] and Kai Ling Chin ⓘ[4]

[1]*Rehabilitation Medicine Unit, Faculty of Medicine & Health Sciences, Universiti Malaysia Sabah, Kota Kinabalu, Malaysia*
[2]*Department of Rehabilitation Medicine, Faculty of Medicine, Universiti Teknologi MARA, Sg. Buloh, Malaysia*
[3]*Department of Surgery, Faculty of Medicine & Health Sciences, Universiti Malaysia Sabah, Kota Kinabalu, Malaysia*
[4]*Department of Biomedical Sciences, Faculty of Medicine & Health Sciences, Universiti Malaysia Sabah, Kota Kinabalu, Malaysia*

Correspondence should be addressed to Fatimah Ahmedy; fatimahmedy@ums.edu.my

Academic Editor: Elisa Rubino

Stroke is one of the most deliberating causes of mortality and disability worldwide. Studies have implicated *Val66Met* polymorphism of the brain-derived neurotrophic factor (BDNF) gene as a genetic factor influencing stroke recovery. Still, the role of BDNF polymorphism in poststroke aphasia is relatively unclear. This review assesses the recent evidence on the association between the BDNF polymorphism and aphasia recovery in poststroke patients. The article highlights BNDF polymorphism characteristics, speech and language interventions delivered, and the influence of BNDF polymorphism on poststroke aphasia recovery. We conducted a literature search through PubMed and Google Scholar with the following terms: "brain derived-neurotrophic factor" and "aphasia" for original articles from January 2000 until June 2020. Out of 69 search results, a detailed selection process produced a total of 3 articles that met the eligibility criteria. All three studies included *Val66Met* polymorphism as the studied human BDNF gene. One of the studies demonstrated insufficient evidence to conclude that BDNF polymorphism plays a role in poststroke aphasia recovery. The remaining two studies have shown that *Met* allele genotype (either single or double nucleotides) was associated with poor aphasia recovery, in either acute or chronic stroke. Carriers of the *Val66Met* polymorphism of BDNF gave a poorer response to aphasia intervention and presented with more severe aphasia.

1. Introduction

Stroke is one of the leading causes of death and acquired disability globally [1]. In addition, many demographic and clinical factors have influenced poststroke recovery, including age, stroke severity, presence of cognitive impairment, and neuropsychological deficits [2]. Thus, there is an emerging interest in studying genetic factors and variations that influence stroke susceptibility and recovery [3]. One genetic variation of interest is the *Val66Met* single-nucleotide polymorphism of the brain-derived neurotrophic factor (BDNF) gene in humans, a potential clinically significant genetic variation associated with stroke risk and prognosis [3]. The BDNF *Val66Met* polymorphism structurally involves the substitution of the amino acid valine (*Val*), to methionine (*Met*), in the $5'$ ori-region of the human BDNF gene [4].

BDNF, being part of the neurotrophin family of growth factors, is believed to influence a wide range of aspects of the nervous system, including but not limited to neuronal migration, dendritic growth, synapse maintenance, and long-term plasticity [5]. However, the number of clinical research studies of the role of BDNF polymorphisms in stroke is limited, and the exact influence of BDNF polymorphisms underpinning the aspects of stroke severity, recovery, and functional outcome is still unclear [6].

The *Val66Met* of the BNDF gene, also known as rs6265, is only known to occur in humans and currently remains one of the most studied single-nucleotide polymorphisms of the BDNF gene [4]. In normal functioning, BDNF plays a significant neurological role in the modulation of hippocampal plasticity and hippocampal-dependent memory in humans and animals [4]. On the other hand, *Val66Met* mutation is associated with a reduction in the hippocampal tissue. Moreover, this mutation is linked hypothetically to several brain diseases, such as memory impairments and neuropsychiatric disorders [7].

The relationship between the language function and variations in the BDNF gene, however, is relatively less prominent. Nevertheless, evidence suggests that BDNF plays a significant role in learning and memory by inducing long-term potentiation (LTP), an essential form of synaptic plasticity [8]. A study by Winter et al. is aimed at investigating the effects of physical exercise and learning performance. They have demonstrated that the peripheral levels of BDNF were increased and sustained more strongly during learning (including language learning) after physical exercise in healthy adults. Here, it proved the role of BDNF as a mediator of exercise-induced learning improvement [9].

The main impetus of the present review is to investigate whether BDNF *Val66Met* polymorphism is associated with language function in people with poststroke aphasia. We hypothesized that the presence of the BDNF *Val66Met* polymorphism would affect the language function outcome after stroke.

2. Material and Methods

2.1. Search Methodology. Two reviewers conducted a literature search in PubMed and Google Scholar, with the following terms: "brain derived-neurotrophic factor" AND "aphasia" AND "stroke" for articles published from January 2011 to December 2020. The search results were then screened based on the subsequent inclusion and exclusion criteria. Any disagreements were resolved by consulting a third reviewer, if necessary.

2.2. Study Selection. The selected articles must be in English. We considered clinical studies that included BDNF evaluation as part of the main variables among adults with stroke (age 18 years and above). Case reports, review articles, technical reports, and thesis dissertation were excluded, as well as abstract-only publications. Studies that exclusively determined nonlanguage cognitive domains outcomes were also excluded.

2.3. Data Extraction and Recording. The following data were extracted and recorded: (i) details of article (title, author, year of publication, study design, and sample size); (ii) demographic and clinical characteristics of the studied population (mean age, type of stroke, and BDNF genotypes); and (iii) study outcomes (researched variables, interventions, outcome measures of assessment, and their corresponding

results). Being a review article, the authors did not request ethical approval as the articles were already published.

3. Results

The electronic search resulted in 10 records. After removing duplicates, screening all the titles and abstracts, and accessing full articles of seven studies, a total of 3 articles were selected based on the eligibility criteria. Figure 1 illustrates the PRISM flowchart on the selection process. Table 1 summarizes the characteristics and key findings of the selected articles.

3.1. BDNF Polymorphism Characteristics. All three studies included *Val66Met* single-nucleotide polymorphism as the studied human BDNF gene [10–12]. de Boer et al. [10] carried out a prospective follow-up study to investigate the effects of the function limiting *Val66Met* polymorphism of BDNF on the recovery of poststroke aphasia in acute stroke. They divided the affected individuals into two groups based on their BDNF genotype, namely, carriers (with at least 1 Met allele) and noncarriers (absence of *Met* allele) [10]. A randomized controlled trial by Fridriksson et al. [11] investigated the response of different carriers of BDNF genotypes on behavioural aphasia treatment in acute stroke, while Kristinsson et al. [12] conducted a cross-sectional study to investigate how BDNF genotype may influence functional brain activation in chronic aphasia. Both divided the groupings of polymorphism into typical and atypical—the former is grouped based on having the *Val66Val* allele, i.e., BDNF polymorphism in the absence of *Met* allele. In contrast, the latter has at least one *Met* allele, either the Val66Met or Met66Met.

3.2. Speech and Language Intervention for Poststroke Aphasia. Only two studies investigated the effect of the intervention on language outcomes [10, 11]. All participants studied by de Boer et al. [10] received 2 to 5 hours of speech and language therapy (SLT) per week throughout the intake period of 2 years. The primary outcomes were measured using the Amsterdam-Nijmegen Everyday Language Tests (ANELT) and Boston Naming Test (BNT), assessed at baseline and discharge, in which both measures demonstrated improvement over time [10]. All acute stroke participants in the study by Fridriksson et al. [11] received 15 computerized language aphasia treatments, which focused on picture-word matching for 45 minutes, five times per week for three weeks. They were randomized to receive either 1 mA of anodal tDCS (transcranial direct stimulation current) or sham tDCS to the left temporoparietal region for the first 20 minutes of each session [11]. The therapeutic response to tDCS was assessed using the Philadelphia Naming Test (PNT), "Naming 80" test, and Western Aphasia Battery (WAB) test at one week, four weeks, and 24 weeks posttreatment [11].

3.3. Influences of BDNF Polymorphism on Poststroke Aphasia Recovery. Even though there were improvements in both ANELT and BNT, de Boer et al. [10] failed to demonstrate significant differences in both performances between the two groups at discharge, despite a large discrepancy in the

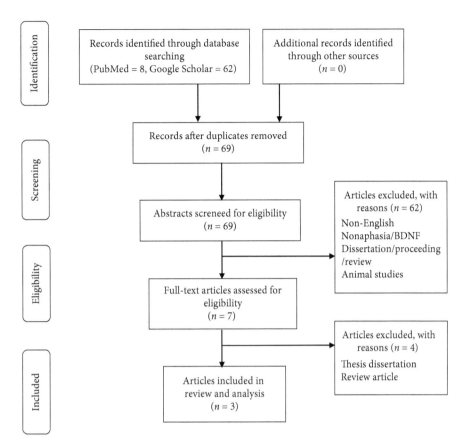

FIGURE 1: PRISM flowchart of the article selection process.

baseline scores and the improvement scores across both groups. The study did not control confounding variables, including stroke severity, conditions for discharge, and social factors in this study [10]. The differences in the improvements of both the ANELT and BNT between both groups were not statistically significant [10]. The findings from this preliminary study suggested that there is insufficient evidence to conclude that BDNF polymorphism plays a role in poststroke aphasia recovery.

Based on the study by Fridriksson et al. [11], the baseline aphasia quotient (AQ) scores from revised Western Aphasia Battery (WAB) demonstrated that atypical BDNF genotype carriers had a more severe aphasia presentation than typical BDNF genotype carriers [11]. This result was consistent with the presumption that the atypical BDNF genotype leads to lower levels of BDNF secretion during activity [11]. Moreover, typical BDNF genotype patients exhibited improvement in naming for both A-tDCS and sham tDCS interventions [11]. Interestingly, contrary to the results from de Boer et al.'s study [10], Fridriksson et al. [11] demonstrated that the BDNF Met allele genotype has an impact on language performance and improvement in stroke. Furthermore, the latter showed that Met allele carriers of the BDNF gene produced a more unsatisfactory response to aphasia treatment than Val66Val and other typical genotype carriers of BDNF, regardless of the language therapy delivered [11]. In addition, Fridriksson et al. found no differences for other factors such as semantic processing, executive func-

tion, stroke severity, age, lesion size, education, or time poststroke between both groups [11].

Kristinsson et al. [12] used functional magnetic resonance imaging (MRI) for visualizing the cortical activation and WAB for measuring language impairment in two groups of participants with chronic stroke based on typical or atypical BNDF polymorphism carrier status [12]. First, the naming-related activation lesion contrast maps showed a relatively lesser activation present in the right hemisphere of the atypical group than the typical group [12]. Following this, they further quantified the MRI finding by obtaining the number of voxels present in predetermined regions of functional naming-related activated regions for each group of participants at the whole-brain level and both the left and right hemispheres, respectively and separately [12]. The typical genotype group demonstrated a higher number of activated voxels than the atypical group at both the whole-brain and right hemispheres [12].

In addition, participants in the atypical BDNF group had an overall greater aphasia severity on the revised-WAB-AQ than that of typical BDNF carriers of chronic stroke [12]. The findings of this study suggest that cortical brain activation is potentially mediated by BDNF genotypes, with reduced cortical activation of Met allele carriers [12]. There were no significant differences between both groups for baseline stroke severity, baseline aphasia severity, and executive functioning [12]. Age, racial distribution, education, lesion size, amount of exercise, or stroke

TABLE 1: A summary of the included studies examining the effect of BDNF Val66Met single-nucleotide polymorphism on the recovery of poststroke aphasia.

Authors, year	Study design, sample size, mean age	Stroke type	BDNF genotypes	Intervention	Outcome assessment	Results/findings
de Boer et al., 2017 [10]	Prospective cohort study, 53 subjects, 58.5 years	Acute (ischemic and hemorrhagic)	(i) Val66Met allele present (ii) Val66Met allele absent	SLT for 2-5 hours per week	(1) ANELT (2) BNT	No significant differences between carriers of both alleles in improvement scores on both the ANELT and BNT
Fridriksson et al., 2018 [11]	Randomized controlled trial, 74 subjects (BDNF genotype available for 67), 61.7 years	Acute (ischemic and hemorrhagic)	(i) Atypical (Val/Met, Met/Met) (ii) Typical (Val/Val)	Received either 1 mA A-tDCS or sham tDCS for 20 mins per session for 5×/week for 3 weeks	(1) Naming 80 (2) PNT (3) WAB-R AQ	Atypical BDNF carriers showed significantly poorer response to A-tDCS than typical BDNF carriers who received both A-tDCS and S-tDCS; Atypical BDNF carriers associated with poorer AQ scores at baseline compared to typical BDNF carriers
Kristinsson et al., 2019 [12]	Cross-sectional study, 87 subjects, 61.7 years	Chronic (ischemic and hemorrhagic)	(i) Atypical (Val66Met, Met66Met) (ii) Typical (Val66Val)	Not applicable	(1) WAB AQ (2) PNT (3) fMRI activation map analysis (4) Activated voxels at the whole-brain level	Atypical BDNF carriers significantly have more severe aphasia on WAB-AQ and performed significantly better in PNT compared to typical BDNF carriers; No group differences between intensity of cortical activation across both groups; The number of activated voxels was significantly lower in atypical BDNF carriers compared to typical BDNF carriers

BDNF: brain-derived neurotrophic factor; SLT: speech and language therapy; ANELT: Amsterdam-Nijmegen Everyday Language Test; BNT: Boston Naming Test; tDCS: transcranial direct current stimulation; A-tDCS: anodal tDCS; S-tDCS: sham tDCS; PNT: Philadelphia Naming Test; WAB: Western Aphasia Battery; WAB-R: Western Aphasia Battery, Revised; AQ: aphasia quotient; MRI: magnetic resonance imaging; fMRI: functional MRI.

severity differed between the two groups but reached non-significant levels [12].

4. Discussion

The majority of the results are primarily in line with established evidence when evaluating the impacts of BDNF polymorphism on poststroke outcomes [3, 6]. Typically, carriers of the *Met* allele of BDNF presented with poorer long-term functional outcomes after stroke [13, 14].

In addition, specific polymorphisms in the human BDNF gene are often linked to greater cognitive performance, including learning and memory, attention, and executive functions [4, 5]. Thus, it would be reasonable to assume that certain genetic variations in the BDNF gene are affiliated with language production and comprehension.

From the literature search performed, only three studies yielded the investigation of the correlation between language impairment or aphasia in stroke and BDNF genotypes, highly suggesting that knowledge in this topic of interest is relatively new and limited. Based on these findings, the *Val66Met* polymorphism of BDNF is linked with more severe aphasia at baseline [11, 12], poorer improvement in language improvement with time [11], and reduced cortical activation [12]. However, the exact role of BDNF polymorphisms in language performance and recovery in stroke may require further investigation.

The findings of de Boer et al. [10] demonstrated that the BDNF genotype is not specific to language performance and improvement, in contrast to the results of the other selected studies, which showed that BDNF genotypes are involved in the language outcome in stroke [13, 14]. Several possible explanations can be stipulated for such discrepancy. First, the study by de Boer et al. [10] received a relatively higher frequency of SLT compared to the intervention in [11]. In contrast, the study by Kristinsson et al. [12] did not account for the presence of SLT. Secondly, there were different standardized aphasia tests to assess aphasia: Dutch [10] and English [11, 12]. Here, the potential effects of bilingualism or multilingualism might require further investigation. Evidence suggests that bilingualism may be protective for adults with aphasia, possibly contributing to cognitive reserve in adults with aphasia [15]. Another consideration in these three prospective studies is the distinction between language recovery and language learning processes during stroke rehabilitation [10]. The significant variation in the improvement scores on the ANT and BNT further complicated the ability to detect significant differences between groups. Lastly, apraxia, which may affect the study results, was not excluded from the study [10].

Although the *Val66Met* allele of BDNF is associated with poorer language performance after tDCS intervention in poststroke aphasia [11], Marangolo et al. [16] demonstrated that the tDCS does not significantly alter the levels of BDNF on chronic aphasia patients. Thus, despite observing improvement in the scores of language performance, BDNF

is not solely responsible for such improvement in language recovery after stroke. Fridriksson et al. [11] have hypothesized that this finding could be due to anodal tDCS (A-tDCS) dependence on baseline levels of BDNF secretion.

Contrary to the current theory that the *Met* allele of BDNF is linked with the defective intracellular secretion of BDNF, Lang et al. [17] have demonstrated that the *Val66Met* polymorphism of BDNF is associated with increased BDNF serum concentrations instead in healthy subjects. Furthermore, Lang et al. [17] postulated that the *Met* allele does not affect the constitutive secretion of BDNF but rather decreases the amount of activity-dependent BDNF secretion. Interestingly, Gajewski et al. [18] have shown that healthy elderly carriers of the Met allele of BDNF *Val66Met* outperformed homozygote (*Val/Val*) carriers of BDNF in task switching based on a cue-based and memory-based task. Their findings hypothesized that the *Met* allele contributes to more efficient cognitive processes under particular circumstances in healthy elderly subjects [18].

In addition, a study by Jasińska et al. [19] investigating the effects of BDNF *Val66Met* polymorphism on reading ability in children has shown that *Met* allele carriers of the BDNF gene experienced greater neural activation in the reading-related regions of the brain during a reading task. The performance of the *Met* allele carriers suggests that the BDNF polymorphism may be associated with phonological working memory, which is crucial in reading ability [19]. Moreover, Freundlieb et al. [20] have failed to find an association between BDNF *Val66Met* polymorphism and implicit short-term associative language learning paradigms in healthy adults.

Despite appreciating many established associations between variations of BDNF gene in stroke [3] with cognitive impairment and psychiatric disorders [7], the pondering question is whether BDNF can be considered a "disease susceptibility gene". For stroke, BDNF *Val66Met* polymorphism is associated with long-term functional outcomes, with *Met* allele carriers exhibiting poorer modified Rankin scale scores [14, 15]. Nevertheless, there were weak associations between the BNDF gene and psychiatric conditions such as bipolar disorder [21]. Petryshen et al. [21] suggested that the variability in BDNF associations with psychiatric disorders could be attributed to the differences in population genetic structure. Hence, the diversity of BDNF polymorphism among worldwide populations would provide important implications for the implementation of further studies on poststroke aphasia. Furthermore, Kim et al. [13] have suggested that ethnic variability in the frequency of distribution of alleles may affect the positive findings to detect associations between BDNF genotypes and stroke outcomes.

Therefore, the BDNF gene may show a significant association with aphasia recovery after stroke, with the *Met* allele of the gene linked to poorer language recovery. In conclusion, some evidence suggests that polymorphism in the BDNF gene may modulate language recovery in poststroke aphasia. However, future research would be required to understand better the relationship between BDNF genetic variations and poststroke aphasia.

4.1. Study Limitations. The current review has several limitations. Firstly, there are a relatively limited number of original articles on the topic of BDNF polymorphism and poststroke aphasia-related outcomes, most prominently in the scope of BDNF genotypes. Hence, making strong inferences from a limited set of results concerning a topic as complex as the role of genetic polymorphism in aphasia would be challenging. In addition, there is variability in the parameters, interventions, and outcome measures utilized by the researchers. Finally, certain uncontrolled variables such as time of onset after stroke, type of aphasia, and presence and intensity of SLT have rendered the study populations as heterogeneous groups, which may have led to insufficient evidence for further statistical meta-analysis. These limitations justify future studies to explore the association between BDNF polymorphism and poststroke aphasia especially considering the emergence of neuromodulation therapy that promotes language improvement. In addition, establishing a more objective connection between these genotyping and the recovery of aphasia after stroke would enhance a better patients' selection for better utilization of resources.

5. Conclusion

There is some evidence suggesting that the *Met* allele of BDNF is associated with poorer language outcome in post-stroke patients, in both acute and chronic stages. Further works are warranted to investigate this association to explore future treatments and strategies, which may produce therapeutic effects more efficiently for stroke patients. Employing an assumption that BDNF *Val66Met* polymorphism influences the severity and recovery of aphasia, identifying specific alleles of BDNF as a predictor for aphasia severity and recovery may be the next step targeting selective therapeutic strategies in stroke patients. However, our current understanding of the influence of specific genes in aphasia recovery is still relatively limited. Based on the findings of the selected articles, it seems that a correlation between BDNF polymorphism and aphasia recovery exists, although the exact mechanisms underpinning this effect are still unclear. Advancement in the study of the genetic influencers of aphasia may provide more efficient therapies for people with aphasia, therefore potentially improving the current prognosis of aphasia.

Acknowledgments

This work is supported by a research grant from Universiti Malaysia Sabah (grant number: GUG4581/2020).

References

[1] G. A. Donnan, M. Fisher, M. Macleod, and S. M. Davis, "Stroke," *The Lancet*, vol. 371, no. 9624, pp. 1612–1623, 2008.

[2] M. Kotila, O. Waltimo, M. L. Niemi, R. I. Laaksonen, and M. A. Lempinen, "The profile of recovery from stroke and factors influencing outcome," *Stroke*, vol. 15, no. 6, pp. 1039–1044, 1984.

[3] M. Balkaya and S. Cho, "Genetics of stroke recovery: BDNF val66met polymorphism in stroke recovery and its interaction with aging," *Neurobiology of Disease*, vol. 126, pp. 36–46, 2019.

[4] M. F. Egan, M. Kojima, J. H. Callicott et al., "The BDNF val66-met polymorphism affects activity-dependent secretion of BDNF and human memory and hippocampal function," *Cell*, vol. 112, no. 2, pp. 257–269, 2003.

[5] A. K. McAllister, "BDNF," *Current Biology*, vol. 12, no. 9, article R310, 2002.

[6] T. M. Stanne, A. Tjärnlund-Wolf, S. Olsson, K. Jood, C. Blomstrand, and C. Jern, "Genetic variation at the BDNF locus: evidence for association with long-term outcome after ischemic stroke," *PLoS One*, vol. 9, no. 12, article e114156, 2014.

[7] K. G. Bath and F. S. Lee, "Variant BDNF (Val66Met) impact on brain structure and function," *Cognitive, Affective, & Behavioral Neuroscience*, vol. 6, no. 1, pp. 79–85, 2006.

[8] C. Cunha, R. Brambilla, and K. L. Thomas, "A simple role for BDNF in learning and memory?," *Frontiers in Molecular Neuroscience*, vol. 3, p. 1, 2010.

[9] B. Winter, C. Breitenstein, F. C. Mooren et al., "High impact running improves learning," *Neurobiology of Learning and Memory*, vol. 87, no. 4, pp. 597–609, 2007.

[10] R. G. de Boer, K. Spielmann, M. H. Heijenbrok-Kal, R. van der Vliet, G. M. Ribbers, and W. M. van de Sandt-Koenderman, "The role of the BDNF Val66Met polymorphism in recovery of aphasia after stroke," *Neurorehabilitation and Neural Repair*, vol. 31, no. 9, pp. 851–857, 2017.

[11] J. Fridriksson, J. Elm, B. C. Stark et al., "BDNF genotype and tDCS interaction in aphasia treatment," *Brain Stimulation*, vol. 11, no. 6, pp. 1276–1281, 2018.

[12] S. Kristinsson, G. Yourganov, F. Xiao et al., "Brain-derived neurotrophic factor genotype-specific differences in cortical activation in chronic aphasia," *Journal of Speech, Language, and Hearing Research*, vol. 62, no. 11, pp. 3923–3936, 2019.

[13] J. M. Kim, R. Stewart, M. S. Park et al., "Associations of BDNF genotype and promoter methylation with acute and long-term stroke outcomes in an East Asian cohort," *PLoS One*, vol. 7, no. 12, article e51280, 2012.

[14] J. Zhao, H. Wu, L. Zheng, Y. Weng, and Y. Mo, "Brain-derived neurotrophic factor G196A polymorphism predicts 90-day outcome of ischemic stroke in Chinese: a novel finding," *Brain Research*, vol. 1537, pp. 312–318, 2013.

[15] M. Dekhtyar, S. Kiran, and T. Gray, "Is bilingualism protective for adults with aphasia?," *Neuropsychologia*, vol. 139, p. 107355, 2020.

[16] P. Marangolo, V. Fiori, F. Gelfo et al., "Bihemispheric tDCS enhances language recovery but does not alter BDNF levels in chronic aphasic patients," *Restorative Neurology and Neuroscience*, vol. 32, no. 2, pp. 367–379, 2014.

[17] U. E. Lang, R. Hellweg, T. Sander, and J. Gallinat, "The Met allele of the BDNF Val66Met polymorphism is associated with

increased BDNF serum concentrations," *Molecular Psychiatry*, vol. 14, no. 2, pp. 120–122, 2009.

[18] P. D. Gajewski, J. G. Hengstler, K. Golka, M. Falkenstein, and C. Beste, "The Met-allele of the BDNF Val66Met polymorphism enhances task switching in elderly," *Neurobiology of Aging*, vol. 32, no. 12, pp. 2327.e7–2327.e19, 2011.

[19] K. K. Jasińska, P. J. Molfese, S. A. Kornilov et al., "The BDNF Val66Met polymorphism influences reading ability and patterns of neural activation in children," *PLoS One*, vol. 11, no. 8, article e0157449, 2016.

[20] N. Freundlieb, S. Philipp, S. A. Schneider et al., "No association of the BDNF Val66met polymorphism with implicit associative vocabulary and motor learning," *PLoS One*, vol. 7, no. 11, article e48327, 2012.

[21] T. L. Petryshen, P. C. Sabeti, K. A. Aldinger et al., "Population genetic study of the brain-derived neurotrophic factor (*BDNF*) gene," *Molecular Psychiatry*, vol. 15, no. 8, pp. 810–815, 2010.

18

Maladaptive Plasticity in Aphasia: Brain Activation Maps Underlying Verb Retrieval Errors

Kerstin Spielmann,[1,2] **Edith Durand,**[3] **Karine Marcotte,**[4] **and Ana Inés Ansaldo**[3,4]

[1]*Rijndam Rehabilitation Institute, P.O. Box 23181, 3001 KD Rotterdam, Netherlands*
[2]*Erasmus MC, University Medical Center Rotterdam, Department of Rehabilitation Medicine, P.O. Box 2040, 3000 CA Rotterdam, Netherlands*
[3]*Centre de Recherche de l'Institut Universitaire de Gériatrie de Montréal, 4565 Chemin Queen-Mary, Montréal, QC, Canada H3W 1W5*
[4]*École d'Orthophonie et d'Audiologie, Université de Montréal, 7077 Avenue du Parc, Montréal, QC, Canada H3N 1X7*

Correspondence should be addressed to Kerstin Spielmann; kspielmann@rijndam.nl

Academic Editor: Malgorzata Kossut

Anomia, or impaired word retrieval, is the most widespread symptom of aphasia, an acquired language impairment secondary to brain damage. In the last decades, functional neuroimaging techniques have enabled studying the neural basis underlying anomia and its recovery. The present study aimed to explore maladaptive plasticity in persistent verb anomia, in three male participants with chronic nonfluent aphasia. Brain activation maps associated with semantic verb paraphasia occurring within an oral picture-naming task were identified with an event-related fMRI paradigm. These maps were compared with those obtained in our previous study examining adaptive plasticity (i.e., successful verb naming) in the same participants. The results show that activation patterns related to semantic verb paraphasia and successful verb naming comprise a number of common areas, contributing to both maladaptive and adaptive neuroplasticity mechanisms. This finding suggests that the segregation of brain areas provides only a partial view of the neural basis of verb anomia and successful verb naming. Therefore, it indicates the importance of network approaches which may better capture the complexity of maladaptive and adaptive neuroplasticity mechanisms in anomia recovery.

1. Introduction

Anomia, or impaired word retrieval, is the most prominent and widespread symptom of aphasia, an acquired language impairment that can result from a focal brain lesion [1]. In the context of oral word retrieval, different types of errors (i.e., paraphasia) can occur, including phonemic paraphasia, semantic paraphasia, neologisms, and circumlocutions (i.e., using devious ways to describe words) [2].

The present study focuses on semantic paraphasia in the context of verb retrieval. Verbs carry a critical meaning since they have important functions in the structural formulation of sentences [3]. Therefore, verb paraphasia has a considerable impact on an individual's capacity to convey meaning, which can lead to a substantial handicap. Semantic verb paraphasia occurs when a target verb is replaced by a semantically related verb [4], such as saying "running" instead of "walking." Research on the cognitive mechanisms underlying the production of semantic paraphasia shows that these may result from impaired phonological processing or impaired semantic processing or a combination of both [5].

Functional neuroimaging techniques allow studying the neural basis underlying verb production and anomia and its recovery. The neural substrate of verb production involves a left frontal cortical network, including the left prefrontal cortex [6], the left superior parietal lobule, the left superior temporal gyrus [7], the left superior frontal gyrus [8], and the primary motor cortex, in the posterior portion of the precentral gyrus [9–11]. In the context of verb anomia, the production of semantic paraphasia may reflect damage of these language-related areas, as well as an attempt to compensate for the impairments resulting from this brain damage as there is a semantic relation between the target and response [12]. This attempt to compensate can be related to the concept of neuroplasticity which refers to a number of brain mechanisms involved in learning and relearning and can be reflected by changes in brain activation patterns highlighted by functional magnetic resonance imaging (fMRI).

Two main forms of neuroplasticity have been studied: functional reactivation, which occurs when previously damaged and inactive areas recover their function after a latency period [13], and functional reorganization, which reflects compensation of the permanent damage of specific brain areas by the recruitment of some other areas not previously involved in language processing [12]. Different types of neuroplasticity may occur during anomia recovery: if this results in functional recovery (as reflected by successful word retrieval), neuroplasticity is defined as adaptive, whereas when errors (such as paraphasia) persist neuroplasticity is considered to be maladaptive [14, 15].

There is an ongoing debate regarding the functional reorganization in anomia recovery and whether these compensatory processes reflect adaptive or maladaptive plasticity. The left cerebral hemisphere (LH) is considered the dominant hemisphere in language processing, at least in right-handed individuals [17]. The fMRI literature has many reports in which LH damage is followed by a shift of language processing to the right cerebral hemisphere (RH), that is, laterality shift [18–21]. However, the extent to which this RH shift reflects adaptive or maladaptive neuroplasticity remains controversial. Some studies focus on the benefits of RH recruitment [22] and emphasize the role of the RH in language processing in healthy subjects [23]. Others suggest that RH recruitment leads to persistent errors, reflecting maladaptive plasticity [24]. Compared to the LH, the RH may have broad overlapping semantic maps: in this case, lexical selection processing would be less semantically specified and would be associated with semantic paraphasia [25]. Another view is that RH recruitment could be beneficial in the short term whereas, in the long term, it could contribute to an incomplete or less efficient improvement compared with a better recovery sustained by the reactivation of LH language processing areas [19–21, 26–28]. Moreover, the extent to which RH recruitment is adaptive or maladaptive may depend on lesion size [12, 27]. These latter authors argue that while minimal damage to core language processing areas leads to maladaptive RH recruitment, extended LH lesions may trigger adaptive RH recruitment by release of the RH potential to process language. Overall, the literature presents a largely negative view on the impact of RH recruitment in the context of aphasia and anomia recovery, in particular in cases of moderate LH damage.

One way of examining the extent of LH and RH recruitment in anomia recovery is by calculating a lateralization index (LI) using fMRI data. The LI reflects hemispheric dominance in terms of the number of activated voxels observed in the context of a specific language task [29]. This index can express the relative contribution of either hemisphere to the processing of specific information, which can be linked to behavioral performance. Several studies have examined the relative contribution of either cerebral

hemisphere to anomia recovery within the context of specific and intensive language therapy and by reference to principles of experience-dependent neuroplasticity, derived from animal research [14, 15]. These studies investigated the neurofunctional markers of adaptive plasticity and link right and left hemisphere performance to posttherapy behavior by correlating activation patterns to posttherapy scores on naming tasks [30, 31].

Other studies used noninvasive brain stimulation techniques to modulate cortical excitability in either hemisphere, using repetitive transcranial magnetic stimulation (rTMS) and transcranial direct current stimulation (tDCS). rTMS generates magnetic fields and this can either activate or inhibit neurons. rTMS inhibiting RH areas can significantly reduce speech-error production in nonfluent aphasia [32, 33]. Inhibiting the right pars triangularis (part of the right inferior frontal gyrus) with rTMS improves naming accuracy and decreases naming latency, while activating the right pars opercularis decreases naming accuracy and improves naming latency [33]. With tDCS, a low current can be applied to the brain and, depending on the polarity, it can either enhance (anodal tDCS) or inhibit neural activity (cathodal tDCS) in a certain area. Studies using tDCS mostly combine tDCS with word-finding therapy and find an additional effect of tDCS on naming performance [34, 35]. In summary, rTMS/tDCS studies aim to modulate adaptive plasticity, either by inhibiting RH areas or by enhancing LH areas.

In general, most of the fMRI literature on the recovery from anomia adopts a segregation approach in the analysis of fMRI activation patterns. This is a within-area approach, based on activation changes occurring in isolation [36]. For example, a brain area found to be critical in successful naming is the left Brodmann area 22, which includes the superior temporal gyrus [12, 37]. Another perspective, the integration perspective, gathers brain activation patterns within coherent networks supporting a specific behavior; for example, functional connectivity analysis can be used to study networks of language processing in healthy and brain-damaged populations [38, 39].

In summary, research on the neural basis of anomia recovery has mostly focused on segregating brain areas whose activation is associated either with persistent anomia (i.e., paraphasia), reflecting maladaptive neuroplasticity, or with recovery (i.e., successful naming), reflecting adaptive neuroplasticity. Within this perspective, rTMS/tDCS has been used to modulate RH takeover by inhibiting RH areas, traditionally associated with maladaptive neuroplasticity, or by enhancing LH areas related to adaptive neuroplasticity. However, there is limited knowledge regarding the specific areas whose activation is associated either with the production of paraphasia or with successful naming.

The present study aims to examine maladaptive and adaptive neuroplasticity processes in the context of verb anomia recovery in aphasia. Three participants with nonfluent chronic aphasia were examined in the context of a picture-naming task during event-related fMRI scanning. Activation patterns related to the production of semantic paraphasia were obtained and compared with our previous study that

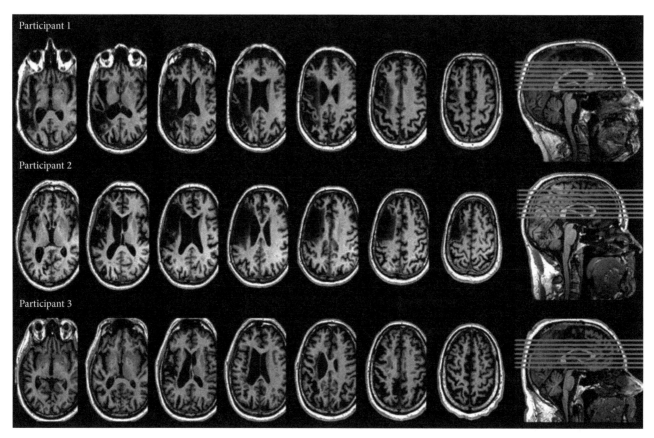

FIGURE 1: Lesion location for Participant 1, Participant 2, and Participant 3.

focused on adaptive plasticity, that is, successful verb naming [16]. The relative contribution of the LH and RH to semantic paraphasia and successful naming is explored by calculating an LI.

2. Materials and Methods

2.1. Experimental Design. The fMRI blood oxygenation level-dependent (BOLD) responses associated with the production of semantic paraphasia produced in the context of verb naming were compared to those related to successful verb naming. BOLD responses were collected in the context of an oral picture-naming verb task within an event-related fMRI paradigm.

2.2. Participants. Three male participants from the sample of Marcotte et al. [40], diagnosed with moderate to severe Broca's aphasia, were examined. Inclusion criteria were as follows: (1) a single LH stroke, (2) a diagnosis of moderate to severe aphasia, according to the Montreal-Toulouse battery [41], (3) the presence of anomia in a standardized naming task [42], (4) having French as their mother tongue, and (5) being right-handed prior to the stroke. Exclusion criteria were as follows: (1) the presence of a neurological or psychiatric diagnosis other than stroke, (2) incompatibility with fMRI testing, or (3) a diagnosis of mild cognitive impairment or dementia prior to stroke, based on medical charts, speech-pathology

TABLE 1: Demographic characteristics of the three participants (adapted from Durand [16]).

	Participant 1	Participant 2	Participant 3
Age (years)	67	67	66
Gender	Male	Male	Male
Months after stroke	72	54	241
Years of education	20	15	12
Lesion volume (cm^3)	167.84	117.84	84.77

reports, and information from the family. The study was approved by the Ethics Committee of the Regroupement Neuroimagerie/Québec (Canada); all participants provided written informed consent.

Lesion location differed between the participants. Participant 1 (P1) presented a left frontoparietal-temporal lesion, whereas Participants 2 (P2) and 3 (P3) presented a left frontotemporal lesion (Figure 1).

Table 1 presents demographic data; participants were comparable in terms of age and chronic status, and all had extended brain lesions in the left hemisphere (chi-square test: age, $p = 0.223$; months after stroke, $p = 0.199$; years of education, $p = 0.199$; lesion volume, $p = 0.199$).

2.3. Procedure

2.3.1. Language Assessment.
Aphasia profiles were determined with the Montreal-Toulouse 86 [41]. To ensure stable performance, two baseline naming assessments were obtained before the fMRI study. This baseline assessment was used to select stimuli for the Semantic Feature Analysis therapy, in order to provide personalized therapy (for details, see Marcotte et al. [40]). The selection was done on the basis of individual performance on the Snodgrass and Vanderwart items [42], including object images, and ColorCards® [43], including pictures depicting action verbs.

The present study focused on the ColorCards [43] which included 120 pictures. A total of 80 pictures (60 incorrectly named verbs and 20 correctly named verbs) were selected for the oral picture-naming task during the fMRI session. In addition, 20 digitally distorted images of a subset of these pictures were added as control stimuli.

2.3.2. fMRI Session: Stimuli and Procedure.
Participants underwent a practice session in the mock scanner to become accustomed to the scanner noise and environment during the fMRI session. During this session, they were also trained to avoid head movements while naming the stimuli. The stimuli for the picture-naming task (ColorCards) and the control stimuli (i.e., computerized distorted pictures) were projected on a white background by means of a series of mirrors and in a random fashion. Each picture was presented for 4500 ms with an interstimulus interval ranging from 4500 to 8500 ms. Participants were asked to name the pictures representing verbs as accurately as possible, avoiding head movements. In the control condition, participants had to say "BABA" when a computerized distorted picture was presented. Oral and event-related BOLD responses were collected.

2.3.3. Functional Neuroimaging Parameters.
Images were acquired using a 3T MRI Siemens Trio scanner, with a standard 8-channel head coil. The image sequence was a $T2^*$-weighted pulse sequence (TR = 2200 ms; TE = 30 ms; matrix = 64 × 64 voxels; FOV = 192 mm; flip angle = 90°; slice thickness = 3 mm; acquisition = 36 slides in the axial plane, with a distance factor of 25%, so as to scan the whole brain, including the cerebellum). A high-resolution structural image was obtained before the two functional runs using a 3D T1-weighted pulse sequence (TR = 2300 ms; TE = 2.91 ms; 160 slices; matrix = 256 × 256 mm; voxel size = 1 × 1 × 1 mm; FOV = 256 mm). The protocol was designed in an event-related fashion so that BOLD responses corresponding to each image could be identified.

2.4. Data Analysis

2.4.1. Behavioral and fMRI Data Analysis.
Average response times and error rates were calculated for four subtypes of errors: semantic paraphasia, phonological paraphasia, neologism, and circumlocutions. Only semantic paraphasia was produced in a sufficient number to perform fMRI data analysis for all three participants. Therefore, the event-related fMRI responses to semantic paraphasia were analyzed

TABLE 2: Error rates and the type of paraphasia produced by each participant.

	Participant 1	Participant 2	Participant 3
Semantic paraphasia	60	15	47
Phonological paraphasia	0	0	0
Neologism	0	0	0
Circumlocution	0	32	0

following the same procedures as described by Marcotte et al. [40] and Durand [16]. Activation maps were obtained for each participant by subtracting BOLD responses in the control condition from those obtained in the trials where the answer provided was semantic paraphasia. t-tests, performed on each voxel, were considered significant with a cluster size $(k) \geq 10$ voxels and a p value < 0.005. Individual activation maps, including significantly activated brain areas, were determined within the framework of the Talairach atlas [44] and transformed from Talairach space to the spatial coordinates in the Montreal Neurological Institute space [45]. BOLD responses on successful verb naming were examined in our previous study that included the same three participants [16]. In this previous study, BOLD responses in the control condition were subtracted from those obtained in the trials where the answer provided was a correct answer.

Furthermore, an LI [29] was calculated for each participant to estimate the relative contribution of the LH and the RH to the production of semantic paraphasia and successful naming, respectively. Regarding successful naming, data from Durand [16] were used. We applied Lehéricy's algorithm [29], as follows: (LH − RH)/(LH + RH), by which a positive LI corresponds to a LH dominant contribution; strong left lateralization is represented by an LI ranging from 0.5 to 1.0, and weak left lateralization is represented by an LI ranging from 0.25 to 0.5. A negative LI corresponds to a predominant RH contribution; strong right lateralization is represented by an LI ranging from −1.0 to −0.5, and weak right lateralization is represented by an LI ranging from −0.5 to −0.25. An LI ranging from −0.25 to 0.25 represents a symmetric contribution of the left and right hemispheres to processing.

3. Results and Discussion

3.1. Behavioral Results.
Average response times were calculated for paraphasia production; however, due to technical issues these data were not available for analysis. For the 80 pictures, Table 2 presents the error rates and the types of paraphasia produced by each participant during the event-related fMRI study. P1 produced 60 semantic paraphasias and 20 correct responses; P2 produced 15 semantic paraphasias, 32 circumlocutions, and 33 correct responses; and P3 produced 47 semantic paraphasias and 33 correct responses. Only semantic paraphasias were produced in a sufficient number to perform fMRI data analysis for all three participants.

3.2. fMRI Results

3.2.1. Single-Subject Brain Activation Maps. Brain activation maps corresponding to maladaptive plasticity, that is, production of semantic paraphasia, in each participant are summarized in Tables 3(a)–3(c). In P1, the production of semantic paraphasia was observed concurrently with significant activation of the precentral gyrus bilaterally, the left superior frontal gyrus (SFG), the inferior frontal gyrus (IFG) bilaterally, the cerebellum (culmen bilaterally, right cerebellar tonsil), the left middle frontal gyrus (MFG), the left brain stem (pons), the left postcentral gyrus, the left fusiform gyrus, the right posterior cingulate cortex, and the right superior temporal gyrus (STG). In P2, the production of semantic paraphasia was observed concurrently with significant activation of the left thalamus (ventral lateral nucleus), the left inferior temporal gyrus (ITG), the cerebellum (left inferior semilunar lobule, right tuber), the right cuneus, the right MFG, the right IFG, the right STG, the right precuneus, the right precentral gyrus, the right middle temporal gyrus (MTG), and the right posterior cingulate cortex. Finally, in P3, the production of semantic paraphasia was observed concurrently with significant activation of the MTG bilaterally, the IFG bilaterally, the left superior parietal lobule, the left inferior parietal lobule, the right precentral gyrus, the right cingulate gyrus, the right SFG, the right putamen, the right MFG, and the right insula.

Table 4 summarizes brain activation maps corresponding to adaptive plasticity (i.e., successful naming) in each participant, adapted from Durand [16]. Successful naming was observed concurrently with significant activation of the MFG bilaterally and the precentral gyrus bilaterally. For the LH, successful naming was observed concurrently with significant activation of the IFG, the SFG, the middle occipital gyrus, the lingual gyrus, the superior parietal lobule, the precuneus, and the pons. For the RH, successful naming was observed concurrently with significant activation of the STG, the MTG, the ITG, the cerebellum (tuber and inferior semilunar lobule), the fusiform gyrus, the sulcus callosomarginalis, and the caudate nucleus.

A comparison was made between brain activation maps associated with semantic paraphasia and those associated with successful naming. In all participants, brain activation maps associated with semantic paraphasia and those associated with successful naming included a number of common significant activation patterns. These common significant activation patterns are highlighted in Tables 3(a)–3(c). In P1, the areas significantly activated with both semantic paraphasia and successful naming included the precentral gyrus bilaterally, the left brainstem (pons), and the right STG. In P2, the areas significantly activated with both semantic paraphasia and successful naming included the cerebellum (tuber), the right STG, and the right MTG. Finally, in P3, the areas significantly activated with both semantic paraphasia and successful naming included the left IFG and the left superior parietal lobule.

3.2.2. Lateralization Indexes. Table 5 presents the LI for the brain activation maps related to maladaptive plasticity (production of semantic paraphasia) and adaptive plasticity (successful naming) for each participant.

The three participants showed bilateral significant activation patterns for both semantic paraphasia and successful naming. Regarding the production of semantic paraphasia, two distinct patterns were observed. Whereas P1 presented a symmetric activation pattern (−0.11), P2 and P3 showed strong predominant LH activation (0.69 and 0.89, resp.). Regarding successful verb naming, P1 showed a symmetric activation pattern (−0.21), P2 showed strong predominant LH activation (0.76), and P3 showed weak predominant LH activation (0.36).

3.3. Discussion.

The present study aimed to explore maladaptive plasticity, defined as the production of semantic paraphasia, in oral verb naming. Three participants with nonfluent chronic aphasia were examined in the context of a picture-naming task during event-related fMRI scanning. Activation patterns related to the production of semantic paraphasia were obtained and compared to our previous study on adaptive plasticity, that is, successful verb naming [16]. For each participant, the relative contribution of the RH and LH to the production of semantic paraphasia and successful verb naming was determined by calculating an LI.

Results show that the production of semantic paraphasia was associated with the significant activation of right and left hemisphere areas in all three participants. All of these areas are reported to sustain normal language processing in healthy adults [46] and particularly verb production [6–11]. The recruitment of these areas may reflect the attempt to find the correct target verb; however, the attempt to compensate for the system's damaged components is not sufficient and leads to semantic paraphasia that is in some way related to the target word. In addition, the production of semantic paraphasia was associated with specific activation patterns in all participants. This may reflect the impact of individual factors such as lesion location and extension, time elapsed after stroke, age, and education level, all of which have been shown to influence language representation and processing [47–51]. Also, specificities in the mechanisms underlying the production of semantic paraphasia between participants may explain these differences. For example, research on cognitive mechanisms underlying the production of semantic paraphasia shows that these may result from impaired phonological processing or impaired semantic processing or a combination of both impairments [5]. In the present study, we did not examine the degree of relative impairment at either of these processing levels in each participant. Therefore, we cannot exclude the possibility that the mechanisms underlying the production of semantic paraphasia may have differed between participants; this may explain why each participant showed specific activation patterns in relation to the production of paraphasia.

The present study also compared the activation patterns related to the production of semantic paraphasia to our previous study on adaptive plasticity, that is, successful verb naming [16]. In each participant, a number of common activation patterns were observed for semantic paraphasia and successful naming. For P1, these included the precentral

TABLE 3: Significantly activated areas associated with the production of semantic verb paraphasia in participant 1 (a), participant 2 (b), and participant 3 (c).

(a)

Left hemisphere

Region	BA	X	Y	Z	T-score	Cluster size
Frontal lobe, precentral gyrus	4	-16	-28	76	3.00	43
Frontal lobe, superior frontal gyrus	6	-20	2	76	2.97	15
Frontal lobe, inferior frontal gyrus	47	-36	22	-18	2.93	18
Cerebellum, culmen		-34	-50	-22	4.03	163
Frontal lobe, middle frontal gyrus	47	-46	40	-12	3.46	38
Frontal lobe, middle frontal gyrus		-62	10	36	3.07	23
Brainstem, pons		-4	-22	-36	4.92	32
Frontal lobe, postcentral gyrus		-58	-10	50	4.72	132
Occipital lobe, fusiform gyrus		-44	-76	-20	4.10	53

Right hemisphere

Region	BA	X	Y	Z	T-score	Cluster size
Limbic lobe, posterior cingulate cortex	29	2	-50	8	3.89	74
Cerebellum, culmen		44	-50	-40	3.74	14
Frontal lobe, precentral gyrus	4	66	-2	18	3.70	34
Cerebellum, cerebellar tonsil		26	-44	-44	3.47	19
Frontal lobe, inferior frontal gyrus	47	38	22	-20	3.37	12
Temporal lobe, superior temporal gyrus	22	70	-34	12	5.92	332
Frontal lobe, precentral gyrus	6	66	-12	40	4.07	155

(b)

Left hemisphere

Region	BA	X	Y	Z	T-score	Cluster size
Thalamus, ventral lateral nucleus		-14	-10	4	3.20	10
Temporal lobe, inferior temporal gyrus	19	-48	-76	-6	8.64	5520
Cerebellum, inferior semilunar lobule		-18	-70	-48	4.66	338

Right hemisphere

Region	BA	X	Y	Z	T-score	Cluster size
Occipital lobe, cuneus	19	18	-86	34	3.15	19
Frontal lobe, middle frontal gyrus	6	40	0	44	3.11	22
Frontal lobe, inferior frontal gyrus	13	34	16	-22	3.06	33
Temporal lobe, superior temporal gyrus	22	58	-8	2	2.96	17
Parietal lobe, precuneus	7	16	-74	56	2.94	11
Frontal lobe, precentral gyrus	4	16	-36	72	2.93	13
Temporal lobe, middle temporal gyrus	22	64	-36	2	2.90	23
Limbic lobe, posterior cingulate cortex		10	-70	12	2.86	22
Occipital lobe, cuneus	18	12	-86	18	2.85	16
Cerebellum, tuber		50	-56	-36	5.36	679
Temporal lobe, superior temporal gyrus	22	56	12	-6	5.28	141
Temporal lobe, middle temporal gyrus	21	66	-50	2	4.21	91

(c)

Left hemisphere

Region	BA	X	Y	Z	T-score	Cluster size
Temporal lobe, middle temporal gyrus	39	-62	-60	8	2.90	16
Frontal lobe, inferior frontal gyrus	45	-54	20	18	6.90	16933
Parietal lobe, superior parietal lobule	7	-36	-72	46	5.67	510
Parietal lobe, inferior parietal lobule	40	-50	-52	48	3.74	169

Right hemisphere

Region	BA	X	Y	Z	T-score	Cluster size
Frontal lobe, precentral gyrus	6	48	0	48	3.28	95
Limbic lobe, cingulate gyrus	24	6	4	30	3.26	25
Frontal lobe, superior frontal gyrus	9	18	48	32	3.10	53
Lentiform nucleus, putamen		30	2	-10	3.00	25
Frontal lobe, inferior frontal gyrus	45	64	12	20	2.99	25
Frontal lobe, middle frontal gyrus		52	34	16	2.92	36
Insula		38	22	-4	4.40	745
Temporal lobe, middle temporal gyrus	21	48	8	-40	3.41	11

TABLE 4: Participant 1, 2, and 3: significantly activated areas associated with successful verb naming (adapted from Durand [16]).

		Left hemisphere							Right hemisphere						
				Results SPM							Results SPM				
	Region	BA	X	Y	Z	T-score	Cluster size	Region	BA	X	Y	Z	T-score	Cluster size
Participant 1	Middle frontal gyrus	6	−38	0	62	4.07	608	Superior frontal gyrus	6	10	2	64	4.54	608
	Precentral gyrus	4	−56	−8	50	4.64	129	Precentral gyrus	6	66	−12	40	4.21	506
	Precentral gyrus	4	−16	−28	72	4.3	111	Middle frontal gyrus	6	28	−6	54	3.98	153
	Pons		−2	−22	−36	4.87	57	Superior temporal gyrus	22	70	−36	12	4.01	64
								Middle temporal gyrus	21	70	−32	4	3.64	64
Participant 2	Middle occipital gyrus	18	−48	−76	−8	7.13	3404	Middle frontal gyrus	6	2	−2	70	6.33	637
	Lingual gyrus	18	−10	−72	−8	6.14	3404	Cerebellum, tuber		50	−56	−36	5.84	83
	Superior parietal lobule	7	−6	−66	60	4.23	116	Fusiform gyrus	37	45	−56	−24	3.9	83
	Precuneus	7	−15	−72	45	3.88	116	Cerebellum, inferior semilunar lobule		12	−70	−48	4.29	74
								Superior temporal gyrus	22	54	14	−6	4.68	54
								Superior frontal gyrus	9	2	52	40	3.91	22
								Middle temporal gyrus	21	66	−50	2	3.8	22
Participant 3	Inferior frontal gyrus	45	−54	22	18	6.05	2028	Sulcus callosomarginalis	8	10	18	48	5.82	1858
	Inferior frontal gyrus	44	−40	10	20	5.84	2028	Middle frontal gyrus	8	6	32	36	4.75	1858
	Middle frontal gyrus	6	−46	12	48	5.25	2028	Middle frontal gyrus	8	36	20	48	3.66	266
	Middle frontal gyrus	6	−22	14	44	4.67	1858	Caudate nucleus		18	−20	22	4.17	205
	Middle frontal gyrus	6	−28	48	18	4.68	449	Inferior temporal gyrus	37	48	−56	−14	4.07	17
	Superior frontal gyrus	9	−8	50	30	3.75	449							
	Superior parietal lobule	7	−36	−72	46	5.17	167							

TABLE 5: Lateralization indexes related to maladaptive plasticity, that is production of semantic paraphasia, and adaptive plasticity, that is, successful naming, for each participant. A lateralization index ranging from −0.25 to 0.25 represents a symmetric contribution of the left and right hemispheres to processing (participant 1), whereas a positive value indicates a predominant RH contribution to processing (participants 2 and 3) [29].

	Participant 1	Participant 2	Participant 3
Brain activation map for semantic paraphasia	−0.11	0.69	0.89
Brain activation map for successful naming	−0.21	0.76	0.36

gyrus bilaterally, the left brainstem (pons), and the right STG; for P2, these included the right cerebellum (tuber), the right STG, and the right MTG; and for P3, these included the left IFG and the left superior parietal lobule.

Interestingly, also these areas are known for their contribution to language processing in healthy adults and, particularly, sustaining verb production. Some of these areas are known to be involved in lexicosemantic processing. The precentral gyrus is known for its role in action semantics [9–11] and the left precentral gyrus is part of a well-known left-lateralized semantic processing circuit [52–54]. The left IFG is involved in lexicosemantic processing [55] and significant activation of the left superior parietal lobule is related to verb production [7]. Further, the right homologue of the left STG is involved in verb production [7]. Besides these areas involved in lexicosemantics, there are common areas for semantic paraphasia and successful naming that are involved in phonological encoding, articulation, and motor speech. The left IFG and the left STG are involved in phonological processing [56, 57]. The left IFG, left MTG, and cerebellum, together with the primary motor cortex (part of the precentral gyrus), support articulatory planning in speech [22, 57–59]. Regarding the left brainstem (pons) and the cerebellum (tuber), they are part of a cerebrocerebellar loop, sustaining articulation and motor speech stages of word production [60, 61].

The finding that our three participants showed common significant activation patterns during both semantic paraphasia and successful naming may again reflect an attempt of the system to find the correct target verb; sometimes the attempt is successful, and other times it is not. The production of semantic paraphasia may represent a nonefficient system's attempt to compensate for its damaged components, which leads to the selection of error production that is in some way related to the target word. Conversely, successful naming may reflect a function of the spared tissue or an adaptive compensation for the damaged language components, leading to activation of the correct target word. Moreover, the finding of common significant activation patterns during both semantic paraphasia and successful naming also suggests that segregation of brain areas provides only a partial view of the neural basis of verb anomia and successful verb naming and indicates the need to involve network approaches which

better capture the complexity of neuroplasticity mechanisms in anomia recovery.

Concerning the lateralization of processing, the contributions of the LH and RH to semantic paraphasia and/or to successful naming are still not totally clear. The LI results of the present study show that both hemispheres contribute to the production of semantic paraphasia and successful naming. RH activation not only is related to the production of semantic paraphasia, but can also be related to successful naming. Therefore, in the present study, RH activation may correspond to efficient compensation in the context of adaptive plasticity processes. This is in line with studies reporting RH activation in the context of successful naming in persons with aphasia [18] and also in healthy participants [23].

The finding that the extent of RH recruitment differed between the three participants might be attributed to lesion size [12, 27]. Larger lesions (associated with poor recovery of language functions) are associated with RH contribution, while in the case of small LH lesions the left perilesional cortex can sustain language recovery. This mechanism is supported by the present data. P1 presents a large lesion and shows a symmetric activation pattern during both semantic paraphasia and successful naming. In contrast, the LI of P2 and P3 reflects predominant LH activation in the presence of smaller LH damage and smaller error rates. The observation of a larger number of semantic verb paraphasia types in P1 can also be related to RH semantic processing abilities. Therefore, it is possible that the RH has access to underspecified semantic representations [25] which may favor the production of semantic paraphasia. However, RH activation in the context of aphasia recovery may reflect the system's attempt to compensate for its damaged components and, to some extent, support access to the correct target word. Therefore, in these three participants, the production of semantic verb paraphasia may reflect an attempt to reach the target in the recovery process.

In summary, these results show that while the global activation pattern differs between the participants, the activation patterns related to maladaptive neuroplasticity and adaptive neuroplasticity comprise a number of common areas. Also, the relative contribution of the left and right hemispheres to maladaptive and adaptive plasticity is not totally clear. This finding challenges the dichotomic distinction between the maladaptive and adaptive roles of the right and left hemispheres, respectively. The present results show that RH recruitment may be associated with adaptive plasticity mechanisms supporting recovery from anomia. Therefore, these findings raise questions regarding the generalizability of rTMS/tDCS studies reporting the advantages of selectively inhibiting the RH homologue of Broca's area to trigger anomia recovery [32–35]. The present findings suggest that inhibiting these areas may, at least in some cases, prevent the expression of the adaptive potential of the RH to support anomia recovery and/or abort the emergence of semantic strategies that may contribute to attenuating the effects of anomia in everyday communication.

The present results support a less dichotomic perspective with regard to the contribution of the right and left hemispheres to recovery from anomia and indicate the importance of adopting a wider perspective when examining the neural basis of anomia recovery. In particular, functional connectivity approaches offer an interesting alternative to the segregation perspective, as they allow considering the dynamic changes that occur within a specific brain network, which may be composed of a similar set of areas. The functional connectivity approach highlights changes in network configuration and activity, depending on a variety of factors, such as complexity level and type of task. Future functional connectivity studies on the neural basis of anomia recovery may help unravel the complex mechanisms underlying neuroplasticity in anomia recovery.

A limitation of the present study is the small number of participants and the fact that all of them were males. However, single-case studies provide important information regarding the variety of idiosyncratic activation patterns in paraphasia and successful naming. Nevertheless, larger samples, including males and females, need to be examined to further elucidate the role of right hemisphere areas and circuits in the adaptive or maladaptive mechanisms that sustain anomia recovery.

4. Conclusion

The present study explored maladaptive plasticity in persistent verb anomia by analyzing activation patterns associated with semantic verb paraphasia production in three male participants with chronic nonfluent aphasia. The results show that activation patterns associated with paraphasia production differ across the three participants. This reflects individual factors such as lesion location, time after onset, and the nature of the underlying processing deficits in the context of anomia. The present study also compared the activation patterns related to the production of semantic paraphasia to our previous study on adaptive plasticity, that is, successful verb naming [16]. Interestingly, our three participants showed common significant activation patterns during both semantic paraphasia and successful naming. Finally, the data show that both the LH and the RH are related to the production of semantic paraphasia, thereby questioning the idea of a maladaptive role of the RH. Our findings have implications for future studies aiming at inhibiting or activating specific areas in the context of rTMS/tDCS and suggest that the neural basis of paraphasia and successful naming is not mutually exclusive but may reflect dynamic processes within a relatively limited set of contributing areas.

Competing Interests

The authors declare that there is no conflict of interests regarding the publication of this paper.

Acknowledgments

This study was supported by the Trans-Atlantic Neuroscience Teaching Network (TANTEN).

References

[1] I. Papathanasiou and P. Coppens, *Aphasia and Related Neurogenic Communication Disorders: Basis Concepts and Operational Definitions*, Jones & Bartlett learning, Burlington, Mass, USA, 2013.

[2] M. Laine and N. Martin, *Anomia: Theoretical and Clinical Aspects*, Psychology Press, New York, NY, USA, 2006.

[3] J. Druks, "Verbs and nouns—a review of the literature," *Journal of Neurolinguistics*, vol. 15, no. 3–5, pp. 289–315, 2002.

[4] H. Goodglass and A. Wingfield, *Word-Finding Deficits in Aphasia: Brain-Behaviour Relations and Clinical Symptomatology*, Academic Press, San Diego, Calif, USA, 1997.

[5] A. Caramazza and A. E. Hillis, "Where do semantic errors come from?" *Cortex*, vol. 26, no. 1, pp. 95–122, 1990.

[6] K. A. Shapiro, A. Pascual-Leone, F. M. Mottaghy, M. Gangitano, and A. Caramazza, "Grammatical distinctions in the left frontal cortex," *Journal of Cognitive Neuroscience*, vol. 13, no. 6, pp. 713–720, 2001.

[7] K. A. Shapiro, L. R. Moo, and A. Caramazza, "Cortical signatures of noun and verb production," *Proceedings of the National Academy of Sciences of the United States of America*, vol. 103, no. 5, pp. 1644–1649, 2006.

[8] K. A. Shapiro, F. M. Mottaghy, N. O. Schiller et al., "Dissociating neural correlates for nouns and verbs," *NeuroImage*, vol. 24, no. 4, pp. 1058–1067, 2005.

[9] C. A. Porro, M. P. Francescato, V. Cettolo et al., "Primary motor and sensory cortex activation during motor performance and motor imagery: a functional magnetic resonance imaging study," *The Journal of Neuroscience*, vol. 16, no. 23, pp. 7688–7698, 1996.

[10] F. Pulvermüller, "Brain mechanisms linking language and action," *Nature Reviews Neuroscience*, vol. 6, no. 7, pp. 576–582, 2005.

[11] F. Pulvermüller, O. Hauk, V. V. Nikulin, and R. J. Ilmoniemi, "Functional links between motor and language systems," *European Journal of Neuroscience*, vol. 21, no. 3, pp. 793–797, 2005.

[12] J. Fridriksson, J. M. Baker, and D. Moser, "Cortical mapping of naming errors in aphasia," *Human Brain Mapping*, vol. 30, no. 8, pp. 2487–2498, 2009.

[13] S. F. Cappa, "Recovery from aphasia: why and how?" *Brain and Language*, vol. 71, no. 1, pp. 39–41, 2000.

[14] J. Grafman, "Conceptualizing functional neuroplasticity," *Journal of Communication Disorders*, vol. 33, no. 4, pp. 345–356, 2000.

[15] J. A. Kleim and T. A. Jones, "Principles of experience-dependent neural plasticity: implications for rehabilitation after brain damage," *Journal of Speech, Language, and Hearing Research*, vol. 51, no. 1, pp. S225–S239, 2008.

[16] E. Durand, *Récupération de la capacité à dénommer des actions dans l'aphasie chronique: étude des effets d'une thérapie sémantique auprès de trois participants [M.S. thesis]*, École d'Orthophonie et d'Audiologie, Faculté de Médecine, Université de Montréal, Montreal, Canada, 2011.

[17] L. J. Harris, "Broca on cerebral control for speech in right-handers and left-handers: a note on translation and some further comments," *Brain and Language*, vol. 45, no. 1, pp. 108–120, 1993.

[18] C. Anglade, A. Thiel, and A. I. Ansaldo, "The complementary role of the cerebral hemispheres in recovery from aphasia after stroke: a critical review of literature," *Brain Injury*, vol. 28, no. 2, pp. 138–145, 2014.

[19] C. Code, *Language Aphasia and the Right Hemisphere*, John Wiley & Sons, England, UK, 1987.

[20] W.-D. Heiss, J. Kessler, A. Thiel, M. Ghaemi, and H. Karbe, "Differential capacity of left and right hemispheric areas for compensation of poststroke aphasia," *Annals of Neurology*, vol. 45, no. 4, pp. 430–438, 1999.

[21] D. Saur, R. Lange, A. Baumgaertner et al., "Dynamics of language reorganization after stroke," *Brain*, vol. 129, no. 6, pp. 1371–1384, 2006.

[22] I. K. Christoffels, E. Formisano, and N. O. Schiller, "Neural correlates of verbal feedback processing: an fMRI study employing overt speech," *Human Brain Mapping*, vol. 28, no. 9, pp. 868–879, 2007.

[23] G. Raboyeau, X. De Boissezon, N. Marie et al., "Right hemisphere activation in recovery from aphasia: lesion effect or function recruitment?" *Neurology*, vol. 70, no. 4, pp. 290–298, 2008.

[24] S. C. Blank, H. Bird, F. Turkheimer, and R. J. S. Wise, "Speech production after stroke: the role of the right pars opercularis," *Annals of Neurology*, vol. 54, no. 3, pp. 310–320, 2003.

[25] M. Jung-Beeman, "Bilateral brain processes for comprehending natural language," *Trends in Cognitive Sciences*, vol. 9, no. 11, pp. 512–518, 2005.

[26] L. Bonilha, E. Gleichgerrcht, T. Nesland, C. Rorden, and J. Fridriksson, "Success of anomia treatment in aphasia is associated with preserved architecture of global and left temporal lobe structural networks," *Neurorehabilitation and Neural Repair*, vol. 30, no. 3, pp. 266–279, 2016.

[27] W.-D. Heiss, H. Karbe, G. Weber-Luxenburger et al., "Speech-induced cerebral metabolic activation reflects recovery from aphasia," *Journal of the Neurological Sciences*, vol. 145, no. 2, pp. 213–217, 1997.

[28] A. Thiel, B. Habedank, K. Herholz et al., "From the left to the right: how the brain compensates progressive loss of language function," *Brain and Language*, vol. 98, no. 1, pp. 57–65, 2006.

[29] S. Lehéricy, L. Cohen, B. Bazin et al., "Functional MR evaluation of temporal and frontal language dominance compared with the Wada test," *Neurology*, vol. 54, no. 8, pp. 1625–1633, 2000.

[30] K. Marcotte and A. I. Ansaldo, "The neural correlates of semantic feature analysis in chronic aphasia: discordant patterns according to the etiology," *Seminars in Speech and Language*, vol. 31, no. 1, pp. 52–63, 2010.

[31] P. Vitali, J. Abutalebi, M. Tettamanti et al., "Training-induced brain remapping in chronic aphasia: a pilot study," *Neurorehabilitation and Neural Repair,* vol. 21, no. 2, pp. 152–160, 2007.

[32] P. I. Martin, M. A. Naeser, H. Theoret et al., "Transcranial magnetic stimulation as a complementary treatment for aphasia," *Seminars in Speech and Language*, vol. 25, no. 2, pp. 181–191, 2004.

[33] M. A. Naeser, P. I. Martin, M. Nicholas et al., "Improved picture naming in chronic aphasia after TMS to part of right Broca's area: an open-protocol study," *Brain and Language*, vol. 93, no. 1, pp. 95–105, 2005.

[34] J. Fridriksson, J. D. Richardson, J. M. Baker, and C. Rorden, "Transcranial direct current stimulation improves naming reaction time in fluent aphasia: a double-blind, sham-controlled study," *Stroke*, vol. 42, no. 3, pp. 819–821, 2011.

[35] A. Monti, R. Ferrucci, M. Fumagalli et al., "Transcranial direct current stimulation (tDCS) and language," *Journal of Neurology, Neurosurgery and Psychiatry*, vol. 84, no. 8, pp. 832–842, 2013.

[36] G. Tononi, G. M. Edelman, and O. Sporns, "Complexity and coherency: integrating information in the brain," *Trends in Cognitive Sciences*, vol. 2, no. 12, pp. 474–484, 1998.

[37] L. Cloutman, R. Gottesman, P. Chaudhry et al., "Where (in the brain) do semantic errors come from?" *Cortex*, vol. 45, no. 5, pp. 641–649, 2009.

[38] K. Marcotte, V. Perlbarg, G. Marrelec, H. Benali, and A. I. Ansaldo, "Default-mode network functional connectivity in aphasia: therapy-induced neuroplasticity," *Brain and Language*, vol. 124, no. 1, pp. 45–55, 2013.

[39] L. Ghazi Saidi, V. Perlbarg, G. Marrelec, M. Pélégrini-Issac, H. Benali, and A.-I. Ansaldo, "Functional connectivity changes in second language vocabulary learning," *Brain and Language*, vol. 124, no. 1, pp. 56–65, 2013.

[40] K. Marcotte, D. Adrover-Roig, B. Damien et al., "Therapy-induced neuroplasticity in chronic aphasia," *Neuropsychologia*, vol. 50, no. 8, pp. 1776–1786, 2012.

[41] J.-L. Nespoulous, A. Lecours, D. Lafond, A. Lemay, M. Puel, and Y. Joanette, *Protocole Montréal-Toulouse d'examen linguistique de l'aphasie MT 86. Module standard initial: MIB*, Laboratoire Théophile-Alajouanine, Montréal, Canada, 1986.

[42] J. G. Snodgrass and M. Vanderwart, "A standardized set of 260 pictures: norms for name agreement, image agreement, familiarity, and visual complexity," *Journal of Experimental Psychology: Human Learning and Memory*, vol. 6, no. 2, pp. 174–215, 1980.

[43] S. P. Limited, *ColorCards*, Speechmark, England, UK.

[44] J. L. Lancaster, M. G. Woldorff, L. M. Parsons et al., "Automated talairach atlas labels for functional brain mapping," *Human Brain Mapping*, vol. 10, no. 3, pp. 120–131, 2000.

[45] A. C. Evans, D. L. Collins, S. R. Mills, E. D. Brown, R. L. Kelly, and T. M. Peters, "3D statistical neuroanatomical models from 305 MRI volumes," in *Proceedings of the IEEE Nuclear Science Symposium & Medical Imaging Conference*, pp. 1813–1817, November 1993.

[46] C. J. Price, "The anatomy of language: a review of 100 fMRI studies published in 2009," *Annals of the New York Academy of Sciences*, vol. 1191, pp. 62–88, 2010.

[47] H. Duffau, S. Moritz-Gasser, and E. Mandonnet, "A re-examination of neural basis of language processing: proposal of a dynamic hodotopical model from data provided by brain stimulation mapping during picture naming," *Brain and Language*, vol. 131, pp. 1–10, 2014.

[48] P. J. Eslinger and A. R. Damasio, "Age and type of aphasia in patients with stroke," *Journal of Neurology Neurosurgery and Psychiatry*, vol. 44, no. 5, pp. 377–381, 1981.

[49] S. Jarso, M. Li, A. Faria et al., "Distinct mechanisms and timing of language recovery after stroke," *Cognitive Neuropsychology*, vol. 30, no. 7-8, pp. 454–475, 2013.

[50] P. M. Pedersen, K. Vinter, and T. S. Olsen, "Aphasia after stroke: type, severity and prognosis: the Copenhagen aphasia study," *Cerebrovascular Diseases*, vol. 17, no. 1, pp. 35–43, 2004.

[51] A. C. Laska, A. Hellblom, V. Murray, T. Kahan, and M. Von Arbin, "Aphasia in acute stroke and relation to outcome," *Journal of Internal Medicine*, vol. 249, no. 5, pp. 413–422, 2001.

[52] T. R. Barrick, I. N. Lawes, C. E. Mackay, and C. A. Clark, "White matter pathway asymmetry underlies functional lateralization," *Cerebral Cortex*, vol. 17, no. 3, pp. 591–598, 2007.

[53] M. Catani, D. K. Jones, and D. H. Ffytche, "Perisylvian language networks of the human brain," *Annals of Neurology*, vol. 57, no. 1, pp. 8–16, 2005.

[54] E. Durand and A. I. Ansaldo, "Recovery from anomia following semantic feature analysis: therapy-induced neuroplasticity
relies upon a circuit involving motor and language processing
areas," *Mental Lexicon*, vol. 8, no. 2, pp. 195–215, 2013.

[55] J.-F. Démonet, F. Chollet, S. Ramsay et al., "The anatomy of
phonological and semantic processing in normal subjects,"
Brain, vol. 115, no. 6, pp. 1753–1768, 1992.

[56] S. Bookheimer, "Functional MRI of language: new approaches
to understanding the cortical organization of semantic processing," *Annual Review of Neuroscience*, vol. 25, pp. 151–188, 2002.

[57] R. Mayeux and E. Kandel, *Natural Language, Disorders of Language, and Other Localizable Disorders of Cognitive Function*,
Elsevier, New York, NY, USA, 1985.

[58] F. H. Guenther, "Cortical interactions underlying the production of speech sounds," *Journal of Communication Disorders*,
vol. 39, no. 5, pp. 350–365, 2006.

[59] P. Indefrey and W. Levelt, *The Neural Correlates of Language
Production*, MIT Press, Cambridge, Mass, USA, 2000.

[60] J. D. Schmahmann and D. N. Pandyaf, "The cerebrocerebellar
system," *International Review of Neurobiology*, vol. 41, pp. 31–60,
1997.

[61] E. V. Sullivan, "Compromised pontocerebellar and cerebel-
lothalamocortical systems: speculations on their contributions
to cognitive and motor impairment in nonamnesic alcoholism,"
Alcoholism: Clinical and Experimental Research, vol. 27, no. 9,
pp. 1409–1419, 2003.

19

Taking Sides: An Integrative Review of the Impact of Laterality and Polarity on Efficacy of Therapeutic Transcranial Direct Current Stimulation for Anomia in Chronic Poststroke Aphasia

Margaret Sandars, Lauren Cloutman, and Anna M. Woollams

Neuroscience and Aphasia Research Unit, School of Psychological Sciences, 3rd Floor, Zochonis Building, University of Manchester, Brunswick Street, Manchester M13 9PL, UK

Correspondence should be addressed to Anna M. Woollams; anna.woollams@manchester.ac.uk

Academic Editor: Chul-Hee Choi

Anomia is a frequent and persistent symptom of poststroke aphasia, resulting from damage to areas of the brain involved in language production. Cortical neuroplasticity plays a significant role in language recovery following stroke and can be facilitated by behavioral speech and language therapy. Recent research suggests that complementing therapy with neurostimulation techniques may enhance functional gains, even amongst those with chronic aphasia. The current review focuses on the use of transcranial Direct Current Stimulation (tDCS) as an adjunct to naming therapy for individuals with chronic poststroke aphasia. Our survey of the literature indicates that combining therapy with anodal (excitatory) stimulation to the left hemisphere and/or cathodal (inhibitory) stimulation to the right hemisphere can increase both naming accuracy and speed when compared to the effects of therapy alone. However, the benefits of tDCS as a complement to therapy have not been yet systematically investigated with respect to site and polarity of stimulation. Recommendations for future research to help determine optimal protocols for combined therapy and tDCS are outlined.

1. Introduction

Aphasia is an acquired disorder that affects the way in which an individual produces and/or understands language [1]. Language is an essential aspect of communication and aphasia can impact significantly on the daily functioning and quality of life of stroke survivors [2]. The neural network supporting speech production is extensive [3] and hence easily disrupted by damage, such as a stroke. It is therefore perhaps unsurprising that anomia, or word finding difficulty, is the most common and persistent symptom across all types of aphasia [4]. Indeed, those with more severe acute deficits tend to recover to this level [5] and, consequently, amelioration of anomia is a frequent aim in poststroke rehabilitation. The typical approach to the treatment of anomia is impairment-based behavioral speech and language therapy, which focuses on helping the patient to "relearn" words they are unable to retrieve or produce. This type of therapy can improve both

object naming [6] and everyday communicative abilities [7, 8]. Yet it can be time-consuming to even achieve small gains. Consequently, researchers have begun to investigate more innovative new treatments based on neuroscientific principles. Recent research has suggested that neurostimulation techniques, such as transcranial Direct Current Stimulation (tDCS), can be used to optimize therapeutic gains.

The purpose of this review is to evaluate current research on the use of tDCS in the treatment of chronic poststroke anomia to determine what has been learnt so far regarding its application and efficacy, with particular reference to the important factors of polarity (whether stimulation is positive or negative) and site of stimulation (notably, left hemisphere versus right hemisphere). Critical gaps in the literature are identified, and recommendations for future research into this combined therapeutic approach are outlined. In contrast to previous reviews on this topic (e.g., [9–14]), the present review will specifically focus on studies that have examined the effects of tDCS on confrontation naming of noun and verb pictures in chronic aphasia via a range of research designs, with reference to current neuroscientific models of speech processing and aphasia recovery.

2. Naming and Recovery

2.1. The Neural Naming Network. Models of language production propose that a number of interrelated tasks are necessary in order to produce speech, involving processing at semantic, phonological, and articulatory levels [15, 16]. Thus, some models of confrontation naming propose that, when presented with a picture of an object and asked to state the object's name, individuals must first map the visual stimulus onto a stored conceptual representation of the object (visual object recognition and semantic access), then retrieve its name (lexical retrieval) and phonological form (phonological code retrieval and phonological encoding), and create a phonetic representation of the name (phonetic encoding), before generating a motor articulatory sequence of the phonetic representation for the vocal tract to follow (articulation) [15, 17].

The brain areas believed to be involved in normal speech comprehension and production have been conceptualized within the dual-stream framework proposed by Hickok and Poeppel [3, 18]. A version of this framework has also been implemented as a neuro-computational model by Ueno et al. [19]. According to the dual stream model, two distinct pathways link language-related regions: the dorsal stream and the ventral stream. The left-dominant dorsal stream is primarily responsible for mapping sensory input and phonological information onto the articulatory network. This pathway extends anteriorly from area Spt (a left-dominant area in the planum temporale, named according to its location in the Sylvian fissure at the parietotemporal boundary) via the arcuate fasciculus to the posterior inferior frontal gyrus (IFG, including Broca's area), the anterior insula, and areas of the premotor cortex. The ventral stream consists predominantly of bilateral structures in the posterior and anterior parts of the temporal lobes surrounding the middle temporal gyrus (MTG) and inferior temporal sulcus (ITS). Both the dorsal and ventral pathways are linked to other cortical areas that play important roles in speech and language tasks, including the bilateral superior temporal gyrus (STG), superior temporal sulcus (STS), and areas of the frontal cortex. The left STG and ventral stream structures incorporate what is commonly referred to as Wernicke's area [20]. The role of the ventral stream is mapping sounds onto meanings and meanings onto spoken output. Consequently, the ventral stream is believed to be involved in a variety of semantically mediated tasks, including auditory comprehension and picture recognition. Consequently, oral picture naming relies on elements of both the dorsal and ventral streams.

Research has shown that naming, alongside other speech production tasks, is typically lateralized to the left hemisphere in healthy individuals [21]. More specifically, neuroimaging studies of healthy adults have shown picture naming to be associated with left lateralized activation in the MTG, posterior STG, thalamus, posterior IFG (namely, pars opercularis,

BA44, pars triangularis, BA45 and BA46) [22–24]. When the naming context is manipulated to make word finding more or less demanding, additional regions are recruited in both hemispheres, such as the bilateral fusiform gyri for less familiar items and the bilateral premotor cortex for items with longer names [25]. Imaging studies of stroke survivors also support the dual stream model. For example, Butler et al. [26] localized phonological and semantic deficits to damage to the dorsal and ventral pathways, respectively. More specifically, voxel-based lesion-symptom mapping (VLSM) studies have revealed that lesions to the left orbital IFG (BA47) and posterior MTG are significantly correlated with impaired picture naming [27] and, correspondingly, that lack of damage to the left midposterior MTG and underlying white matter tracts is critical for successful oral picture naming [28]. Piras and Marangolo [29] further highlighted the complexity of the neural network underpinning naming. In their study, impaired noun naming was associated with lesions to the left STG and MTG, while impaired verb naming was more strongly associated with a wider range of lesion sites, extending from BA45 to the anterior temporal lobe (BA22, BA38).

2.2. Language Recovery. Despite damage to language processing areas, most individuals who have suffered a left hemisphere stroke are able to recover at least some language skills, both spontaneously and following therapy, even many years after onset [30]. Language recovery following stroke can be considered to take place during three overlapping temporal stages: acute (hours to days), subacute (weeks to months), and chronic (months to years) [30]. This recovery is facilitated by several different mechanisms that play key roles during different stages, such as the restoration of blood flow during the acute stage (e.g., [31, 32]), the functional recovery of intact, temporarily dysfunctional brain regions during the subacute stage (e.g., [33]), and the brain's ability to undergo significant structural and functional reorganization following damage, that is, neuroplasticity, well into the chronic stage.

2.2.1. Neural Regions Associated with Spontaneous Recovery. Researchers have attempted to explore the evolution of changes in spontaneous (re)organization of language function within the brain, particularly in relation to the relative influence of the impaired left hemisphere versus the intact right hemisphere. Saur and colleagues [34] found that different temporal stages were associated with different patterns of cerebral activation. In their longitudinal study, participants were scanned using fMRI and completed an aphasia test battery at three points (acute: 0–4 days, subacute: 2 weeks, and chronic: 4–12 months after onset) during their first year after stroke. Compared to age-matched controls, the stroke survivors showed reduced activation in the left IFG during the acute stage, with better initial language performance correlated with higher activation in this region. In contrast, two weeks later, strong bilateral activation was observed, and early relative improvement in language abilities was associated with increased activation in regions within the *right* IFG and adjacent insular cortex and the right supplementary motor area. At the final assessment point, however, language activation had shifted back to areas including the left IFG and

MTG was associated with further, significant improvement in language abilities.

The precise timings of changes in hemispheric dominance may vary between individuals (e.g., [35]). Nevertheless, this sequence of brain reorganization is supported by a recent review by Anglade et al. [36], and research confirms that, by the chronic stage, stroke survivors with the most favorable language recovery appear to be those who, like healthy individuals, demonstrate predominantly left lateralized language functions (e.g., [37]). When critical left hemisphere language areas are irretrievably damaged, compensatory recruitment of undamaged regions immediately surrounding the damaged areas ("perilesional" areas) is consistently linked to improvement in language abilities in chronic aphasia [38]. For example, Fridriksson et al. [39] found that stroke survivors with better naming ability showed greater activation than both control participants and patients with poorer naming ability in areas perilesional to Broca's area, including BA32 (anterior cingulate gyrus) and BAs 10 and 11/47 (medial and middle frontal gyrus). The role of the right hemispheric activation in the chronic stage remains more controversial [40]. One theory maintains that damage to the left hemisphere can lead to transcallosal disinhibition, meaning that homologous areas in the right hemisphere that are normally inhibited by the left during language tasks become overactive and, in turn, may impose greater inhibition on the left hemisphere language regions [41]. In support of this hypothesis, a number of fMRI studies have shown that individuals with chronic poststroke aphasia do indeed have higher activation in areas such as the right IFG and right STG than healthy controls when carrying out a range of language tasks (e.g., [42, 43]). Activation in the right IFG has, however, been associated with errors of omission and semantic paraphasias in picture naming [4]. One potential explanation for such findings is that hyperactivation in the right hemisphere may prevent recruitment of perilesional areas in the left hemisphere, hindering long-term recovery from aphasia [44].

2.2.2. Neural Regions Associated with Therapeutic Recovery. Further neuroimaging studies indicate that speech and language therapy can facilitate recruitment of perilesional language areas in the left hemisphere (such as the left precentral and supramarginal gyri) in individuals with chronic poststroke aphasia, resulting in improved oral picture naming ability and a reduction in both semantic and phonological errors [45–49]. In contrast, those who respond less favorably to therapy tend to activate a greater number of diverse areas in the left and right hemispheres during naming tasks [45]. Like spontaneous relateralization, left hemisphere rerecruitment following anomia therapy is likely to be a dynamic process. For instance, Menke et al. [50] found that, immediately following a computer-based intervention program, correct naming was related to increased bilateral and right hemisphere activity in regions including the bilateral parahippocampal gyri, right precuneus, cingulate gyrus, and both occipital lobes. However, by eight months after therapy, as naming ability was consolidated, success on trained items was associated with increased activity in left perilesional middle and superior temporal areas, along with some increased

activity in the right hemisphere Wernicke's homologue. The authors suggest that the residual right hemisphere activity at eight months after therapy could have been functionally beneficial for particular individuals in their study, who had large left hemisphere lesions that made full left relateralization of language function unfeasible (see also [51]).

To conclude, stroke survivors with damage to the left hemisphere may activate homologous areas in the right hemisphere in order to recapture some degree of language ability at varying stages in the recovery process. In the longer term, this is likely to be a less effective strategy than recruitment of perilesional areas in the left hemisphere, with research strongly suggesting that left hemisphere relateralization (as far as possible) is most beneficial for language recovery [51]. Behavioral speech and language therapy can increase activity in the left hemisphere, and such activation is associated with superior outcomes from a variety of poststroke treatment programs. However, all these studies have incorporated intensive treatment protocols, which are not always available in clinical settings and do not suit all patients [12]. Consequently, researchers have begun to investigate the potential of neurostimulation techniques, namely, Transcranial Magnetic Stimulation (TMS) and transcranial Direct Current Stimulation (tDCS), to facilitate the language recovery process.

3. Neurostimulation to Enhance Recovery

3.1. Transcranial Magnetic Stimulation (TMS). TMS involves the delivery of rapidly alternating magnetic fields to the underlying cortical tissue via an electromagnetic coil placed on the scalp. The effects of TMS vary according to the frequency of electromagnetic pulses. High frequency, or fast, TMS ($\geq$5 Hz) can induce increases in cortical excitability. In contrast, low frequency, or slow, TMS (typically 1 Hz) is associated with cortical inhibition [14]. The majority of studies investigating the therapeutic effects of TMS on poststroke anomia have involved the application of low frequency TMS to the right hemisphere. This is based on the rationale discussed above that language deficits persist due to right hemispheric inhibition of perilesional left hemisphere language regions [10]. Consequently, inhibiting this inhibition via the application of TMS should theoretically lead to improvements in naming ability.

In support of this theory, Naeser and colleagues [52, 53] demonstrated, across a series of studies, that applying repetitive slow (inhibitory) TMS to the right hemisphere of patients with chronic aphasia had beneficial effects on their language skills. In the first study, three nonfluent participants all with lesions involving damage to Broca's area received single ten-minute sessions of 1 Hz TMS either in the right Broca's homologue (pars triangularis, BA45) or in the mouth area of the motor cortex [52]. The researchers found that only stimulation to the pars triangularis portion of the right Broca's homologue significantly increased picture naming accuracy, thus supporting the notion that dysfunctional right hemisphere overactivation had previously been adversely affecting naming skills. These effects were, however, short-lived and disappeared within 30 minutes. In an attempt to produce longer lasting effects, the same research group administered 1 Hz

TMS to the pars triangularis of the right Broca's homologue of four stroke survivors (two with Broca's aphasia, one with Broca's aphasia recovered to Anomic/Conduction aphasia, and one with Global aphasia) for 20 minutes a day, five days a week, for two weeks [53]. Language abilities were assessed at baseline and again at two weeks, two months, and eight months after TMS. As in Naeser et al.'s earlier study, TMS resulted in significantly better naming ability for all four participants, this time in terms of both naming accuracy and speed. Furthermore, for three of the four participants, these effects were maintained for eight months following stimulation. This suggests that multiple stimulation sessions led to long-term brain reorganization, although the authors did not use brain imaging tools to confirm this hypothesis.

One criticism of Naeser et al.'s studies is that all participants received only active TMS. Although unlikely, it is possible that the observed effects on naming abilities were not the direct result of the suppression of right hemispheric activation, but due to an unidentified factor related to the presence of the TMS equipment. To clarify this issue, Barwood and colleagues [54] recruited a dozen individuals with long-standing aphasia of varying severities. Half of the participants received 1 Hz TMS to the right pars triangularis, while the other half acted as a control group, receiving sham stimulation instead. Only active stimulation resulted in significant increases in naming accuracy and speed both immediately and one week after the stimulation sessions, thus supporting the view that inhibition of right hemisphere activation was responsible for improvements at single word production level.

The results of the TMS studies outlined above suggest that poststroke language production skills are optimized when activation in right frontal regions (and in particular the right pars triangularis) is reduced. However, as is the case with spontaneous recovery, individual differences play a significant role in a person's potential for language recovery following TMS. Factors shown to influence language recovery in aphasia include lesion site, lesion size, age, gender, handedness, and premorbid intelligence levels [55]. The particular importance of lesion site was demonstrated by Martin et al. [41], who administered ten sessions of slow TMS to the right pars triangularis of two individuals with chronic, nonfluent aphasia. Patient 1 (P1) responded well behaviorally to the TMS treatment. He named more object pictures and used longer phrases during an elicited speech task 3, 16, and 46 months after TMS than he had done before. In line with these increases in language performance, P1 also showed increased left hemisphere activation in perilesional sensorimotor cortical regions following TMS. In contrast, TMS had no significant effects on P2's measured language abilities. Nor did he demonstrate any new and lasting perilesional activation in the left hemisphere after stimulation. The authors suggest that the differences in response to TMS between P1 and P2 were likely to be related to their lesion sites. While both participants had lesions to Broca's and Wernicke's areas, unlike P1, P2 had additional lesions in the left motor and prefrontal cortices and regions both inferior and posterior to Wernicke's area. The additional left hemispheric damage to P2's extended language network may have prevented him from

activating perilesional areas following inhibitory TMS to the right hemisphere.

In each of the studies above, participants received only low frequency TMS in isolation. It is possible that administering TMS followed by behavioral speech and language therapy may be more efficient than either TMS or therapy alone in increasing language abilities in individuals with aphasia [56]. To examine the potential enhancing effect of TMS on speech and language therapy, Weiduschat and colleagues [57] applied up to 1 Hz low frequency TMS to either the right pars triangularis or the vertex (as a sham condition) of small groups of subacute stroke survivors with different types of aphasia, five days a week for two weeks. In each session, 20 minutes of stimulation was immediately followed by 45 minutes of individually tailored speech and language therapy. Results showed that while language abilities including single word naming increased in both groups of participants after intervention, this increase was only significant for the participants who had received TMS to the right pars triangularis. This finding indicates that therapy sessions that combine inhibitory right hemisphere TMS with more traditional speech and language therapy can result in greater therapeutic gains when compared to therapy alone, at least for subacute stroke survivors. Other research suggests that combining enhancing activity in the left hemisphere via excitatory TMS with speech and language therapy can also convey therapeutic benefits. For instance, Cotelli et al. [56] gave three patients with chronic aphasia 25 minutes of high frequency TMS to the left dorsolateral prefrontal cortex, immediately followed by 25 minutes of therapy designed to increase noun naming ability. TMS targeted a region whose excitatory stimulation has been shown to facilitate naming in both healthy controls [58] and individuals with Alzheimer's disease [59]. All patients received at least a fortnight of real TMS plus therapy. In line with expectations based on these previous findings, two weeks of combined TMS and anomia therapy led to significant improvements in the percentage of correctly named objects. This effect generalized to untreated items and persisted for both treated and untreated items until the final follow-up, 48 weeks after intervention.

In summary, applying low frequency TMS to the right hemisphere or high frequency TMS to the left hemisphere appears to have some therapeutic benefit for individuals with subacute or chronic poststroke anomia, whether administered alone or in conjunction with behavioral speech and language therapy. More research is required to tease out the relative effects of TMS and behavioral therapy. However, the practical appeal of TMS as a therapeutic tool is somewhat limited. For instance, TMS can cause muscle twitching which, as well as being unpleasant for patients, may hinder verbal responses if their facial muscles are affected [60]. Additionally, the noise of the stimulator may make it difficult for patients to complete therapy tasks. Consequently, it is not generally feasible to apply TMS concurrently with behavioral speech and language therapy or create effective sham conditions. To overcome these issues, research has increasingly focused on an alternative technique that shows particular promise as a therapeutic tool, transcranial Direct Current Stimulation (tDCS) [61].

3.2. Transcranial Direct Current Stimulation (tDCS). tDCS is a noninvasive neurostimulation technique that uses a battery pack to deliver weak electrical currents to the brain via two saline-soaked electrodes. The active electrode is placed on the scalp over a particular region of interest, stimulating the cortex underneath, while the reference electrode is usually placed on the contralateral supraorbital or contralateral shoulder [48]. Positive (anodal) stimulation is associated with increased neuronal excitability while negative (cathodal) stimulation is associated with inhibition of neuronal activity [62].

3.2.1. Neurobiology of tDCS-Induced Excitability Changes. Research has shown that the effects of tDCS on brain activation and task performance are determined by multiple factors, including the number of stimulation sessions, the strength, and duration of the current applied, as well as the task in hand [63]. After effects have been found to be potentially long-lasting, persisting up to twelve months after stimulation [64], the physiological mechanisms underlying the effects of tDCS are not yet fully understood. However, unlike TMS, the currents generated by tDCS are considered insufficient to directly induce action potentials [14], and different processes are believed to be responsible for changes in cortical activation during and after stimulation [61]. During stimulation, tDCS is thought to indirectly alter neuronal excitability by temporarily affecting membrane polarity: anodal stimulation causes neuronal depolarization (increased sodium and calcium ion channel activity), whereas cathodal stimulation causes neuronal hyperpolarization (decreased sodium and calcium ion channel activity) [65, 66]. This proposition is supported by the observation that blocking sodium channels (using carbamazepine, or CBZ) and calcium channels (using flunarizine, or FLU) prior to stimulation reduces the excitatory effects of anodal tDCS, but it does not impact the effects of cathodal stimulation [65, 66].

While the short-term effects of tDCS appear to rely on transient changes in membrane potential, poststimulation effects are believed to be the result of longer-lasting changes in synaptic strength [61]. One likely mechanism by which tDCS may act to modulate synaptic strength is long-term potentiation (LTP). LTP is based on the Hebbian principle [67] that when pre- and postsynaptic neurons repeatedly fire together, metabolic changes occur which make the firing of one neuron more likely to result in the firing of the other in future. The result of LTP (and its reverse process, long-term depression, or LTD) is stable changes in synaptic activation that persist over many months or even years [68]. The inducement of LTP or LTD is dependent on the levels of specific neurotransmitters and neuromodulators (neurochemicals that can potentiate or attenuate the responses evoked by neurotransmitters) [63]. In particular, tDCS appears to involve the regulation of the excitatory neurotransmitter glutamate and the inhibitory neurotransmitter GABA, plus the neuromodulators dopamine, acetylcholine, and serotonin [61]. To examine the relationship between tDCS and changes in cortical neurotransmitter concentrations, Stagg and colleagues [69] administered 1 mA of anodal, cathodal, and sham tDCS to the left primary motor cortex of 11 healthy adults in three separate

sessions, at least seven days apart, and examined the effects using magnetic resonance spectroscopy (MRS). These MRS results showed that anodal stimulation led to significant decreases in GABA concentration. In comparison, cathodal stimulation led to significant decreases in glutamate levels as well as correlated decreases in GABA concentration. This latter finding may initially appear at odds with expectations; however, GABA is synthesized from glutamate and, therefore, reducing the amount of available glutamate via inhibitory tDCS will result in corresponding decreases in GABA [69]. Taken together, Stagg et al.'s results indicate that the after effects of anodal tDCS are mediated, at least in part, by a reduction in GABAergic inhibition, while the after effects of cathodal stimulation are related to a reduction in glutamatergic neurotransmission. Other researchers have shown that, as well as glutamate and GABA themselves, NMDA receptors also play an important role in the development of tDCS-induced after effects. For example, Nitsche and colleagues [65, 66] demonstrated that administration of the glutamate antagonist dextromethorphan (DMO), which acts to block NMDA glutamate receptors, abolished the after effects of both anodal simulation and cathodal stimulation.

With respect to neuromodulators, acetylcholine has been found to have an adverse impact on potential tDCS-induced alterations in neuronal excitability. In one study, increasing acetylcholine levels by administering the acetylcholinesterase inhibitor rivastigmine eliminated the after effects of anodal tDCS and reduced the after effects of cathodal tDCS [70]. In comparison, increasing serotonin levels via the use of the selective serotonin reuptake inhibitor citalopram both enhanced and prolonged the excitatory after effects of anodal tDCS and reversed the inhibitory after effects of cathodal tDCS to produce excitation [71]. Conversely, increasing dopamine via its precursor L-DOPA turned anodal tDCS-induced excitability to inhibition and extended cathodal tDCS-induced reductions in excitability by several days [72]. Thus, serotonin appears to facilitate excitatory stimulation while dopamine facilitates inhibitory stimulation. However, the impact of neuromodulator levels on tDCS effects is complex, and they do not appear to follow simple, linear relationships. For example, in a study examining the influence of dopamine on cathodal after effects, Monte-Silva and colleagues [73] found that only intermediate doses (0.5 mg) of ropinirole (a D_2 dopamine receptor agonist) increased the inhibitory after effects of cathodal tDCS, with low (up to 0.25 mg) and high doses (1.0 mg) actually abolishing the effects instead. Further investigation is required to clarify the intricate interactions between neurotransmitters and neuromodulators in inducing and sustaining the behavioral effects of tDCS.

An important caveat to acknowledge regarding the use of tDCS is that applying an electrical current to the brain transcranially (as opposed to directly stimulating the cortex) may mean that the underlying cortex fails to receive the expected dose of stimulation, resulting in the recipient failing to demonstrate the desired behavioral consequences. One reason for this is the dispersion of current before it reaches the target cortex. For example, Miranda et al. [74] modelled the spatial distribution of 2 mA anodal tDCS delivered to four different cortical regions. Their results revealed that the intensity of current on the scalp directly underneath the anode varied, in that the current density was observed to be higher at the perimeters than in the center of the electrode. Although current density was more uniform once it reached the brain surface, between 41% and 61% of the current did not penetrate through the skull to the cortex underneath. Research has also revealed that, even once current reaches the cortex, the effects of tDCS on brain activity may not be restricted to areas directly under the active electrode, but they can extend to a wider network of functionally related brain regions via excitatory and inhibitory neural pathways [75]. For instance, in one study, anodal tDCS to the dorsal lateral prefrontal cortex of ten healthy volunteers led to increased synchronous activity between distal frontal and parietal areas [76]. Finally, it is important to note that studies that have examined the neurobiological basis of tDCS have generally only considered its effects on healthy humans, or even on animal subjects. It is possible that the neurological activation patterns and subsequent behavioral effects may not be the same in stroke-damaged human brains as they are in healthy ones [77]. In support of this, Datta et al. [78] modelled the current flow as a result of anodal stimulation to the left frontal cortex (BA6) in a nonfluent patient who had responded favorably to an intervention program combining tDCS and computerized anomia therapy. Their analysis revealed that current flow in this particular individual was indeed altered from the pattern observed in a healthy brain due to the presence of the lesion, with the current found to be most concentrated in deep, perilesional brain regions. Furthermore, they observed that current flow was also influenced by the positioning of the reference cathode, with different electric fields associated with contralateral shoulder, contralateral mastoid, contralateral supraorbital, and contralateral cortical homologue cathodes. As such, all of these factors should be borne in mind when designing protocols that aim to modify individuals' behavior with tDCS.

3.2.2. Potential Advantages of tDCS as a Therapeutic Tool. Despite the caveats noted above, a growing body of evidence indicates that tDCS can have significant positive behavioral effects on a wide variety of cognitive and motor tasks in both healthy individuals and stroke survivors (e.g., [79–82]). From a practical viewpoint, tDCS has a number of key characteristics that make it a viable therapeutic tool for use within the poststroke population. tDCS is considered safe when administered in accordance with the established conventions and, unlike TMS, it is not associated with an increased seizure risk [65, 66, 83–85]. It is generally well tolerated, although individuals undergoing tDCS occasionally report side effects such as localized tingling, itching, burning, pain, and headaches, related to stimulation itself and to the bands used to hold electrodes in position. These effects are typically mild and fade within 30 seconds to 1 minute of stimulation [86, 87]. Side effects can also be reduced by soaking the sponge electrodes in a 15–140 mM saline solution [88]. Moreover, studies have not found any physiological differences in participants' systolic and diastolic blood pressure, heart rate, or rated mood between stimulation and sham (no stimulation) conditions,

further indicating the comfort and safety of tDCS [86, 89] and confirming that changes in arousal do not mediate the effects of tDCS on performance. Furthermore, as tDCS does not result in action potentials, it does not induce the muscle twitches associated with TMS. Taken together, these factors make tDCS an ideal method by which one can administer stimulation in conjunction with speech and language therapy, both "online" (with therapy and stimulation administered concurrently) and "offline" (with therapy following stimulation). The lack of physiological changes and the diminishing of the sensations associated with stimulation within one minute after onset also mean that recipients are often unable to distinguish sham (where active stimulation is administered for approximately 30 seconds to produce the initial sensations, before slowly being turned off) from longer periods of active stimulation (e.g., [86]). The potential to include this no stimulation control condition enables the studies to compare the effectiveness of behavioral speech and language therapy in conjunction with tDCS with that of behavioral speech and language therapy alone. Finally, tDCS equipment is relatively inexpensive and easily portable, making it theoretically possible for clinicians to administer tDCS to people with aphasia in a variety of contexts, including patients' own homes [79].

4. Therapeutic Effects of tDCS on Naming Ability in Aphasia

In order to thoroughly assess the therapeutic effects of tDCS on the naming performance of individuals with chronic stroke-induced aphasia, comprehensive searches of databases and other sources were carried out at several time points to obtain details of all relevant studies. Electronic databases (CINAHL Plus, Medline, and PubMed) were searched periodically between July 2013 and October 2014 to identify possible papers, published in English in peer-reviewed journals. The search terms used were "tDCS," "transcranial direct current stimulation," "stimulation," or "neurostimulation" in combination with "language," "aphasia," or "anomia." Although broad, these search terms were chosen to maximize identification of all relevant studies. No specific publication dates were imposed. In addition, the "related citations" suggested by PubMed and the reference lists of relevant papers were also checked. All generated papers were then closely examined to confirm that they involved the use of tDCS rather than alternative brain stimulation techniques, such as TMS, and that any therapy provided and any outcome measures used focused primarily on single word confrontation naming of object and/or action pictures. Studies were only included if some or all of the participants were adult stroke survivors with chronic aphasia, meaning that studies that involved language production in healthy participants and/or stroke survivors in the acute or subacute stages alone were omitted [103–107].

Following the literature search, 14 studies that directly investigated the therapeutic effects of tDCS on single noun or verb picture naming in individuals with chronic poststroke aphasia, both as a stand-alone technique and in conjunction with behavioral speech and language therapy, emerged. These studies are summarized in Table 1. Studies are grouped by stimulation hemisphere: left, right, and bilateral, and their findings are discussed with reference to previously described TMS results.

4.1. Left Hemisphere Stimulation. Two studies investigated the effects of left hemisphere tDCS alone on naming ability in individuals with aphasia [90, 91]. In a preliminary study, Monti et al. [90] administered tDCS to eight chronic non-fluent aphasic individuals. In the first part of their study, all participants received one ten-minute session of sham tDCS to Broca's area. In addition, six participants received a further session of 2 mA anodal stimulation and six received a further session of 2 mA cathodal stimulation to Broca's area (four participants received all three types of stimulation). Picture naming was assessed before and immediately after each stimulation session. In the second part of the study, carried out two months later, all eight participants received single sessions of both cathodal and sham stimulations to the occipital lobe (2 cm above the inion). The results of both studies revealed that only cathodal tDCS to Broca's area significantly improved noun picture naming accuracy, which the authors attributed to a decreased excitability of inhibitory circuits within the left hemisphere. However, this result was obtained with a very limited sample size and, in contrast to studies showing the effectiveness of TMS alone in improving anomia [41, 52–54], other studies involving the application of tDCS to the left hemisphere in the absence of concomitant therapy tasks have shown little benefit, even when the overall dose of stimulation is greatly increased. For instance, within a diverse group of eight stroke survivors with chronic mild to moderate aphasia, Volpato and colleagues [91] demonstrated that, with the exception of one individual with severe anomia, 20 minutes of 2 mA anodal stimulation to Broca's area once a day for two weeks had no significant effects on either object or action naming.

In contrast to the application of tDCS alone, a number of studies have found evidence for the efficacy of anodal stimulation to the left hemisphere in conjunction with speech and language therapy in improving naming abilities in individuals with poststroke aphasia. For example, Baker et al. [92] gave ten patients with chronic stroke-induced aphasia (six fluent, four nonfluent) five consecutive days of anodal tDCS (1 mA for 20 minutes) and five consecutive days of sham tDCS. Participants completed a computerized matching task (following [108]) at the same time as receiving stimulation. This involved showing a series of color noun pictures, each immediately followed by an audio video clip of a man's mouth saying an object name. After each coupled presentation, patients were required to indicate whether the image and the associated video clip referred to the same item or not. Therapy runs were separated by a seven-day rest period to avoid carryover effects and the order of runs was counterbalanced across participants. During therapy, care was taken to ensure that the active electrode was placed over structurally intact perilesional cortex that had previously shown the most activation during a pretherapy naming assessment during fMRI. Consequently, electrode positioning varied slightly for each individual, although, across all participants, the active electrode was placed over either the left precentral gyrus or parts of the left frontal gyrus.

The study found that both the anodal and sham stimulation conditions resulted in increased numbers of correctly named treated items compared to baseline for the majority of participants. However, these increases were only significant in the anodal tDCS condition, with this effect maintained at follow-up, one week after therapy ceased. The number of correctly named untreated items also increased in the anodal tDCS condition, although this increase failed to reach statistical significance at either time point. More detailed inspection of Baker et al.'s results reveals that four participants (two fluent and two nonfluent) performed significantly better on the noun naming measure following anodal stimulation than following sham stimulation, indicating that they benefited more from active tDCS than the remaining six participants. This variability in therapeutic response was unrelated to aphasia severity. However, all four good responders had damage to the left frontal cortex, meaning that the perilesional stimulation was applied especially near to their lesion sites. It is possible that targeting intact tissue situated very close to damaged regions is critical to the effectiveness of tDCS as an adjunct to behavioral anomia therapy. Utilizing the same electrode positioning and therapy protocol as Baker et al. [92], Fridriksson et al. [93] showed that anodal tDCS plus computerized anomia treatment was significantly more effective in improving treated noun picture naming speed in a group of eight patients with chronic fluent aphasia, both immediately after treatment and at the three-week follow-up. Due to the location of their participants' lesions, the active electrodes were placed more posteriorly in Fridriksson et al.'s study than Baker et al.'s in order to stimulate regions close to Wernicke's area, again demonstrating the importance of proximal perilesional stimulation for maximal therapeutic outcomes. The results of these two studies also indicate that when used in conjunction with behavioral language therapy, anodal tDCS applied to intact perilesional cortical areas in the left hemisphere can benefit individuals with anomia associated with both fluent aphasia and nonfluent aphasia, demonstrating its wide clinical applicability.

The observation that anodal tDCS to the left hemisphere can enhance naming ability is further supported by four studies conducted by Fiori and colleagues [94, 95], Marangolo et al. [96], and Vestito et al. [97]. In the first of these studies, three individuals with chronic nonfluent aphasia completed two runs of therapy (each of five consecutive days), during which they were asked to name pictures of objects while receiving 20 minutes of 1 mA anodal or sham stimulation to Wernicke's area [94]. During therapy, written labels were provided when participants were unable to spontaneously name any item within 15 seconds. Results revealed that unsupported confrontation naming was faster and more accurate following anodal rather than sham stimulation. These observations held true for two individuals (one with moderate and one with severe nonfluent aphasia) who completed the final follow-up three weeks after therapy. More recently, Fiori et al. [95] extended their earlier work by investigating the effects of tDCS plus therapy on both noun naming and verb naming. Seven nonfluent patients took part in two three-week

TABLE 1: tDCS studies of naming ability of individuals with chronic poststroke aphasia. Images are supplied to illustrate key aspects of the protocol. Ovals represent stimulation site, with size reflecting electrode size. Red ovals represent anodal stimulation, blue ovals represent cathodal stimulation, and grey ovals represent sham stimulation. Symbols on the ovals indicate target site; symbols alone indicate reference electrodes.

Study	tDCS protocol	Number of participants	Months after stroke	Aphasia profile	Concurrent therapy	Outcome measures	Initial results (mean values)	Length of follow-up
Monti et al. 2008 [90]	2 mA, 10 mins, single sessions, electrodes 35 cm². *Experiment 1* At least a week between anodal or/and cathodal and sham. *Experiment 2* (2 months later) Time between cathodal and sham not reported	8 in total; 4 + 2 also cathodal; 4 + 2 also anodal	24–96	Left hemisphere; 4 × Broca's; 4 × Global	None	Noun picture naming accuracy and reaction time	Naming accuracy increased significantly (+33.6%) following cathodal stimulation but not after anodal or sham stimulation. There were no significant changes in reaction time following anodal, cathodal or sham stimulation. There were no significant changes in either naming accuracy or reaction time following cathodal or sham stimulation	N/A
Volpato et al. 2013 [91]	2 mA, 20 minutes × 5 days for 2 weeks, electrodes 35 cm². Time between anodal and sham not reported. Reference electrode on contralateral shoulder.	8	6–126	2 × Anomic; 1 × Broca's; 1 × Conduction; 1 × Transcortical motor; 1 × Transcortical sensory; 2 × Wernicke's mild-moderate	None	Noun and verb picture naming accuracy and reaction time	Anodal tDCS significantly improved verb picture naming accuracy (+184.62%) and reduced reaction time (−32.68%) for only 1 ppt, with the most severe anomia. There were no significant effects of stimulation on noun picture naming accuracy and speed	N/A
Baker et al. 2010 [92]	1 mA, 20 mins × 5 days for 1 week, electrodes 25 cm². At least one week between anodal and sham	10	10–242	6 × Anomic; 4 × Broca's. Wide ranging severity of aphasia	Computerized noun naming therapy	Noun picture naming accuracy. Treated and untreated items	Anodal tDCS significantly improved the naming accuracy of treated items and numerically increased (from 27.3 to 40/50 after treatment) the number of untreated items named correctly	1 week: the significant effect of anodal stimulation was maintained and the number of untreated items named correctly increased further (42/50, still n.s.)

TABLE 1: Continued.

Study	tDCS protocol	Number of participants	Months after stroke	Aphasia profile	Concurrent therapy	Outcome measures	Initial results (mean values)	Length of follow-up
Fridriksson et al. 2011 [93]	1 mA, 20 mins × 5 days for 1 week, electrodes 25 cm^2 3 weeks between anodal and sham	8	10–150	Fluent	Computerized noun naming therapy	Noun picture naming reaction time Treated and untreated items	Anodal tDCS significantly reduced reaction times (−455.57 ms) for 7/8 ppts on treated items versus sham tDCS (−281.17 ms) There were no significant effects of stimulation on untreated items	3 weeks: all 8 ppts now showed reduced reaction times for treated items after anodal tDCS (−430.6 ms) and not after sham tDCS (−265.86 ms)
Fiori et al. 2011 [94]	1 mA, 20 mins × 5 days for 1 week, electrodes 35 cm^2 One week between anodal and sham	3	21–71	Nonfluent (1 × mild, 1 × moderate, 1 × severe)	Computerized noun naming therapy	Noun picture naming accuracy and reaction time Treated items only	Naming accuracy significantly increased (+21% more than sham) and reaction time significantly reduced following anodal tDCS rather than sham tDCS (1486 ms versus 1763 ms)	1 and 3 weeks (only 2/3 ppts): some reduction in naming accuracy from the end of therapy to 1 week follow-up (still significant) effects on reaction times maintained
Fiori et al. 2013 [95]	1 mA, 20 mins × 5 days for 1 week, electrodes 35 cm^2 Six days between anodal Wernicke's, anodal Broca's and sham, one month between noun cycle and verb cycle	7	7–84	Nonfluent with noun and verb retrieval deficits	Computerized noun and verb naming therapy	Noun and verb picture naming accuracy Treated items only	Anodal tDCS to Broca's area significantly improved verb naming accuracy (Broca's versus Wernicke's = +24%, Broca's versus sham = +22%). Anodal tDCS to Wernicke's area significantly improved noun naming accuracy (Wernicke's versus Broca's = +17%, Wernicke's versus sham = +24%)	1 and 4 weeks: significant effects of Broca's stimulation on verb naming and of Wernicke's stimulation on noun naming persisted
Marangolo et al. 2013 [96]	1 mA, 20 mins × 5 days for 1 week, electrodes 35 cm^2 Six days between anodal Wernicke's, anodal Broca's and sham	7	7–84	Nonfluent with verb retrieval deficits	Computerized verb naming therapy	Verb picture naming accuracy Treated items only	Anodal tDCS to Broca's area significantly improved verb naming accuracy. (% correct responses: Broca's = 33% Wernicke's = 24% Sham = 23%)	1 and 4 weeks (only 6/7 ppts): effects maintained

Table 1: Continued.

Study	tDCS protocol	Aphasia profile	Months after stroke	Number of participants	Concurrent therapy	Outcome measures	Initial results (mean values)	Length of follow-up
Vestito et al. 2014 [97]	1.5 mA, 20 mins × 5 days for 2 weeks, electrodes 25 cm². Anodal one hour after sham	2 × nonfluent (1 × high, 1 × very high severity) 1 × Anomic (moderate severity)	20–64	3	Noun and verb naming therapy. Therapy task difficulty was increased for the second week (different item set with increased number of lower frequency words)	Noun and verb picture naming accuracy. Treated items only. Boston Naming Test (BNT), Aachen Aphasia Test (AAT) (naming, oral/written comprehension)	Anodal stimulation significantly increased the number of items correctly named from baseline, with initial increases following the first session and further increases over the remaining sessions each week for ppt 1 (week 1 5/24/28, week 2 8/24/30) and ppt 3 (26/30/35, week 2 27/31/36), and for week 2 for ppt 2 (16/22/26). Therapy task difficulty was unrelated to naming outcomes. Anodal stimulation increased % correct responses for all ppts on the BNT (ppt 2 and ppt 3 n.s.) and AAT (ppt 3 n.s.)	4, 8, 12, 16, and 21 weeks: effects on number of correct responses persisted significantly for all ppts to 16 weeks and persisted up to 21 weeks (n.s.). % correct responses on the AAT and BNT persisted significantly up to 12 weeks and persisted up to 21 weeks (n.s.)
		Right hemisphere						
Kang et al. 2011 [98]	2 mA, 20 mins × 5 days for 1 week (starting 10 minutes into each 30-minute training session) electrodes 25 cm². One week between cathodal and sham	2 × Anomic 3 × Global 4 × nonfluent 1 × Transcortical motor	6–180	10	Individually tailored computerized noun retrieval therapy	Noun picture naming accuracy (including % cued responses) and reaction time on Korean version of BNT	Trend for increased naming accuracy following cathodal tDCS versus sham ($p = 0.058$)	1 hour: trend still apparent
Rosso et al. 2014 [99]	1 mA, 15 mins × single sessions, electrodes 35 cm². Two hours between cathodal and sham	Picture naming deficits. Range of severity of aphasia. 11 ppts with lesions involving Broca's area (B+), 14 with lesions not involving Broca's area (B−)	>3 (mean = 15)	25	None	Noun picture naming accuracy (calculated as a function of the number of correct and partially correct (e.g., containing one phonemic error) responses)	Naming accuracy of B+ ppts increased significantly following cathodal tDCS, naming accuracy of 13/14 of B− ppts decreased or remained the same following cathodal stimulation. Greater improvements in naming were also associated with greater integrity of the arcuate fasciculus	N/A
Flöel et al. 2011 [89]	1 mA, 20 mins × twice per day for 3 days (at start of each training hour), electrodes 35 cm². 3 weeks between anodal, cathodal and sham	2 × Anomic 7 × Broca's 1 × Global 1 × Wernicke's 1 × not classified	14–260	12	Computerized noun naming therapy involving a decreasing cueing hierarchy	Noun picture naming accuracy. Treated items only	All conditions resulted in increased naming ability (= 83%), but anodal tDCS led to significantly greater improvements than cathodal or sham stimulation. Ppts with more severe anomia showed the greatest therapy gains	2 weeks: effects persisted

TABLE 1: Continued.

Study	tDCS protocol	Number of participants	Months after stroke	Aphasia profile	Concurrent therapy	Outcome measures	Initial results (mean values)	Length of follow-up
				Bilateral				
Lee et al. 2013 [100]	2 mA, 30 mins, single sessions, electrodes 25 cm², therapy given during last 15 minutes of stimulation >24 hours between anodal + sham and bilateral conditions. Reference electrodes were placed over the ipsilateral buccinator muscles	11	6+	4 × Broca's 2 × Transcortical motor 5 × Anomic	Picture naming and reading short paragraphs	Noun picture naming accuracy and reaction time on Korean version of the BNT. Verbal fluency	Naming accuracy significantly increased in both conditions. Reaction time decreased in both conditions, but this was only significant for the bilateral stimulation condition. Stimulation had no effect on verbal fluency	N/A
Manenti et al. 2015 [101]	2 mA, 25 minutes × 5 days for 4 weeks, electrodes 35 cm². Anodal and cathodal delivered simultaneously	1	8	Mild nonfluent	None. 25 minutes of semantic-phonological therapy given directly after each stimulation session	Nonverbal reasoning, verbal fluency, Aachen Aphasia Test (AAT), Battery for the Analysis of Aphasia Deficits (BADA), Stroke and Aphasia Quality of Life Scale-39 (SAQOL-39), noun and verb picture naming accuracy. Treated and untreated items	There were a number of significant changes at 4 weeks after stimulation. Phonemic fluency: significant increase. SAQOL-39: significant increases in psychosocial/mood and communication scales. Verb naming: significant increases in % named correctly (treated and untreated items) and significant decreases in number of "circumlocution" and "replacement with noun" errors	12, 24, and 48 weeks of phonemic fluency: further increases at 48 weeks. SAQOL-39: effects on psychosocial/mood scale maintained at 24 weeks and on communication scale at 48 weeks. Verb naming: effects on % named correctly maintained at 48 weeks and effects on error type maintained at 24 weeks

TABLE 1: Continued.

Study	tDCS protocol	Number of participants	Months after stroke	Aphasia profile	Concurrent therapy	Outcome measures	Initial results (mean values)	Length of follow-up
Costa et al. 2015 [102]	1 mA, 20 minutes, electrodes 16 cm² / *Pilot study* / 3 single sessions, one week between conditions	1	30	Severe nonfluent Possible crossed aphasia	None	Scores on a noun and verb naming task (calculated as a function of correct responses without cues and with one/two letter phonological cues)	Naming scores were significantly higher than baseline following anodal left/cathodal right stimulation than following either cathodal left/anodal right or sham stimulation ($p = 0.017$) There was no significant difference between noun and verb naming	N/A
	1 month later / *Experiment 1* / *20 minutes × 5 days for 2 weeks* / 9 days between simultaneous and sham				None	Scores on the noun and verb naming task	Naming scores were significantly higher than baseline following active than following sham stimulation ($p < 0.05$) There was no significant difference between noun and verb naming	Scores taken every three days after stimulation; effect maintained for 9 days
	4 months later / *Experiment 2* / *20 minutes × 5 days for 2 weeks* / 9 days between simultaneous and sham				None	Scores on the noun and verb naming tas	There was no significant difference in naming scores following active or sham stimulation There was no significant difference between noun and verb naming	N/A
	4 months later / *Experiment 3* / *20 minutes × 5 days for 2 weeks* / 9 days between simultaneous and sham				None	Scores on the noun and verb naming task	Naming scores were significantly higher than baseline following active than following sham stimulation ($p < 0.05$) There was no significant difference between noun and verb naming	Scores taken every three days after stimulation; effect maintained for 6 days

long therapy cycles, during which they received anodal stimulation to Broca's area, anodal stimulation to Wernicke's area, and sham stimulation over either Broca's (three participants) or Wernicke's (four participants) areas. Therapy involved individuals being asked to name depicted items or enacted actions that appeared on a computer screen, initially without cues. Objects and actions were matched for imageability, length, frequency, and age of acquisition. As in Fiori et al.'s previous study, in the event of failure to name the image within 15 seconds, participants were briefly presented with the written name. To minimize the potential impact of practice effects, the order of therapy cycles was counterbalanced across participants. The main finding from this study was an interaction between anodal stimulation location and lexical class in that tDCS to Broca's area significantly improved verb naming while tDCS to Wernicke's area significantly improved noun naming. These effects were still clearly evident at four weeks after therapy. Fiori et al.'s [95] findings are supported by a similar study carried out by Marangolo et al. [96] in which anodal tDCS to Broca's but not Wernicke's area was again associated with significant increases in verb naming accuracy for a diverse group of patients with nonfluent aphasia, both immediately after therapy and four weeks later.

Taken together, Fiori et al.'s [95] and Marangolo et al.'s [96] results indicate that the most effective site of stimulation depends on the lexical class of the treatment items. This finding is in line with VLSM work, linking noun naming to activity in the STG and MTG and verb naming to activity in the IFG and more anterior regions of the temporal lobe [29]. However, Vestito and colleagues [97] did not find the effects of frontal anodal stimulation to be qualified by lexical class. In their study, three individuals with nonfluent aphasia received 20 minutes of sham tDCS followed by 20 minutes of 1.5 mA anodal tDCS to Broca's area (with an hour's rest period between stimulation sessions) each weekday for a fortnight. Concurrently, with all tDCS sessions, participants were asked to name a total of 40 nouns and verbs in the absence of any cues or feedback. Separate treatment sets were used each week, with the second week incorporating increased numbers of lower frequency words in order to increase the task difficulty. Over both intervention weeks, the number of items correctly named by all participants increased significantly from baseline only following active stimulation. These significant effects were maintained for 16 weeks after stimulation and persisted, although they are no longer significant, until the final follow-up 5 weeks after this. Contrary to Fiori et al.'s and Marangolo et al.'s results, participants showed similar relative increases in both noun and verb naming following anterior stimulation.

The studies discussed above provide increasing evidence that combining anodal stimulation to the left hemisphere with concurrent speech and language therapy may significantly improve picture naming accuracy and/or speed in individuals with chronic anomia. This is in line with the findings obtained by Cotelli et al. [56], who noted that high frequency TMS to the left hemisphere facilitated correct noun naming in patients with chronic anomia for up to 48 weeks after therapy. In comparison, outcomes from unilateral left hemisphere tDCS studies have been maintained for up to 21

weeks after intervention, the longest follow-up reported. Stimulating both left frontal and temporal regions has been shown to be effective, with precise results likely to be dependent on individual patient characteristics, including lesion site, and also the word class targeted in therapy.

4.2. Right Hemisphere Stimulation. Akin to research into the therapeutic effects of TMS, studies have also investigated whether beneficial effects on naming may be obtained by using cathodal tDCS to inhibit supposedly dysfunctional activation in the right hemisphere and encourage left activation during language tasks. One such study was carried out by Kang et al. [98], who administered five consecutive days of 2 mA cathodal tDCS or sham tDCS to the undamaged right Broca's homologue of ten participants with differing aphasia diagnoses. Participants received 30 minutes of noun retrieval therapy each day, with tDCS applied for 20 minutes during each session. In line with previous TMS studies (e.g., [52–54]), Kang et al. found that cathodal stimulation was more effective than sham in increasing scores on a Korean version of the BNT [109], although this trend failed to reach statistical significance.

More recently, a larger, exploratory study carried out by Rosso and colleagues [99] reported significant increases in naming accuracy after lower intensity (1 mA) cathodal tDCS to the same right IFG site. Rosso et al. recruited 11 Anomic participants with lesions involving Broca's area (B+ participants) and 14 with lesions that left Broca's area intact (B− participants). All participants received single 15-minute sessions of both sham and cathodal tDCS to the undamaged right Broca's homologue, with the order of sessions counterbalanced across participants. Despite the facts that active and sham sessions were separated by only a two-hour washout period and patients did not complete a therapy task alongside stimulation, differences between conditions were significant. Results showed that changes in noun picture naming ability following cathodal tDCS were strongly related to lesion site in that naming accuracy of all B+ participants increased significantly while, for all but one of the B− participants, naming accuracy decreased or remained the same. This pattern of results is consistent with the notion that excessive inhibition by the undamaged right Broca's homologue on the damaged left hemisphere had been hindering naming abilities in the B+ participants until this inhibition was itself inhibited via cathodal stimulation (e.g., [10, 41]). Consequently, these findings support previous TMS studies in which inhibitory stimulation to the same cortical area significantly increased stroke survivors' naming abilities (e.g., [52–54]). Rosso et al. also discovered that individuals who demonstrated the greatest improvements in naming ability were those with the greatest integrity of the arcuate fasciculus, thus providing further support for the dual steam model and VLSM studies that posit Broca's area and the arcuate fasciculus as two neural components crucial for successful oral picture naming (e.g., [3, 27]).

Although Rosso et al. [99] did not include a concurrent therapy task, both this and Kang et al.'s [98] study suggest that cathodal stimulation to the undamaged hemisphere may be therapeutically beneficial for certain individuals with poststroke anomia. However, Kang et al. only collected outcome measures up to one hour after stimulation and Rosso et al. did not incorporate any follow-up period, making it impossible to know whether their interventions had any significant lasting effects, an important aim of most therapy programs. Furthermore, since cathodal tDCS to the right hemisphere was not compared to any other form of tDCS in either study, the relative effectiveness of each cannot be considered. In contrast, Flöel et al. [89] compared the effects of 1 mA anodal and cathodal applied tDCS to the right Wernicke's homologue of a mixed group of seven fluent and nonfluent participants while they carried out a computerized anomia therapy task. During therapy, participants were asked to name object pictures presented multiple times per session. Initially the pictures were shown alongside semantic, auditory, and graphemic cues, but these were gradually reduced as participants' naming abilities improved (following [50]). For each condition, participants received two one-hour therapy sessions per day for three consecutive days, with tDCS administered for the first 20 minutes of each session. At odds with Kang et al.'s and Rosso et al.'s findings, anodal rather than cathodal stimulation resulted in a significantly higher average percentage of correct, noncued naming of trained objects, with the effects being still evident two weeks after therapy. For the cathodal condition, although there was a significant improvement in naming compared to sham immediately after training, this positive effect was not maintained at the two-week follow-up. One key difference between this study and those of Kang et al. and Rosso et al., which could account for the discrepant results, is the location of stimulation. The expressive language functions associated with Broca's area are strongly left lateralized; however, the lexical-semantic functions associated with Wernicke's area are less, with the right Wernicke's homologue proposed to play a role in normal language processing (see e.g., [50]). As such, while a reduction of activation in Broca's homologue via cathodal stimulation may help restore left hemisphere functional dominance, leading to beneficial gains in naming performance, enhanced activation of the right Wernicke's homologue may help this region to better functionally compensate for the damaged left hemisphere, consistent with the findings of Menke et al. [50].

In summary, to date, a trio of studies have directly explored the effects of applying tDCS to the right hemisphere on noun naming ability with conflicting results. Both Kang et al.'s [98] and Rosso et al.'s [99] findings indicating that cathodal tDCS can improve naming ability are in line with previous TMS studies, while Flöel et al.'s [89] support for anodal rather than cathodal stimulation is consistent with a positive role for posterior right hemisphere activation in naming in some patients. Alongside varying patient characteristics, there are a number of differences between studies that may account for these discrepancies in results. For instance, Kang et al. and Rosso et al. chose more anterior stimulation sites, and the intervention protocols differed between all three studies. The current used was also stronger in Kang et al.'s study than in the two other studies. Further research is needed to clarify the effects of anodal and cathodal stimulation to anterior and posterior regions of the right hemisphere for participants with differing aphasic and lesion profiles and to directly compare the effects of right with left hemispheric stimulation.

4.3. Bilateral Stimulation. Lee et al. [100] investigated the added benefits of bilateral stimulation over unilateral stimulation. In their study, 11 aphasic individuals (six nonfluent and five fluent) received two 30-minute sessions of 2 mA tDCS. In one session, anodal tDCS over the left IFG was applied with concurrent sham stimulation over the right IFG. In the other session, simultaneous anodal tDCS over the left IFG and cathodal tDCS over the right IFG were applied, with the order of sessions counterbalanced across participants. During both sessions, reference electrodes were placed over the ipsilateral buccinator muscles. Speech and language therapy (involving picture naming and short paragraph reading) was provided during the last 15 minutes of stimulation of each session. Participants were tested immediately before and after each type of stimulation. Results showed that correct object picture naming scores on the short version of the Korean-BNT [109] increased significantly following both unilateral and bilateral stimulations. Only bilateral stimulation led to significant decreases in mean reaction time, although a nonsignificant reduction in mean reaction time was also noted following unilateral stimulation. In addition to changes in single object naming ability, Lee et al. measured pre- and postintervention verbal fluency in terms of the number of syllables produced during a picture description task. However, neither type of stimulation had any significant effects on this measure. Lee et al.'s findings suggest that bilateral left excitatory and right inhibitory stimulation of the IFG may be more effective than left excitatory IFG stimulation alone in improving confrontation object naming performance, yet they did not carry out any follow-up testing to check for longevity of the treatment effect. Nor did they include a sham condition. Furthermore, participants received only 15 minutes of speech and language therapy in each condition. This limited amount of input may, in part at least, explain why Lee et al. failed to support previous results reported by Fridriksson et al. [93] and Fiori et al. [94] who both found that unilateral anodal stimulation to the left hemisphere significantly reduced object naming reaction time following five 20-minute therapy plus tDCS sessions.

More recently, Manenti et al. [101] administered simultaneous bilateral stimulation to a 49-year-old woman with mild nonfluent aphasia for 25 minutes every weekday for four weeks. While stimulation was delivered offline in this study, each tDCS application was immediately followed by 25 minutes of semantic phonological action naming therapy (which required the participant to repeat the name of each verb three times and answer a series of questions regarding its semantic and phonological attributes), with the rationale that the neurostimulation may prime the resting language network for subsequent learning. The electrode montage used was similar to that adopted by Lee et al. [100], with anodal stimulation directed at the left dorsolateral prefrontal cortex and cathodal stimulation directed at the same area in the right hemisphere. The authors subsequently assessed the effects of the intervention program on a wide range of outcome measures. Results showed posttherapy gains in naming both treated and untreated verbs, indicating some degree of generalization, although the effects were greater for treated items. The percentage of correctly named verbs was unrelated to psycholinguistic characteristics such as frequency and number of syllables. Contrary to Lee et al.'s findings, Manenti et al.'s intervention program resulted in improvements in the participant's phonemic fluency, as well as her self-reported quality of life. Crucially, many of these effects were still evident at the 24- and 48-week follow-up periods, demonstrating the potential long-term benefits of tDCS-enhanced speech and language therapy programs.

There are a number of noteworthy features of Manenti et al.'s methodology that could be adopted in future research, such as their use of a diverse and extensive range of outcome measures, the length of their follow-up, and the provision of individualized therapy for their participant's verb naming deficit. However, the results generated in this study pertain to only a single individual with relatively mild language impairments, meaning that one cannot attempt to generalize the findings to the wider aphasic population. Moreover, the absence of a sham condition means that it is unclear what proportion of the observed gains can be attributed to tDCS relative to the contribution of the large number of therapy sessions provided. In addition, the participant received only one form of bilateral stimulation, making it impossible to state whether anodal stimulation to the left hemisphere or cathodal stimulation to the right hemisphere individually would actually have been more effective than both combined. It is also unclear whether concurrent (online) stimulation with therapy would also have had even greater positive effects.

The final study identified via the literature search describes three interrelated experiments involving a single individual with suspected crossed aphasia [102], a condition which occurs when a right handed individual presents with severe aphasia in the absence of structural damage to the left hemisphere [110]. Thus, the case studied by Costa and colleagues acquired her aphasia following a right middle cerebral artery (MCA) stroke, which resulted in damage to the right frontal, temporal, and parietal lobes. While it is also unclear from this case study whether combining bilateral stimulation with therapy would have enhanced the effects of stimulation (as again no concurrent therapy task was included), the authors investigated a wider range of bilateral electrode positions than either Lee et al. [100] or Manenti et al. (2013). Prior to their main experiments, Costa et al. carried out a brief pilot study, during which simultaneous anodal stimulation to Broca's area and cathodal stimulation to the right Broca's homologue were found to be more effective in increasing baseline scores on a noun and verb naming task than either simultaneous cathodal stimulation to Broca's area and anodal stimulation to the right Broca's homologue, or sham stimulation. Experiment 1 extended the findings of the pilot study by showing not only that simultaneous anodal tDCS to Broca's area and cathodal tDCS to the right Broca's homologue led to significantly higher naming scores but also that this effect was maintained for nine days. Experiments 2 and 3 followed the same procedure as Experiment 1, except that the electrodes were placed more posteriorly, in order to target Wernicke's area and the right Wernicke's homologue. In Experiment 2, anodal stimulation was delivered to the left hemisphere at the same time as cathodal stimulation to the right hemisphere, whereas Experiment 3 investigated the effects of the inverse electrode montage. Results showed that only the electrode arrangement in Experiment 3 led to significant increases in naming ability (this time maintained for six days after stimulation), indicating that, within this particular participant, the optimal simultaneous stimulation polarities for oral picture naming differed according to which cortical regions were targeted. Anodal stimulation to the intact (in this case, left) frontal lobe plus cathodal stimulation to the damaged (right) frontal lobe, and cathodal stimulation to the left temporal lobe plus anodal stimulation to the right temporal lobe were both linked to increased noun and verb picture naming ability. These findings are, however, difficult to interpret with respect to other studies, given that they pertain to just one individual with atypical language lateralization.

The three studies discussed above indicate that bilateral stimulation (comprising anodal tDCS to the left hemisphere and cathodal tDCS to the right hemisphere) may enhance naming ability in individuals with chronic anomia. Although Costa et al. [102] incorporated a range of bilateral stimulation montages in their case study, it is still unclear from the current studies whether bilateral stimulation is more effective than sham, unilateral left anodal, and/or unilateral right cathodal stimulation, and whether the effects hold true for larger groups of participants with typical left hemisphere language dominance.

5. Recommendations for Future Research

From the discussions above, it is clear that there is a growing body of evidence in support of the use of tDCS as an adjunct to enhance behavioral therapy in individuals with poststroke aphasia. However, it is also evident that this support is limited by its lack of systematicity and by the highly varied protocols used across studies [11, 13, 111]. As a consequence, a number of key issues regarding the methodological application of tDCS remain unresolved, including the individualization of electrode placement given different lesion locations, the exploration of a greater range of stimulation conditions and locations, and therapy delivery in relation to timing, tasks, targets, and outcome assessment.

Studies have varied regarding whether electrode placement was determined on a patient by patient basis, considering lesion size and location, or on a consistent target location basis, with the same key brain regions stimulated for all individuals. For example, Baker et al. [92] and Fridriksson et al. [93] used fMRI to determine electrode placement to ensure that stimulation targeted structurally intact cortex which had demonstrated the greatest activation associated with correct naming on a pretherapy naming task. However, in the majority of studies examined in the current review, a less individualized approach to electrode placement was used and, instead, electrodes were positioned over the same target brain regions in all participants, regardless of lesion location and extent, even when MRI scans showing precise lesion locations were available (e.g., [89, 95, 102]). A possible consequence of this more general approach is that certain participants may not have benefitted as anticipated from tDCS due to electrodes being placed over areas with insufficient viable underlying brain tissue. Some authors argue that precise placement is unnecessary as the effects of tDCS are generally fairly diffuse as a result of the size of active electrodes typically used (approximately 25–35 cm^2) [74, 112]. Moreover, it is cheaper, simpler, and less demanding of patients if they are not required to undergo scanning prior to participation. Nevertheless, research has consistently highlighted the importance of recruitment of intact perilesional areas in poststroke recovery (e.g., [44]) and tDCS results have indicated that therapeutic benefits may be limited if stimulation does not target perilesional areas sufficiently close to patients' lesion sites [92]. Consequently, it would seem prudent to use scanning data, whenever available, to place electrodes where stimulation is believed to result in the best possible therapy outcomes.

Related to the issue of stimulation site, the current review found that, in the majority of the studies discussed, participants were given only one type of active stimulation to one region, while, in others, only one further condition (altering the polarity or location of stimulation) was included. This means that it is impossible to determine whether an alternative active stimulation condition would have led to even greater gains than those reported. The effects of cathodal tDCS to right contralesional areas remain generally underresearched compared to the effects of both anodal tDCS to the left hemisphere and TMS to the right pars triangularis. While one must caution against assuming that the effects of tDCS and TMS are equivalent [12], given the significant language benefits repeatedly observed after inhibiting right hemisphere activation using TMS, the role of cathodal tDCS to the right hemisphere warrants greater attention. Similarly, the effects of stimulation to posterior language regions (e.g., those surrounding Wernicke's area) are underrepresented relative to the effects on more frontal regions.

With the exception of Rosso and colleagues [99], who highlighted the differential effects of utilizing the same stimulation parameters with individuals with/out Broca's area intact, none of the reviewed studies explicitly compared the effects of stimulation on individuals with nonfluent and fluent aphasia following damage to different parts of the left hemisphere. Existing knowledge suggests that anodal stimulation applied to left frontal regions and/or cathodal stimulation applied to right frontal regions will yield the best results for individuals with nonfluent aphasia associated with frontal lesions and that anodal stimulation applied to left or right posterior regions will yield the best results for individuals with fluent aphasia associated with more posterior lesions. However, additional research is required to thoroughly investigate potential interactions between aphasia type and stimulation site/polarity. Furthermore, additional research should aim to clarify the relationship between aphasia severity and therapeutic effectiveness. In two studies [89, 91], the participants who showed the greatest gains from tDCS plus therapy were those with the most severe deficits. Fridriksson et al.'s [93] results support the notion that tDCS is more likely to increase naming speed than naming accuracy of patients with less severe aphasia, whose pretherapy accuracy may be

near ceiling. It may be that tDCS has the potential to benefit individuals representing the full spectrum of symptom severities, but the optimum stimulation parameters for these individuals differ. This possibility should be addressed via more comprehensive research designs incorporating a range of participants and stimulation montages.

While several studies have suggested that tDCS can help to enhance naming for certain individuals in the absence of concurrent behavioral therapy [90, 91, 99], the majority of the studies indicate that combining tDCS with a therapy task leads to more consistent gains. The therapy tasks utilized vary across studies, making direct comparison impossible, although all tasks required participants to take an active role by matching stimuli, producing item names, or answering questions regarding items' properties. It may be the case that the particular therapy task is less important to the success of tDCS plus therapy interventions than the location and polarity of stimulation; however, this is another factor that could be explored in the future. The therapeutic protocols adopted by previous studies also differ in terms of the number of sessions, the length of any follow-up, and the outcome measures adopted. Regarding the frequency of tDCS plus therapy sessions, the majority of studies have incorporated fairly intensive and often extensive therapy schedules, with clients receiving stimulation every day for three to 20 days. As mentioned previously, this type of schedule can be difficult to maintain in clinical practice for various reasons [12]. Within the domain of behavioral language therapy, studies have found that both intensive and nonintensive anomia therapies may lead to similarly significant improvements in naming ability. Indeed, there is evidence that long-term retention may actually be greater when equal hours of therapy are distributed over five rather than two weeks [113]. Consequently, future research could investigate whether the observed beneficial effects of tDCS and speech and language therapy can be achieved using less frequent sessions, reducing the demands on clinicians and patients alike. On a related note, the longer that therapy effects remain evident, the less often any potentially time-consuming and costly repeat or "top up" treatment needs to be administered. Despite research with healthy adults indicating that beneficial effects of tDCS on cognitive abilities can remain significant for at least twelve months [64], many of the studies discussed above failed to investigate any possible lasting effects of intervention. When participants were tested following a posttreatment interval, other than Manenti et al.'s [101] notable case study and Vestito et al.'s small pilot study, the longest follow-up was four weeks after therapy. Further, larger studies involving much longer follow-ups are clearly required to investigate how long any significant outcomes following tDCS plus anomia therapy persist in the majority of individuals.

Predictably, given the scope of the literature search, the primary outcome measure in all of the above studies was unassisted confrontation naming of noun and/or verb pictures. In the majority of studies, only noun naming was examined, although Fiori et al. [95] revealed an interesting potential interaction between stimulation site and word class: anodal tDCS to Broca's area resulted in significantly better verb naming and anodal tDCS to Wernicke's area resulted in significantly better noun naming. The observation that anodal tDCS to frontal regions may particularly enhance verb naming is supported by Marangolo et al. [96] but not Vestito et al. [97]. Given the small number of studies and patients involved, more research involving within-participant designs is clearly indicated. Regardless of whether nouns, verbs, or both were considered, almost all studies looked only at improvements in naming treated items rather than the effects of therapy on naming both treated and untreated items. It is, of course, impossible to treat all words that individuals with anomia have difficulty with in therapy; therefore, it is crucial that therapies have the potential to generalize from treated to untreated items. Such generalization has been documented in the behavioral anomia therapy literature (e.g., [114]) and the small number of the existing tDCS studies to address generalization has suggested that stimulation plus therapy may lead to some increases in naming of untreated items [92, 101]. However, future research designs could further investigate the potential for significant generalization by incorporating testing of both treated and untreated items at baseline and all follow-up time points.

Additionally, within the field of aphasia rehabilitation, there is a general consensus that single noun and verb naming ability can be influenced by the psycholinguistic properties of the words involved, such as age of acquisition, frequency, familiarity, imageability, concreteness, length, typicality, and animacy (e.g., [115, 116]). As mentioned in Section 2, there is also a growing body of evidence to suggest that different cortical regions may be involved in naming words with certain properties [25, 27]. Given the apparent importance of psycholinguistic properties for naming, it is perhaps surprising to note that there is a current paucity of evidence regarding potential interactions between such variables and the observed effects of tDCS on confrontation naming ability. Several studies, which included treated and untreated word sets or a number of treated sets, explicitly stated that sets were matched on the basis of particular psycholinguistic variables. For example, Baker et al.'s [92] treated and untreated noun sets were matched for frequency (low/medium/high), semantic category, and word length. However, only one study [101] provided further discussion regarding which words benefited most from tDCS. In this study, Manenti and colleagues [101] found that psycholinguistic properties had no effects on verb naming in their study, although their findings pertain to a single case with mild aphasia. More detailed examination of the impact of psycholinguistic variables on the effectiveness of tDCS-based therapeutic interventions in the wider patient population is undoubtedly warranted.

Finally, it is important that statistically significant increases in picture naming performance translate into meaningful changes to patients' everyday communication [7, 117, 118]. Thus, while two existing studies assessed verbal fluency [100, 101], no studies to date have measured the potential effects of therapy on functional, real-life conversational abilities. Moreover, given the known adverse impact of aphasia on individuals' well-being and social interactions [2], it is perhaps surprising that the majority of previous studies (again with the exception of [101]) have also failed to include any outcome measures related to these factors. It is clear that ongoing research would benefit from the inclusion of a variety of outcome measures designed to assess the effects of tDCS plus anomia therapy intervention programs on functional communication and socioemotional factors.

5.1. Summary. While there is growing evidence that tDCS can enhance the effects of behavioral speech and language therapy for anomia, further research is required to segregate the effects of varying the polarity, site, timing, and frequency of stimulation in order to determine optimal tDCS parameters for maximal benefits. In particular, future studies should

(1) consider the effects of tDCS on naming ability with concurrent speech and language therapy tasks as this approach seems to provide the most consistent gains;

(2) utilize within-participants study designs, with individuals receiving sham stimulation as a control condition;

(3) consider the effects of stimulation in the context of the patient's lesion site, stage of recovery, and behavioral profile/severity of anomia;

(4) optimize electrode placement by exploiting neuroimaging data, using new head models that take into account the extent to which individual lesions affect current flow;

(5) consider systematically the polarity (anodal versus cathodal) and laterality (left and/or right hemisphere) of stimulation to determine which electrode montage leads to the greatest improvements in picture naming ability;

(6) examine directly the effects of tDCS in relation to both word class (nouns versus verbs) and the psycholinguistic properties of targeted items;

(7) vary the number and frequency of tDCS plus therapy sessions to determine whether similar gains can be achieved via less intensive treatment protocols;

(8) explore the longevity of tDCS effects by incorporating postintervention follow-ups greater than four weeks;

(9) highlight any potential generalization by assessing the effects of tDCS on naming both treated and untreated items;

(10) incorporate a more extensive range of outcome measures to assess not only accuracy and speed of confrontation naming, but also effects on connected speech tasks and quality of life measures. This would facilitate fuller understanding of the range of potential gains from tDCS plus therapy intervention programs.

6. Conclusion

Successful picture naming is a complex task that relies on multiple, interconnected brain regions, many of which are left lateralized in healthy individuals. Anomia arises when parts of the normal naming network are damaged, for example, by a stroke. Long-term recovery from poststroke anomia is facilitated by a number of cortical mechanisms and, in particular, by spontaneous and/or therapy-induced relateralization of language skills to the left hemisphere. Behavioral speech and language therapy can promote relateralization; however, research increasingly supports the use of neurostimulation techniques in lieu of, or in conjunction with, naming therapy to aid this process. Applying inhibitory TMS to the right Broca's homologue can significantly enhance naming performance in individuals with chronic aphasia, both as a standalone approach or when immediately followed by behavioral therapy. There is also limited evidence that administering excitatory TMS to left hemisphere language areas followed by such therapy produces similar benefits. However, tDCS offers increased patient comfort and safety over TMS and, consequently, may be the more useful therapeutic tool. Studies have revealed significant effects of tDCS and concurrent speech and language therapy on the naming ability of stroke survivors, in particular demonstrating that anodal (excitatory) stimulation to the left hemisphere and/or cathodal (inhibitory) stimulation to the right hemisphere can significantly increase naming accuracy and speed. To determine optimal therapeutic protocols, future research should incorporate more comprehensive designs in terms of polarity, site, frequency, and timing of stimulation for patients with different lesion sites at different stages of language recovery. A greater number of well-designed studies could one day help to translate the potential of tDCS as an adjunct to behavioral speech and language therapy into clinical practice, resulting not only in increased naming ability but also in improved quality of life for those with chronic anomia.

Acknowledgments

This work was supported by a Stroke Association Junior Training Fellowship Award (2013/01). The authors are grateful to Emma Wells for her contribution to the early stages of this review.

References

[1] H. Goodglass and E. Kaplan, *The Assessment of Aphasia and Related Disorders*, Lee & Febiger, Philadelphia, Pa, USA, 1972.

[2] K. Hilari, J. J. Needle, and K. L. Harrison, "What are the important factors in health-related quality of life for people with aphasia? A systematic review," *Archives of Physical Medicine and Rehabilitation*, vol. 93, no. 1, supplement, pp. S86–S95.e4, 2012.

[3] G. Hickok and D. Poeppel, "The cortical organization of speech processing," *Nature Reviews Neuroscience*, vol. 8, no. 5, pp. 393–402, 2007.

[4] W. A. Postman-Caucheteux, R. M. Birn, R. H. Pursley et al., "Single-trial fMRI shows contralesional activity linked to overt naming errors in chronic aphasic patients," *Journal of Cognitive Neuroscience*, vol. 22, no. 6, pp. 1299–1318, 2010.

[5] P. M. Pedersen, K. Vinter, and T. S. Olsen, "Aphasia after stroke: type, severity and prognosis," *Cerebrovascular Diseases*, vol. 17, no. 1, pp. 35–43, 2004.

[6] M. A. Lambon Ralph, C. Snell, J. K. Fillingham, P. Conroy, and K. Sage, "Predicting the outcome of anomia therapy for people with aphasia post CVA: both language and cognitive status are key predictors," *Neuropsychological Rehabilitation*, vol. 20, no. 2, pp. 289–305, 2010.

[7] W. Best, J. Grassly, A. Greenwood, R. Herbert, J. Hickin, and D. Howard, "A controlled study of changes in conversation following aphasia therapy for anomia," *Disability and Rehabilitation*, vol. 33, no. 3, pp. 229–242, 2011.

[8] P. Conroy, K. Sage, and M. L. Ralph, "Improved vocabulary production after naming therapy in aphasia: can gains in picture naming generalize to connected speech?" *International Journal of Language & Communication Disorders*, vol. 44, no. 6, pp. 1036–1062, 2009.

[9] V. de Aguiar, C. L. Paolazzi, and G. Miceli, "tDCS in post-stroke aphasia: the role of stimulation parameters, behavioral treatment and patient characteristics," *Cortex*, vol. 63, pp. 296–316, 2015.

[10] V. Costa, "Use of noninvasive cerebral stimulation techniques in aphasia: an updating," *Acta Medica Mediterranea*, vol. 28, no. 2, pp. 105–108, 2012.

[11] B. Elsner, J. Kugler, M. Pohl, and J. Mehrholz, "Transcranial direct current stimulation (tDCS) for improving aphasia in patients after stroke," *The Cochrane Database of Systematic Reviews*, vol. 6, Article ID CD009760, 2013.

[12] R. Holland and J. Crinion, "Can tDCS enhance treatment of aphasia after stroke?" *Aphasiology*, vol. 26, no. 9, pp. 1169–1191, 2012.

[13] A. Monti, R. Ferrucci, M. Fumagalli et al., "Transcranial direct current stimulation (tDCS) and language," *Journal of Neurology, Neurosurgery and Psychiatry*, vol. 84, no. 8, pp. 832–842, 2013.

[14] J. Torres, D. Drebing, and R. Hamilton, "TMS and tDCS in post-stroke aphasia: Integrating novel treatment approaches with mechanisms of plasticity," *Restorative Neurology and Neuroscience*, vol. 31, no. 4, pp. 501–515, 2013.

[15] G. S. Dell, M. F. Schwartz, N. Martin, E. M. Saffran, and D. A. Gagnon, "Lexical access in aphasic and nonaphasic speakers," *Psychological Review*, vol. 104, no. 4, pp. 801–838, 1997.

[16] W. J. M. Levelt, A. Roelofs, and A. S. Meyer, "A theory of lexical access in speech production," *Behavioral and Brain Sciences*, vol. 22, no. 1, pp. 1–38, 1999.

[17] P. Indefrey, "The spatial and temporal signatures of word production components: a critical update," *Frontiers in Psychology*, vol. 2, article 255, Article ID Article 255, 2011.

[18] G. Hickok and D. Poeppel, "Dorsal and ventral streams: a framework for understanding aspects of the functional anatomy of language," *Cognition*, vol. 92, no. 1-2, pp. 67–99, 2004.

[19] T. Ueno, S. Saito, T. T. Rogers, and M. A. Lambon Ralph, "Lichtheim 2: synthesizing aphasia and the neural basis of language in a neurocomputational model of the dual dorsal-ventral language pathways," *Neuron*, vol. 72, no. 2, pp. 385–396, 2011.

[20] I. DeWitt and J. P. Rauschecker, "Wernicke's area revisited: parallel streams and word processing," *Brain and Language*, vol. 127, no. 2, pp. 181–191, 2013.

[21] S. Knecht, B. Dräger, M. Deppe et al., "Handedness and hemispheric language dominance in healthy humans," *Brain*, vol. 123, no. 12, pp. 2512–2518, 2000.

[22] P. Indefrey and W. J. M. Levelt, "The neural correlates of language production," in *The New Cognitive Neurosciences*, M. S. Gazzaniga, Ed., pp. 845–865, MIT Press, Cambridge, Mass, USA, 2000.

[23] C. J. Price, "The anatomy of language: a review of 100 fMRI studies published in 2009," *Annals of the New York Academy of Sciences*, vol. 1191, no. 1, pp. 62–88, 2010.

[24] C. J. Price, "A review and synthesis of the first 20 years of PET and fMRI studies of heard speech, spoken language and reading," *NeuroImage*, vol. 62, no. 2, pp. 816–847, 2012.

[25] S. M. Wilson, A. L. Isenberg, and G. Hickok, "Neural correlates of word production stages delineated by parametric modulation of psycholinguistic variables," *Human Brain Mapping*, vol. 30, no. 11, pp. 3596–3608, 2009.

[26] R. A. Butler, M. A. L. Ralph, and A. M. Woollams, "Capturing multidimensionality in stroke aphasia: mapping principal behavioural components to neural structures," *Brain*, vol. 137, no. 12, pp. 3248–3266, 2014.

[27] I. Henseler, F. Regenbrecht, and H. Obrig, "Lesion correlates of patholinguistic profiles in chronic aphasia: comparisons of syndrome-, modality- and symptom-level assessment," *Brain*, vol. 137, no. 3, pp. 918–930, 2014.

[28] J. V. Baldo, A. Arévalo, J. P. Patterson, and N. F. Dronkers, "Grey and white matter correlates of picture naming: evidence from a voxel-based lesion analysis of the Boston Naming Test," *Cortex*, vol. 49, no. 3, pp. 658–667, 2013.

[29] F. Piras and P. Marangolo, "Noun-verb naming in aphasia: a voxel-based lesion-symptom mapping study," *NeuroReport*, vol. 18, no. 14, pp. 1455–1458, 2007.

[30] E. B. Marsh and A. E. Hillis, "Recovery from aphasia following brain injury: the role of reorganization," *Progress in Brain Research*, vol. 157, pp. 143–156, 2006.

[31] A. E. Hillis, J. T. Kleinman, M. Newhart et al., "Restoring cerebral blood flow reveals neural regions critical for naming," *The Journal of Neuroscience*, vol. 26, no. 31, pp. 8069–8073, 2006.

[32] A. E. Hillis, L. Gold, V. Kannan et al., "Site of the ischemic penumbra as a predictor of potential for recovery of functions," *Neurology*, vol. 71, no. 3, pp. 184–189, 2008.

[33] C. J. Price, E. A. Warburton, C. J. Moore, R. S. J. Frackowiak, and K. J. Friston, "Dynamic diaschisis: anatomically remote and context-sensitive human brain lesions," *Journal of Cognitive Neuroscience*, vol. 13, no. 4, pp. 419–429, 2001.

[34] D. Saur, R. Lange, A. Baumgaertner et al., "Dynamics of language reorganization after stroke," *Brain*, vol. 129, no. 6, pp. 1371–1384, 2006.

[35] S. Jarso, M. Li, A. Faria et al., "Distinct mechanisms and timing of language recovery after stroke," *Cognitive Neuropsychology*, vol. 30, no. 7-8, pp. 454–475, 2013.

[36] C. Anglade, A. Thiel, and A. I. Ansaldo, "The complementary role of the cerebral hemispheres in recovery from aphasia after stroke: a critical review of literature," *Brain Injury*, vol. 28, no. 2, pp. 138–145, 2014.

[37] J. P. Szaflarski, J. B. Allendorfer, C. Banks, J. Vannest, and S. K. Holland, "Recovered vs. not-recovered from post-stroke aphasia: the contributions from the dominant and non-dominant hemispheres," *Restorative Neurology and Neuroscience*, vol. 31, no. 4, pp. 347–360, 2013.

[38] P. E. Turkeltaub, S. Messing, C. Norise, and R. H. Hamilton, "Are networks for residual language function and recovery consistent across aphasic patients?" *Neurology*, vol. 76, no. 20, pp. 1726–1734, 2011.

[39] J. Fridriksson, L. Bonilha, J. M. Baker, D. Moser, and C. Rorden, "Activity in preserved left hemisphere regions predicts anomia severity in aphasia," *Cerebral Cortex*, vol. 20, no. 5, pp. 1013–1019, 2010.

[40] P. E. Turkeltaub, H. B. Coslett, A. L. Thomas et al., "The right hemisphere is not unitary in its role in aphasia recovery," *Cortex*, vol. 48, no. 9, pp. 1179–1186, 2012.

[41] P. I. Martin, M. A. Naeser, M. Ho et al., "Overt naming fMRI pre- and post-TMS: two nonfluent aphasia patients, with and without improved naming post-TMS," *Brain & Language*, vol. 111, pp. 20–35, 2009.

[42] D. Perani, S. F. Cappa, M. Tettamanti et al., "A fMRI study of word retrieval in aphasia," *Brain & Language*, vol. 85, no. 3, pp. 357–368, 2003.

[43] M. A. Naeser, P. I. Martin, E. H. Baker et al., "Overt propositional speech in chronic nonfluent aphasia studied with the dynamic susceptibility contrast fMRI method," *NeuroImage*, vol. 22, no. 1, pp. 29–41, 2004.

[44] R. H. Hamilton, E. G. Chrysikou, and B. Coslett, "Mechanisms of aphasia recovery after stroke and the role of noninvasive brain stimulation," *Brain and Language*, vol. 118, no. 1-2, pp. 40–50, 2011.

[45] K. Marcotte, D. Adrover-Roig, B. Damien et al., "Therapy-induced neuroplasticity in chronic aphasia," *Neuropsychologia*, vol. 50, no. 8, pp. 1776–1786, 2012.

[46] M. Meinzer, T. Flaisch, C. Breitenstein, C. Wienbruch, T. Elbert, and B. Rockstroh, "Functional re-recruitment of dysfunctional brain areas predicts language recovery in chronic aphasia," *NeuroImage*, vol. 39, no. 4, pp. 2038–2046, 2008.

[47] J. Fridriksson, "Preservation and modulation of specific left hemisphere regions is vital for treated recovery from anomia in stroke," *The Journal of Neuroscience*, vol. 30, no. 35, pp. 11558–11564, 2010.

[48] J. Fridriksson, "Measuring and inducing brain plasticity in chronic aphasia," *Journal of Communication Disorders*, vol. 44, no. 5, pp. 557–563, 2011.

[49] J. Fridriksson, J. D. Richardson, P. Fillmore, and B. Cai, "Left hemisphere plasticity and aphasia recovery," *NeuroImage*, vol. 60, no. 2, pp. 854–863, 2012.

[50] R. Menke, M. Meinzer, H. Kugel et al., "Imaging short- and long-term training success in chronic aphasia," *BMC Neuroscience*, vol. 10, article118, 2009.

[51] W.-D. Heiss and A. Thiel, "A proposed regional hierarchy in recovery of post-stroke aphasia," *Brain & Language*, vol. 98, no. 1, pp. 118–123, 2006.

[52] M. Naeser, T. Hugo, M. Kobayashi et al., "Modulation of cortical areas with repetitive transcranial magnetic stimulation to improve naming in nonfluent aphasia," *NeuroImage*, vol. 16, no. 2, abstract 13, 2002, Proceedings of the 8th International Conference on Functional Mapping of the Human Brain.

[53] M. A. Naeser, P. I. Martin, M. Nicholas et al., "Improved picture naming in chronic aphasia after TMS to part of right Broca's area: an open-protocol study," *Brain & Language*, vol. 93, no. 1, pp. 95–105, 2005.

[54] C. H. S. Barwood, B. E. Murdoch, B.-M. Whelan et al., "The effects of low frequency Repetitive Transcranial Magnetic Stimulation (rTMS) and sham condition rTMS on behavioural language in chronic non-fluent aphasia: short term outcomes," *NeuroRehabilitation*, vol. 28, no. 2, pp. 113–128, 2011.

[55] R. M. Lazar and D. Antoniello, "Variability in recovery from aphasia," *Current Neurology and Neuroscience Reports*, vol. 8, no. 6, pp. 497–502, 2008.

[56] M. Cotelli, A. Fertonani, A. Miozzo et al., "Anomia training and brain stimulation in chronic aphasia," *Neuropsychological Rehabilitation*, vol. 21, no. 5, pp. 717–741, 2011.

[57] N. Weiduschat, A. Thiel, I. Rubi-Fessen et al., "Effects of repetitive transcranial magnetic stimulation in aphasic stroke: a randomized controlled pilot study," *Stroke*, vol. 42, no. 2, pp. 409–415, 2011.

[58] S. F. Cappa, M. Sandrini, P. M. Rossini, K. Sosta, and C. Miniussi, "The role of the left frontal lobe in action naming: rTMS evidence," *Neurology*, vol. 59, no. 5, pp. 720–723, 2002.

[59] M. Cotelli, R. Manenti, S. F. Cappa, O. Zanetti, and C. Miniussi, "Transcranial magnetic stimulation improves naming in Alzheimer disease patients at different stages of cognitive decline," *European Journal of Neurology*, vol. 15, no. 12, pp. 1286–1292, 2008.

[60] J. A. Kaminski, F. M. Korb, A. Villringer, and D. V. M. Ott, "Transcranial magnetic stimulation intensities in cognitive paradigms," *PLoS ONE*, vol. 6, no. 9, Article ID e24836, 2011.

[61] C. J. Stagg and M. A. Nitsche, "Physiological basis of transcranial direct current stimulation," *The Neuroscientist*, vol. 17, no. 1, pp. 37–53, 2011.

[62] M. A. Nitsche and W. Paulus, "Excitability changes induced in the human motor cortex by weak transcranial direct current stimulation," *Journal of Physiology*, vol. 527, no. 3, pp. 633–639, 2000.

[63] L. F. Medeiros, I. C. C. de Souza, L. P. Vidor et al., "Neurobiological effects of transcranial direct current stimulation: a review," *Frontiers in Psychiatry*, vol. 3, article 110, Article ID Article 110, 2012.

[64] C. A. Dockery, R. Hueckel-Weng, N. Birbaumer, and C. Plewnia, "Enhancement of planning ability by transcranial direct current stimulation," *The Journal of Neuroscience*, vol. 29, no. 22, pp. 7271–7277, 2009.

[65] M. A. Nitsche, K. Fricke, U. Henschke et al., "Pharmacological modulation of cortical excitability shifts induced by transcranial direct current stimulation in humans," *Journal of Physiology*, vol. 553, no. 1, pp. 293–301, 2003.

[66] M. A. Nitsche, D. Liebetanz, N. Lang et al., "Safety criteria for transcranial direct current stimulation (tDCS) in humans," *Clinical Neurophysiology*, vol. 114, no. 11, pp. 2220–2223, 2003.

[67] D. O. Hebb, *The Organization of Behavior*, Wiley, New York, NY, USA, 1949.

[68] T. V. P. Bliss and T. Lomo, "Long lasting potentiation of synaptic transmission in the dentate area of the anaesthetized rabbit following stimulation of the perforant path," *The Journal of Physiology*, vol. 232, no. 2, pp. 331–356, 1973.

[69] C. J. Stagg, J. G. Best, M. C. Stephenson et al., "Polarity-sensitive modulation of cortical neurotransmitters by transcranial stimulation," *Journal of Neuroscience*, vol. 29, no. 16, pp. 5202–5206, 2009.

[70] M.-F. Kuo, J. Grosch, F. Fregni, W. Paulus, and M. A. Nitsche, "Focusing effect of acetylcholine on neuroplasticity in the human motor cortex," *Journal of Neuroscience*, vol. 27, no. 52, pp. 14442–14447, 2007.

[71] M. A. Nitsche, M.-F. Kuo, R. Karrasch, B. Wächter, D. Liebetanz, and W. Paulus, "Serotonin affects transcranial direct current-induced neuroplasticity in humans," *Biological Psychiatry*, vol. 66, no. 5, pp. 503–508, 2009.

[72] M.-F. Kuo, W. Paulus, and M. A. Nitsche, "Boosting focally-induced brain plasticity by dopamine," *Cerebral Cortex*, vol. 18, no. 3, pp. 648–651, 2008.

[73] K. Monte-Silva, M.-F. Kuo, N. Thirugnanasambandam, D. Liebetanz, W. Paulus, and M. A. Nitsche, "Dose-dependent inverted U-shaped effect of dopamine (D2-like) receptor activation on focal and nonfocal plasticity in humans," *The Journal of Neuroscience*, vol. 29, no. 19, pp. 6124–6131, 2009.

[74] P. C. Miranda, M. Lomarev, and M. Hallett, "Modeling the current distribution during transcranial direct current stimulation," *Clinical Neurophysiology*, vol. 117, no. 7, pp. 1623–1629, 2006.

[75] X. Zheng, D. C. Alsop, and G. Schlaug, "Effects of transcranial direct current stimulation (tDCS) on human regional cerebral blood flow," *NeuroImage*, vol. 58, no. 1, pp. 26–33, 2011.

[76] C. Peña-Gómez, R. Sala-Lonch, C. Junqué et al., "Modulation of large-scale brain networks by transcranial direct current stimulation evidenced by resting-state functional MRI," *Brain Stimulation*, vol. 5, no. 3, pp. 252–263, 2012.

[77] K. Suzuki, T. Fujiwara, N. Tanaka et al., "Comparison of the after-effects of transcranial direct current stimulation over the motor cortex in patients with stroke and healthy volunteers," *International Journal of Neuroscience*, vol. 122, no. 11, pp. 675–681, 2012.

[78] A. Datta, J. M. Baker, M. Bikson, and J. Fridriksson, "Individualized model predicts brain current flow during transcranial direct-current stimulation treatment in responsive stroke patient," *Brain Stimulation*, vol. 4, no. 3, pp. 169–174, 2011.

[79] J. P. Brasil-Neto, "Learning, memory and transcranial direct current stimulation," *Frontiers in Psychiatry*, vol. 3, article 80, 2012.

[80] A. J. Butler, M. Shuster, E. O'Hara, K. Hurley, D. Middlebrooks, and K. Guilkey, "A meta-analysis of the efficacy of anodal transcranial direct current stimulation for upper limb motor recovery in stroke survivors," *Journal of Hand Therapy*, vol. 26, no. 2, pp. 162–171, 2013.

[81] F. Fregni, P. S. Boggio, C. G. Mansur et al., "Transcranial direct current stimulation of the unaffected hemisphere in stroke patients," *NeuroReport*, vol. 16, no. 14, pp. 1551–1555, 2005.

[82] R. Holland, A. P. Leff, O. Josephs et al., "Speech facilitation by left inferior frontal cortex stimulation," *Current Biology*, vol. 21, no. 16, pp. 1403–1407, 2011.

[83] M. A. Nitsche, L. G. Cohen, E. M. Wassermann et al., "Transcranial direct current stimulation: state of the art 2008," *Brain Stimulation*, vol. 1, no. 3, pp. 206–223, 2008.

[84] C. Poreisz, K. Boros, A. Antal, and W. Paulus, "Safety aspects of transcranial direct current stimulation concerning healthy subjects and patients," *Brain Research Bulletin*, vol. 72, no. 4–6, pp. 208–214, 2007.

[85] S. Rossi, M. Hallett, P. M. Rossini et al., "Safety, ethical considerations, and application guidelines for the use of transcranial magnetic stimulation in clinical practice and research," *Clinical Neurophysiology*, vol. 120, no. 12, pp. 2008–2039, 2009.

[86] A. Flöel, N. Rösser, O. Michka, S. Knecht, and C. Breitenstein, "Noninvasive brain stimulation improves language learning," *Journal of Cognitive Neuroscience*, vol. 20, no. 8, pp. 1415–1422, 2008.

[87] S. K. Kessler, P. E. Turkeltaub, J. G. Benson, and R. H. Hamilton, "Differences in the experience of active and sham transcranial direct current stimulation," *Brain Stimulation*, vol. 5, no. 2, pp. 155–162, 2012.

[88] J. E. Dundas, G. W. Thickbroom, and F. L. Mastaglia, "Perception of comfort during transcranial DC stimulation: effect of NaCl solution concentration applied to sponge electrodes," *Clinical Neurophysiology*, vol. 118, no. 5, pp. 1166–1170, 2007.

[89] A. Flöel, M. Meinzer, R. Kirstein et al., "Short-term anomia training and electrical brain stimulation," *Stroke*, vol. 42, no. 7, pp. 2065–2067, 2011.

[90] A. Monti, F. Cogiamanian, S. Marceglia et al., "Improved naming after transcranial direct current stimulation in aphasia," *Journal of Neurology, Neurosurgery and Psychiatry*, vol. 79, no. 4, pp. 451–453, 2008.

[91] C. Volpato, M. Cavinato, F. Piccione, M. Garzon, F. Meneghello, and N. Birbaumer, "Transcranial direct current stimulation (tDCS) of Broca's area in chronic aphasia: a controlled outcome study," *Behavioural Brain Research*, vol. 247, pp. 211–216, 2013.

[92] J. M. Baker, C. Rorden, and J. Fridriksson, "Using transcranial direct-current stimulation to treat stroke patients with aphasia," *Stroke*, vol. 41, no. 6, pp. 1229–1236, 2010.

[93] J. Fridriksson, J. D. Richardson, J. M. Baker, and C. Rorden, "Transcranial direct current stimulation improves naming reaction time in fluent aphasia: a double-blind, sham-controlled study," *Stroke*, vol. 42, no. 3, pp. 819–821, 2011.

[94] V. Fiori, M. Coccia, C. V. Marinelli et al., "Transcranial direct current stimulation improves word retrieval in healthy and nonfluent aphasic subjects," *Journal of Cognitive Neuroscience*, vol. 23, no. 9, pp. 2309–2323, 2011.

[95] V. Fiori, S. Cipollari, M. Di Paola, C. Razzano, C. Caltagirone, and P. Marangolo, "tDCS stimulation segregates words in the brain: evidence from aphasia," *Frontiers in Human Neuroscience*, vol. 7, article 269, 2013.

[96] P. Marangolo, V. Fiori, M. Di Paola et al., "Differential involvement of the left frontal and temporal regions in verb naming: a tDCS treatment study," *Restorative Neurology and Neuroscience*, vol. 31, no. 1, pp. 63–72, 2013.

[97] L. Vestito, S. Rosellini, M. Mantero, and F. Bandini, "Long-term effects of transcranial direct-current stimulation in chronic post-stroke aphasia: a pilot study," *Frontiers in Human Neuroscience*, vol. 8, article 785, 2014.

[98] E. K. Kang, Y. K. Kim, H. M. Sohn, L. G. Cohen, and N.-J. Paik, "Improved picture naming in aphasia patients treated with cathodal tDCS to inhibit the right Broca's homologue area," *Restorative Neurology and Neuroscience*, vol. 29, no. 3, pp. 141–152, 2011.

[99] C. Rosso, V. Perlbarg, R. Valabregue et al., "Broca's area damage is necessary but not sufficient to induce after-effects of cathodal tDCS on the unaffected hemisphere in post-stroke aphasia," *Brain Stimulation*, vol. 7, no. 5, pp. 627–635, 2014.

[100] S. Y. Lee, H.-J. Cheon, K. J. Yoon, W. H. Chang, and Y.-H. Kim, "Effects of dual transcranial direct current stimulation for aphasia in chronic stroke patients," *Annals of Rehabilitation Medicine*, vol. 37, no. 5, pp. 603–610, 2013.

[101] R. Manenti, M. Petesi, M. Brambilla et al., "Efficacy of semantic-phonological treatment combined with tDCS for verb retrieval in a patient with aphasia," *Neurocase*, vol. 21, no. 1, pp. 109–119, 2015.

[102] V. Costa, G. Giglia, F. Brighina, S. Indovino, and B. Fierro, "Ipsilesional and contralesional regions participate in the improvement of poststroke aphasia: a transcranial direct current stimulation study," *Neurocase*, vol. 21, no. 4, 2015.

[103] Z. Cattaneo, A. Pisoni, and C. Papagno, "Transcranial direct current stimulation over Broca's region improves phonemic and semantic fluency in healthy individuals," *Neuroscience*, vol. 183, pp. 64–70, 2011.

[104] A. Fertonani, S. Rosini, M. Cotelli, P. M. Rossini, and C. Miniussi, "Naming facilitation induced by transcranial direct current stimulation," *Behavioural Brain Research*, vol. 208, no. 2, pp. 311–318, 2010.

[105] V. Fiori, S. Cipollari, C. Caltagirone, and P. Marangolo, "'If two witches would watch two watches, which witch would watch which watch?' tDCS over the left frontal region modulates tongue twister repetition in healthy subjects," *Neuroscience*, vol. 256, pp. 195–200, 2014.

[106] M. Meinzer, S. Jähnigen, D. A. Copland et al., "Transcranial direct current stimulation over multiple days improves learning and maintenance of a novel vocabulary," *Cortex*, vol. 50, pp. 137–147, 2014.

[107] K. E. Polanowska, M. M. Leśniak, J. B. Seniów, W. Czepiel, and A. Członkowska, "Anodal transcranial direct current stimulation in early rehabilitation of patients with post-stroke nonfluent aphasia: a randomized, double-blind, sham-controlled pilot study," *Restorative Neurology & Neuroscience*, vol. 31, no. 6, pp. 761–771, 2013.

[108] J. Fridriksson, J. M. Baker, J. M. Whiteside et al., "Treating visual speech perception to improve speech production in nonfluent aphasia," *Stroke*, vol. 40, no. 3, pp. 853–858, 2009.

[109] H. Kim and D. L. Na, *Korean Version Boston Naming Test*, Hakjisa, Seoul, Republic of Korea, 1997.

[110] P. Mariën, B. Paghera, P. P. De Deyn, and L. A. Vignolo, "Adult crossed aphasia in dextrals revisited," *Cortex*, vol. 40, no. 1, pp. 41–74, 2004.

[111] B. Elsner, J. Kugler, M. Pohl, and J. Mehrholz, "Transcranial direct current stimulation (tDCS) for improving aphasia in patients after stroke," *Cochrane Database of Systematic Reviews*, no. 5, Article ID CD009760, 2015.

[112] A. Datta, V. Bansal, J. Diaz, J. Patel, D. Reato, and M. Bikson, "Gyri-precise head model of transcranial direct current stimulation: Improved spatial focality using a ring electrode versus conventional rectangular pad," *Brain Stimulation*, vol. 2, no. 4, pp. 201.e1–207.e1, 2009.

[113] K. Sage, C. Snell, and M. A. Lambon Ralph, "How intensive does anomia therapy for people with aphasia need to be?" *Neuropsychological Rehabilitation*, vol. 21, no. 1, pp. 26–41, 2011.

[114] W. Best, A. Greenwood, J. Grassly, R. Herbert, J. Hickin, and D. Howard, "Aphasia rehabilitation: does generalisation from anomia therapy occur and is it predictable? A case series study," *Cortex*, vol. 49, no. 9, pp. 2345–2357, 2013.

[115] L. Nickels and D. Howard, "Aphasic naming: what matters?" *Neuropsychologia*, vol. 33, no. 10, pp. 1281–1303, 1995.

[116] C. Rossiter and W. Best, "'Penguins don't fly': an investigation into the effect of typicality on picture naming in people with aphasia," *Aphasiology*, vol. 27, no. 7, pp. 784–798, 2013.

[117] M. Carragher, P. Conroy, K. Sage, and R. Wilkinson, "Can therapy change the everyday conversations of people with aphasia? A review of the literature and future directions," *Aphasiology*, vol. 27, no. 7, pp. 895–916, 2012.

[118] R. Herbert, J. Hickin, D. Howard, F. Osborne, and W. Best, "Do picture-naming tests provide a valid assessment of lexical retrieval in conversation in aphasia?" *Aphasiology*, vol. 22, no. 2, pp. 184–203, 2008.

Permissions

List of Contributors

Tali Bitan
University of Haifa, Haifa, Israel
University of Toronto, Toronto, ON, Canada

Cheryl Jones
University of Toronto, Toronto, ON, Canada

Cristina Saverino, Joanna Glazer and Brenda Collela
Toronto Rehabilitation Institute, Toronto, ON, Canada

Catherine Wiseman-Hakes and Robin Green
University of Toronto, Toronto, ON, Canada
Toronto Rehabilitation Institute, Toronto, ON, Canada

Elizabeth Rochon and Tijana Simic
University of Toronto, Toronto, ON, Canada
Toronto Rehabilitation Institute, Toronto, ON, Canada
Canadian Partnership for Stroke Recovery, Heart and Stroke Foundation, Ottawa, ON, Canada

Sladjana Lukic and Elena Barbieri
Center for the Neurobiology of Language Recovery, Northwestern University, Evanston, IL, USA
Department of Communication Sciences and Disorders, School of Communication, Northwestern University, Evanston, IL, USA

Xue Wang
Center for the Neurobiology of Language Recovery, Northwestern University, Evanston, IL, USA
Department of Radiology, Feinberg School of Medicine, Northwestern University, Chicago, IL, USA

David Caplan
Center for the Neurobiology of Language Recovery, Northwestern University, Evanston, IL, USA
Department of Neurology, Massachusetts General Hospital, Harvard Medical School, Boston, MA, USA

Swathi Kiran
Center for the Neurobiology of Language Recovery, Northwestern University, Evanston, IL, USA
Department of Speech, Language, and Hearing, College of Health & Rehabilitation, Boston University, Boston, MA, USA
Department of Speech Language and Hearing Sciences, Boston University Sargent College, 635 Commonwealth Avenue, Boston, MA 02215, USA

Brenda Rapp
Center for the Neurobiology of Language Recovery, Northwestern University, Evanston, IL, USA
Department of Cognitive Science, Krieger School of Arts & Sciences, Johns Hopkins University, Baltimore, MD, USA

Cynthia K. Thompson
Center for the Neurobiology of Language Recovery, Northwestern University, Evanston, IL, USA
Department of Communication Sciences and Disorders, School of Communication, Northwestern University, Evanston, IL, USA
Department of Neurology, Neurology, Feinberg School of Medicine, Northwestern University, Chicago, IL, USA
Department of Neurology, Feinberg School of Medicine, Northwestern University, Evanston, IL, USA

Xinlei Xu, Jianfeng Hao, Hui Fang, Ping Chen, Zhaohui Li, Yunyun Ji, Qingjie Cai and Fei Gao
Department of Neurological Rehabilitation, Wuxi Tongren Rehabilitation Hospital of Nanjing Medical University, Wuxi, Jiangsu Province, China

Caili Ren
Department of Neurological Rehabilitation, Wuxi Tongren Rehabilitation Hospital of Nanjing Medical University, Wuxi, Jiangsu Province, China Department of Psychiatry, The Affiliated Wuxi Mental Health Center of Nanjing Medical University, Wuxi, Jiangsu Province, China

Guofu Zhang
Department of Psychiatry, The Affiliated Wuxi Mental Health Center of Nanjing Medical University, Wuxi, Jiangsu Province, China

Stephanie M. Awad
Family Medicine Residency Program, Baton Rouge General Medical Center, Baton Rouge, LA 70806, USA

Amer M. Awad
Family Medicine Residency Program, Baton Rouge General Medical Center, Baton Rouge, LA 70806, USA
Baton Rouge Neurology Associates, Baton Rouge General Medical Center, 3600 Florida Boulevard, Baton Rouge, LA 70806, USA

Tamra Ranasinghe and Amelia Adcock
Neurology Department, West Virginia University, USA

SoHyun Boo
Radiology Department, West Virginia University, USA

Xiaotong Zhang, Zhaocong Chen, Na Li, Jingfeng Liang, Huixiang Wu, Zulin Dou and Weihong Qiu
Department of Rehabilitation Medicine, The Third Affiliated Hospital of Sun Yat-sen University, Guangzhou, Guangdong Province, China

Yan Zou and Zhuang Kang
Department of Radiology, The Third Affiliated Hospital of Sun Yat-sen University, Guangzhou, Guangdong Province, China

Isabel Balachandran and Jason Lucas
Department of Speech Language and Hearing Sciences, Boston University Sargent College, 635 Commonwealth Avenue, Boston, MA 02215, USA

Dara Oliver Kavanagh, Conor Lynam, Thorsten Düerk and Paul W. Eustace
Department of Surgery, Mayo General Hospital, Castlebar, Co Mayo, Ireland

Mary Casey
Department of Radiology, Mayo General Hospital, Castlebar, Co Mayo, Ireland

Yasmeen Faroqi-Shah
University of Maryland, College Park, MD, USA

Laura Friedman
University of Wisconsin-Madison, Madison, WI, USA

Berit Arnesveen Bronken and Randi Martinsen
Department of Nursing Science, Faculty of Medicine, Institute of Health and Society, University of Oslo, Blindern, 0318 Oslo, Norway
Department of Nursing and Mental Health, Faculty of Public Health, Hedmark University College, 2418 Elverum, Norway

Kari Kvigne
Department of Nursing and Mental Health, Faculty of Public Health, Hedmark University College, 2418 Elverum, Norway

Marit Kirkevold
Department of Nursing Science, Faculty of Medicine, Institute of Health and Society, University of Oslo, Blindern, 0318 Oslo, Norway
Institute of Public Health, University of Århus, Nordre Ringgade 1, 8000 Århus C, Denmark

Torgeir Bruun Wyller
Faculty of Medicine, Institute of Clinical Medicine, University of Oslo, Blindern, 0318 Oslo, Norway
Department of Geriatric Medicine, Oslo University Hospital, Nydalen, 0424 Oslo, Norway

Shuo Xu, Yongquan Pan and Qing Yang
Department of Rehabilitation Medicine, Huashan Hospital, Fudan University, Shanghai, China

Zhijie Yan
Department of Rehabilitation Medicine, Huashan Hospital, Fudan University, Shanghai, China
Xinxiang Medical University, Xinxiang, China

Zhilan Liu
Department of Rehabilitation Medicine, Shanghai Fourth Rehabilitation Hospital, Shanghai, China

Jiajia Gao
Department of Neurorehabilitation, The Shanghai Third Rehabilitation Hospital, Shanghai, China

Yanhui Yang
Department of Rehabilitation Medicine, Shaanxi Provincial Rehabilitation Hospital, Shaanxi, China

Yufen Wu
Department of Rehabilitation Medicine, Liuzhou Traditional Chinese Medicine Hospital, Guangxi, China

Yanan Zhang
Department of Rehabilitation Medicine, The Third Affiliated Clinical Hospital of Changchun University of Chinese Medicine, Jilin, China

Jianhui Wang
Department of Rehabilitation Medicine, Nanshi Hospital Affiliated to Henan University, Henan, China

Ren Zhuang
Department of Rehabilitation Medicine, Changzhou Dean Hospital, Jiangsu, China

Chong Li
Department of Rehabilitation Medicine, Huashan Hospital, Fudan University, Shanghai, China
Shanghai University of Sport, Shanghai, China

Yongli Zhang
Department of Rehabilitation Medicine, Huashan Hospital, Fudan University, Shanghai, China
Fujian University of Traditional Chinese Medicine, Fujian, China

Jie Jia
Department of Rehabilitation Medicine, Huashan Hospital, Fudan University, Shanghai, China
National Clinical Research Center for Aging and Medicine, Huashan Hospital, Fudan University, China
National Center for Neurological Disorders, Shanghai, China

Narges Radman, Michael Mouthon and Jean-Marie Annoni
Neurology Unit, Department of Medicine, Faculty of Sciences, University of Fribourg, Fribourg, Switzerland

Beatrice Leemann and Marie Di Pietro
Neurorehabilitation Department, University Hospital, University of Geneva, Geneva, Switzerland

Chrisovalandou Gaytanidis
Neurorehabilitation Department, University Hospital, University of Geneva, Geneva, Switzerland
Neuropsychology Unit, Fribourg Cantonal Hospital, Fribourg, Switzerland

Jubin Abutalebi
Center for Neurolinguistics and Psycholinguistics, San Raffaele University and Scientific Institute San Raffaele, Milan, Italy

Matthew Walenski
Center for the Neurobiology of Language Recovery, Northwestern University, Evanston, IL, USA
Department of Communication Sciences and Disorders, School of Communication, Northwestern University, Evanston, IL, USA

YuFen Chen and Todd B. Parrish
Department of Radiology, Feinberg School of Medicine, Northwestern University, Evanston, IL, USA

Kristin Grunewald, Mia Nunez and Richard Zinbarg
Center for the Neurobiology of Language Recovery, Northwestern University, Evanston, IL, USA
Department of Psychology, Weinberg College of Arts and Sciences, Northwestern University, Evanston, IL, USA

Yuping Yan
Shanghai Business School, Room 612, Administrative Building, No.123, Fengpu Avenue, Fengxian District, Shanghai 201400, China

Mingzhe Wang, Wenfei Jiang, Men Xu and Weidong Pan
Department of Neurology, Shuguang Hospital Affiliated to Shanghai University of TCM, No. 528, Zhang-Heng Road, Pu-Dong New Area, Shanghai 201203, China

Liang Zhang
Department of Neurology, Shanghai Seventh Hospital, Shanghai University of Traditional Chinese Medicine, Shanghai 200137, China

Zhenwei Qiu
Department of Emergency, Shuguang Hospital Affiliated to Shanghai University of TCM, No. 528, Zhang-Heng Road, Pu-Dong New Area, Shanghai 201203, China

Xiangjun Chen
Department of Neurology, Hua Shan Hospital Affiliated to Fu Dan University, No. 12, Wu Lu Mu Qi Zhong Road, Shanghai 200040, China

Christian Georgi, Michael Neuß, Viviane Möller, Martin Seifert and Christian Butter
Heart Center Brandenburg-Department of Cardiology and Medical School Brandenburg Theodor Fontane, Bernau bei Berlin, Germany

Ladan Ghazi Saidi
Centre de Recherché de l'Institut Universitaire de Gériatrie de Montréal, 4565 Queen Mary Road, Montréal, QC, Canada

Ana Inés Ansaldo
Centre de Recherché de l'Institut Universitaire de Gériatrie de Montréal, 4565 Queen Mary Road, Montréal, QC, Canada
Speech-Language Pathology and Audiology Department, Faculty of Medicine, University of Montreal, Pavillon 7077 Avenue du Parc, local 3001-1, Montréal, QC, Canada
École d'Orthophonie et d'Audiologie, Université de Montréal, 7077 Avenue du Parc, Montréal, QC, Canada

Nathan T. Lee and Fatimah Ahmedy
Rehabilitation Medicine Unit, Faculty of Medicine & Health Sciences, Universiti Malaysia Sabah, Kota Kinabalu, Malaysia

Natiara Mohamad Hashim
Department of Rehabilitation Medicine, Faculty of Medicine, Universiti Teknologi MARA, Sg. Buloh, Malaysia

Khin Nyein Yin
Department of Surgery, Faculty of Medicine & Health Sciences, Universiti Malaysia Sabah, Kota Kinabalu, Malaysia

Kai Ling Chin
Department of Biomedical Sciences, Faculty of Medicine & Health Sciences, Universiti Malaysia Sabah, Kota Kinabalu, Malaysia

Kerstin Spielmann
Rijndam Rehabilitation Institute, 3001 KD Rotterdam, Netherlands
Erasmus MC, University Medical Center Rotterdam, Department of Rehabilitation Medicine, 3000 CA Rotterdam, Netherlands

Edith Durand
Centre de Recherche de l'Institut Universitaire de Gériatrie de Montréal, 4565 Chemin Queen-Mary, Montréal, QC, Canada

Karine Marcotte
École d'Orthophonie et d'Audiologie, Université de Montréal, 7077 Avenue du Parc, Montréal, QC, Canada

Margaret Sandars, Lauren Cloutman and Anna M. Woollams
Neuroscience and Aphasia Research Unit, School of Psychological Sciences, 3rd Floor, Zochonis Building, University of Manchester, Brunswick Street, Manchester M13 9PL, UK

Index

Phonological, 11, 15, 23, 25, 29, 37, 45-46, 50-53, 59, 88, 114, 134, 163-165, 168-169, 175, 178, 181-182, 185, 188, 190-191, 202, 209

Planum Temporale, 142-143, 145, 147, 190

Positron Emission Tomographic, 25, 29, 33

Posttraumatic Stress Disorder, 72-73

Primary Motor Cortex, 110, 113, 178

Primary Progressive Aphasia, 35, 37

Psychosocial Adjustment Process, 90-91

S

Semantic Switching Score, 58, 60-62, 67

Severe Aphasia, 8, 91-92, 96, 101-102, 116, 137, 171, 173-175, 180, 203-204

Speech Therapist, 71

Superior Frontal Gyrus, 142, 145, 147, 178, 183-184

Superior Parietal Lobule, 142-143, 145, 147, 178, 182-185

Supplementary Motor Area, 6, 9-10, 13, 22, 27, 138, 142-143

Syntactic Processing, 53

T

Thalamus, 15, 40-41, 115, 152, 182-183, 190

Thrombosis, 93, 155, 158

Tissue Segmentation, 17, 141

Transcortical Sensory, 116

Transcranial Direct Current Stimulation, 113, 174, 179, 187, 189, 192-194, 208-209

Transcranial Magnetic Stimulation, 28-29, 33, 179, 191, 207-208

Transfer Of Therapy Effects, 161, 163-164, 168

V

Ventral Stream, 29, 190

Voxel-based Morphometry, 14-15, 17, 20

W

Wernicke's Area, 29, 70-71, 190, 195, 201-202, 204, 206

Western Aphasia Battery, 15, 26, 29, 42-43, 83, 89, 108, 110-112, 137, 139-140, 151-153, 156, 172, 174

Printed in the USA
CPSIA information can be obtained
at www.ICGtesting.com
LVHW082347150324
774517LV00005B/771